Robotic Radiosurgery

Lee E. Ponsky (Editor-in-chief)
Donald B. Fuller
Robert M. Meier
C-M Charlie Ma
(Co-Editors)

Treating Prostate Cancer and Related Genitourinary Applications

Springer

Editor-in-chief
Lee E. Ponsky, M.D.
Associate Professor, Urology
Leo and Charlotte Goldberg Chair in
Advanced Surgical Therapies
Director, Center Urologic Oncology
and Minimally Invasive Therapies
Urology Institute
University Hospitals Case Medical Center
Case Western Reserve University School
of Medicine
Euclid Avenue 11100
44106 Cleveland Ohio
USA
lee.ponsky@uhhospitals.org

Co-Editors
Donald B. Fuller, M.D.
San Diego Cyberknife Center
Radiosurgery Medical Group, Inc.
Ruffin Rd. 5395
92123 San Diego California
USA
dfuller@genhp.com

Robert M. Meier, M.D.
Swedish Cancer Institute at Northwest Ho
Medical Director, Radiation
Oncology
1560 North 115th Street G16
98133 Seattle Washington
USA
bob.meier@swedish.org

C-M Charlie Ma, Ph.D.
Fox Chase Cancer Center
Director, Physics
333 Cottman Avenue
19111-2497 Philadelphia
Pennsylvania
USA
charlie.ma@fccc.edu

ISBN 978-3-662-51960-8 ISBN 978-3-642-11495-3 (eBook)
DOI 10.1007/978-3-642-11495-3
Springer Heidelberg Dordrecht London New York

Printed on acid-free paper

Springer is part of Springer Science+Business Media (www.springer.com)

To Monica, Ilan, Eric, and Maiya who remind me everyday of what is important in life.
To Mimi, who inspires me everyday.
To my parents for their continued support and guidance.
In honor of Mario Fastag, my father-in-law and friend, who taught me about living. Who also taught me more about cancer than any textbook could.

Lee E. Ponsky

Foreword

One of the major problems in the derivation of treatment programs for patients with malignant disease is to accommodate for motion during the course of the radiation therapy event. This has led to major adjustments in terms of the volume to be irradiated and is associated with potential risk of increased complications from the radiation therapy.

The advances in technology have been dramatic over the years, but more so in the last 10–20 years than ever before. In the early 1980s, the National Cancer Institute funded a project including multiple institutions to assess the potential for developing programs for dynamic treatment planning and delivery. The outcome of those studies was that the technology and computers were not advanced enough to deal with dynamic treatment programs that would allow the tumor to be in the field of treatment in a more precise fashion throughout the entire treatment program.

Subsequent to that, efforts were directed toward three-dimensional conformal treatment programs with better immobilization devices leading to the utilization of intensity-modulated radiation therapy, and subsequently, to image-guided radiation therapy, and tomotherapy.

However, when the CyberKnife® system (Accuray Incorporated, Sun-nyvale, CA) became available more than 12 years ago, it was used primarily to treat patients with intracranial lesions. This was a competitive treatment regimen to Gamma Knife® (Elekta AB, Stockholm, Sweden), but robotic radiosurgery offered a more precise definition of the volume being treated, along with the use of multifractions, and the better sparing of surrounding brain tissue. Many of the treatment pro-grams for radiosurgery at that time utilized skull frame immobilization devices such as the BRW ring, and subsequently, the Gibbs-Murray ring, which did not require placing screws into the skull for the frame, as the BRW ring did. With CyberKnife, this painful and cumbersome stereotactic head frame was eliminated, and it was possible to target the brain tumor in a precise manner, with no more than a conventional immobilization mask.

The evolution of events since the development of the prototype stereotactic robotic radiosurgery system (CyberKnife) has been toward developing an increasingly more accurate machine allowing for the table and the treatment head to be in synchrony with built-in diagnostic x-ray units to ensure that the volume being treated is always in the field of treatment. The development and use of fiducials to deal with tumors in other sites in the body has allowed for accommodation for motion, for respiration, and bladder and bowel filling and emptying, in a manner that had not been possible before. It has also allowed for precision to such a degree that hypofractionation techniques have become possible with treatments with single or multiple fractions. Much of these decisions were based on the pioneer work that had been done by Professor

John F. Fowler, indicating that hypofractionation in the appropriate proper circumstances with a high degree of precision would give rise to results that were equivalent to other techniques in radiation therapy, or other techniques that utilize surgical intervention as a treatment program.

This approach has allowed the opportunity for cooperative partnerships between surgeons and radiation oncologists such as that seen with the Gamma Knife and in many prostate brachytherapy programs. This type of cooperative efforts ultimately results in advancements in the field and improved patient care. Combining the surgeon's anatomical perspective with the radiation oncologist's knowledge and expertise in radiation, the potential development and growth of the field of radiosurgery is immense.

With the expansion of this image-guided approach to radiosurgery, the technology could be advanced to include tumors in any location from head to toe. The technology for robotic radiosurgery has now progressed to a point where essentially any tumor in the body could be treated effectively with excellent outcomes and with very little in the way of side effects from the treatment program, and with diminished number of fractions as compared to conventional radiation therapy programs that require 6–8 weeks of treatment on a daily basis.

The CyberKnife system has now taken its position in the armamentarium of the radiation oncologist and surgeon in a manner that is equivalent to, if not better than, other, conventional radiation therapy or surgical techniques.

Philadelphia, PA, USA Luther W. Brady

Introduction

The application of radiosurgery to the field of Urology is just at its infancy, but will play a major role in the treatment of urologic disease of today and the future. The addition of radiosurgery to the armamentarium of treatment options for our urologic patients requires a multi-disciplinary approach as well as an understanding of the role of each discipline within the team. This book presents all aspects of treatment of urologic disease with radiosurgical technology. It is unique to have a book with physicists, radiation oncologists and surgeons all contributing aspects of a treatment from each of their perspectives. While neurosurgeons have been familiar with radiosurgery for many years, urologists have not. This book allows the surgeon, physicist and/or radiation oncologist to understand the different perspectives and roles that they each play in the team approach to treating urologic disease.

Beginning with the background of treating prostate cancer and the evolution of the treatment of this disease helps one understand the progression of the 'era's' of prostate cancer management. It is extremely important for a patient to consider all of their options while deciding how to be treated for their prostate cancer. It is equally as important for the physician to understand the intricacies of the different treatments so he/she can accurately and appropriately explain the advantages and disadvantages of the different modalities and hopefully individualize the treatment recommendations for each patient. Currently, patients are presented with a variety of options and are often overwhelmed by the numerous options to choose from when deciding how to manage their prostate cancer. Radiosurgical management offers very unique advantages to the appropriately selected patient.

It is critical that surgeons involved with radiosurgery have a basic understanding of the physics and radiobiology behind radiosurgery and how it differs from tradition external beam radiation or brachytherapy. While these aspects are not typically taught to urology residents during their training, this book serves as a comprehensive source to understanding all aspects of treating specifically prostate and kidney cancer with radiosurgery. For example, understanding organ motion, the role of markers and tracking are extremely important. The concept of alpha/beta ratio is important to understand when treating prostate cancer particularly when comparing radiosurgery to other radiation options. Understanding the alpha/beta ratio allows the physician to understand the rationale for different doses being used to treat the same disease based on the type of treatment. It is equally important to understand the impact of hypofractionation and how that plays a role in the treatments.

While radiation has been one of the standards of care for prostate cancer for years, that is not the case for kidney tumors. The idea of using radiation to treat renal tumors is essentially unheard of due to the long standing belief that renal tumors are 'radio-resistant'. However, an understanding of the mechanism of ablation as seen with radiosurgery as opposed to traditional external beam radiation is extremely important. Also, an understanding of the previously published and current ongoing work to evaluate the safety and efficacy of radiosurgery for the treatment of renal tumors is critical. As we continue to understand the role and understand the technologies that allow us to deliver radiosurgery, we will likely be able to expand the application to other lesions such as adrenal tumors and bladder.

On behalf of my co-editors and the production team, I would like to invite you to use this book as a resource to understanding radiosurgery, which will be critical to surgeons and radiation oncologists for the treatment of urologic malignancies currently, and even more so in the future.

I would like to personally thank Mikail Gezginci, David Schaal, Pam Commike, and Katherine Striedinger for all of their assistance (and patience) with putting this book together.

Contents

Abbreviations

3D	3-Dimensional
3D-CRT	3-Dimensional conformal radiotherapy
5-ARIs	5α-Reductase inhibitors
5-FU	5-Fluorouracil
5BF	Biochemical failure at 5 years
A	
AD	Adenocarcinoma
ADC	Apparent diffusion coefficient
ADT	Androgen deprivation therapy
AJCC	American joint committee for cancer
AP/PA	Anterior-posterior and posterior-anterior
ART	Adaptive radiation therapy
ARTs	Acute-response tissues
ASTRO	American society for therapeutic radiation oncology
AUA	American urological association
AUC	Area under the curve
AVM	Arteriovenous malformation
B	
B	Biopsy
BAT	Ultrasound B-mode acquisition and targeting ultrasound
BC	Biochemical control
BDFS	Biochemical disease-free survival
BED	Biological equivalent dose
BF	Biochemical failure
BID	Twice a day
BP	Bladder preservation
BPH	Benign Prostatic Hyperplasia
BT	Brachytherapy
C	
CBCT	Cone beam computed tomography
CET	California Endocurietherapy Cancer Center
CGE	Cobalt gray equivalent
cGy	Centigray
CI	Conformity index
Cine-MRI	Cinetographic magnetic resonance imaging
cis-Pt	Cisplatin

CK	CyberKnife
CNS	Central nervous system
CPt	Carboplatin
CRT	Conformal radiotherapy
Cs	Cesium
CSS	Cause-specific survival
CT	Computed tomography
CTC	Common toxicity criteria
CTCAE	Common terminology criteria for adverse events
CTV	Clinical target volume

D

DCE	Dynamic contrast enhanced
DFS	Disease free survival
DIL	Dominant intraprostatic lesion
DM	Distant metastases
DPF	Dose per fraction
DRE	Digital rectal exam
DRRs	Digitally reconstructed radiographs
DVH	Dose volume histogram
DW	Diffusion-weighted
DWI	Diffusion-weighted imaging

E

EBRT	External beam radiotherapy
ECE	Extracapsular extension
ED	Erectile dysfunction
EES	Extravascular extracellular space
EORTC	European Organization for Research and Treatment of Cancer
EPI	Echo planar imaging
EPIC	Expanded prostate cancer index composite
EQD2	Equivalent dose
erMRI	endorectal magnetic resonance imaging
ERSPC	European Randomized Study of Screening in Prostate Cancer
ESTRO	European Society for Therapeutic Radiology and Oncology

F

FA	Fractional anisotropy
FBF	Freedom from biochemical failure
FDM	Freedom from distant metastases
FIGO	Federation of Gynecology and Obstetrics
F/U	Follow up

G

GI	Gastrointestinal
GOG	Gynecologic oncology group
GS	Gleason score
GTV	Gross tumor volume
GU	Genitourinary
GYN	GEC ESTRO Group European de Curitherapie/European Society for Therapeutic Radiology and Oncology

H

HDR	High dose rate
HDRBR	High dose rate brachytherapy
HI	Homogeneity index
HIC	Human investigational committee
HIFU	High intensity focused ultrasound

I

IC-BT	Intracavitary brachytherapy
ICRU	International Commission on Radiation Units & Measurements
IGRT	Image guided radiation therapy
IMRT	Intensity modulated radiation therapy
IORT	Intraoperative radiotherapy
IPSS	International prostate symptom score
Ir-192	Iridium 192
IRB	Institution Review Board
IS-BT	Interstitial brachytherapy

K

KU	Kiel University
kV	CT Kilo voltage computed tomography

L

L	Lymphangiogram
LDR	Low dose rate
LDRBR	Low dose rate brachytherapy
LQ/L-QM	Linear quadratic model
LR	Local recurrence
LRF	Locoregional failure
LRTs	Late-response tissues

M

MDAH	MD Anderson Hospital
Mets	Metastases
MLC	Multileaf collimator
MR	Magnetic resonance
MRI	Magnetic resonance imaging
MRS	Magnetic resonance spectroscopy
MRSi	Magnetic resonance spectroscopy imaging
MSKCC	Memorial Sloan Kettering Cancer Center
MV	Megavoltage
MV	CT Megavoltage computed tomography

N

NCCN	National Comprehensive Cancer Network
NCIC	National Cancer Institute of Canada
NCICT	National Cancer Institute Clinical Trials
NED	No evidence of disease
NF	Normofractionated
NR	Not reported
NS	Not stated

NTD	Normalized total dose
NTD2	Normalized total doses in 2-Gy per fraction
NVB	Neurovascular bundle
O	
OS	Overall survival
OTT	Overall treatment time
P	
PA	Periaortic
PAN	Periaortic nodes or periaortic node region
PCPT	Prostate Cancer Prevention Trial
PDF/mm	Percentage of dose fall-off per millimeter
PDR	Pulse-dose-rate
PET	Positron emission tomography
PFS	Progression free survival
PLCO	Colorectal and ovarian cancer screening
PORTEC	Post-operative radiation therapy in endometrial carcinoma
PROG	Proton Radiation Oncology Group
PSA	Prostate serum antigen
PSADT	PSA doubling time
PSAV	PSA velocity
PTV	Planning target volume
Q	
QD	Every day
QOD	Every other day
QOL	Quality of Life
QUANTEC	Quantitative analysis of normal tissue effects in the clinic
R	
Ra-226	Radium needles
RCC	Renal cell carcinomas
RF	Radiofrequency
RFA	Radiofrequency ablation
R-L	Right-left dimension
RP	Radical prostatectomy
RT	Radiotherapy
RTOG	Radiation Therapy Oncology Group
S	
SBO	Small bowel obstruction
SBRT	Stereotactic body radiotherapy
SCC	Squamous cell carcinoma
SD	Standard deviations
SELECT	Selenium and vitamin E cancer prevention trial
SHIM	Sexual Health Inventory Matrix score/ Sexual Health Inventory for Men
S-I	Superior-inferior dimension
SIB	Simultaneous integrated boosting
SNR	Signal-to-noise ratio
SPECT	Single photon emission computed tomography

SRMs	Small renal masses
SRS	Stereotactic radiosurgery
SV	Seminal vesicle
T	
TNM	Tumor, node, metastases classification
TO	TomoTherapy®
TPOT	Post-treatment potential doubling time
TRUS	Transrectal ultrasound
TURB	Transurethral resection of the bladder
TURP	Transurethral resection of the prostate
U	
UN	Universidad de Navarra in Spain
US	Ultrasound
W	
WHO	World Health Organization
WBH	William Beaumont Hospital

Author Index

Part I

Introduction to Radiosurgery as a Multidisciplinary Practice

Radiosurgery, a Treatment Principle: From Brain to Body

Alexander Muacevic

CONTENTS

1.1 Abstract

Radiosurgery is an increasingly attractive treatment principle, which has traditionally been used for local treatment of brain lesions. During recent years, it has gained relevance worldwide for treatment of tumors throughout the body, such as in the spine, lung, liver, pancreas, and also the prostate. Clinical data is accumulating fast, and early feasibility studies and phase I/II trials show promising results of this technology-driven irradiation technique in selected extracranial cases as an alternative or adjunct to invasive surgical treatment. In this chapter, we aim to provide a brief historical background of radiosurgery during the last century to better understand the fundamental aspects of this application, describe current treatment indications, and have an outlook of future developments in this exciting emerging medical field.

1.2 Introduction

Radiosurgery is defined as the highly localized application of a high dose of radiation to a target, without compromising the surrounding healthy tissue structures. During its early development, radiosurgery was considered to be a surgical technique for treating a sharply defined lesion in the brain by focusing a single, high dose of radiation from external sources onto the target lesion. A narrow radiation beam became, in effect, akin to a new surgical tool, but unlike "real surgery," radiosurgery was a noninvasive technique. This vision was developed by the pioneer Swedish neurosurgeon, Lars Leksell, with the aim of avoiding the necessity of opening the skull and the consequent risk of infection or intracranial bleeding [1]. According to Leksell's own belief, radiosurgery was the ultimate goal of surgery, eliminating intracranial lesions by a noninvasive technique. He called his first system the Gamma Unit (later Gamma Knife) as the radiation came from Cobalt-60 (^{60}Co) sources emitting gamma rays [2, 3].

Radiosurgery is now considered to be an irradiation procedure for producing a radiobiological effect, such as tumor control or vessel obliteration, by focus-

L.E. Ponsky et al. (eds.), *Treating Prostate Cancer and Related Genitourinary Applications*, Robotic Radiosurgery, DOI 10.1007/978-3-642-11495-3_1,

ing radiation from external sources into a stereotactically defined target. Traditionally, radiosurgery was defined as a single-session procedure. Nowadays, frameless systems allow splitting of the dose in cases where tumors are attached to highly eloquent areas, such as the optic system, and up to five sessions may still be regarded as a radiosurgical procedure when done in combination with stereotactic guidance [4]. No matter how many fractions are applied, two main requirements are prerequisites for radiosurgery: precise spatial targeting of the lesion and a steep dose fall-off (gradient) at the border of the target volume.

Over the years, different techniques have been developed by only a handful of scientists around the world. These main protagonists and their technological achievements are briefly covered in this chapter to provide background to some of our readers, who may not be as familiar with the subject matter as others, to better understand the current and upcoming clinical applications.

1.3 History

The first radiation therapy machine to include mechanical rotation was designed and built in 1915 at the Royal Cancer Hospital, London [5]. It was used successfully in the clinic for more than a decade. Because treatment with multiple fixed-field 200-kV X-ray beams was inadequate for many deep-seated tumors, such as those of the esophagus and bronchi, this then new device was developed specifically to deliver large doses of radiation to smaller and deeper-seated target volumes. During the rotational treatment, the external beam apparatus rotated at a constant speed around the stationary patient and continuously irradiated over one or two planned prescribed arcs. This technology, using cross-fired radiation, employed a principle still used today for stereotactic irradiation even in the most modern radiation systems.

Stereotactic radiosurgery and its possible general applications were first described by Leksell who used a stereotactic frame and moved a 280-kV X-ray source along an arc [2]. The target was precisely located at the geometric center of the arc. This first apparatus was employed for precise irradiation of the gasserian ganglion to treat trigeminal neuralgia. However, the high scatter fraction of these low-energy X-ray beams had significant drawbacks.

Larsson et al. studied the effect of 185-MeV protons on cerebral tissue [6]. This method was applied to a select number of patients for whom a small, well-demarcated lesion in the thalamic nuclei was created for the treatment of movement disorders and intractable pain.

In 1959, Raymond Kjellberg initiated a study using Bragg-peak proton irradiation at Harvard University's 186-MeV cyclotron unit. The pituitary gland was selected as the first suitable target. However, in the past, and somewhat also today, proton and heavy ion irradiation proved to be cumbersome and difficult to establish, because of technical and logistical, as well as financial reasons [7].

Trying to overcome the problems encountered with proton radiosurgery, in 1967, Leksell and his colleagues developed the first stereotactic irradiation apparatus designed specifically to perform radiosurgical treatment of intracranial targets [8], the Gamma Unit I. In this device, an array of ^{60}Co sources distributed over a spherical sector of 70° × 160° allowed simultaneous cross-firing with 170 separate beams with high mechanical precision and physical reproducibility. The Gamma Unit I was initially used mainly to treat pain [9]. When radiosurgery's primary indication began shifting toward treatment of intracranial tumors and vascular malformations, the Gamma Unit I proved to be inadequate. Hence, in 1975, the Gamma Unit II was introduced with larger circular collimators, ranging from 4 to 20 mm, which allowed irradiation of larger targets. In the 1970s, Leksell and his colleagues demonstrated the efficacy of Gamma Unit II for the treatment of a variety of intracranial lesions [10]. Ladislau Steiner, in particular, deserves a special mention as a radiosurgery pioneer, as he performed the first successful obliteration of an inoperable cerebral arteriovenous malformation (AVM) and opened up a completely new treatment perspective for otherwise untreatable AVMs [11].

The first report of a linear accelerator radiosurgical technique was published in 1983 by Betti and Derechinsky [12]. In this early adaptation, the procedure employed a number of isocentric, fixed radiation fields in different planes accomplished through the rotation of the patient's head around a transverse axis.

In 1985, Colombo et al. in Italy published a technique, which was based on multiple converging arc irradiations [13]. Hartmann and Sturm in Germany reported a similar technique independently to treat brain metastases [14].

In 1991, the CyberKnife® (Accuray Incorporated, Sunnyvale, CA) radiosurgical system was initially described as a concept by Guthrie and Adler [15]. It incorporated several distinctive features, including image-guided target localization, robotically administered radiation, a small X-band linear accelerator, dynamic compensation for target motion (eventually including motion caused by respiration), and, finally, the potential to use up to 1,600 intersecting beams of therapeutic radiation. This last feature, cross-fired photon beams, was first proposed as early as in 1905 [16]. Thus, in 1994, when the first CyberKnife was installed at Stanford, cross-fired beams had been in routine use for 90 years. Adler quickly realized that the same radiophysical principles of cross-fire could be clinically applicable to targets in the spine, chest, or abdomen, just as readily as they were to intracranial targets. It was also soon obvious that the concept of frame-based targeting embodied by the Gamma Knife® (Elekta AB, Stockholm, Sweden) could not practically be extrapolated to these new potential therapeutic applications.

1.4 Indications for Radiosurgery

Radiosurgery was originally designed to treat small intracranial targets like acoustic neuromas, arteriovenous malformations, or skull base meningiomas. During recent years, the intracranial treatment principles developed through the years started expanding to the spine, and just recently to the rest of the body. Today, radiosurgery's primary application is in the treatment of extracranial indications [17–22]. Usage varies according to the physical and pathological circumstances associated with the particular case at hand. Due to the steep dose fall-off which is achieved, theoretically any lesion with sharply defined borders could be selectively destroyed, provided that an adequate radiation dose is administered.

As stated above, the ultimate prerequisite for radiosurgery is the exact targeting of the lesion. For brain and spine lesions, this is relatively easy to accomplish given that these organs do not move during treatment, and patient movements can be tracked via skeletal structures. It becomes significantly more difficult if the treated tumor moves with respiration, as aiming at such a moving target without harming the surrounding tissue is understandably challenging. To overcome this hurdle, different techniques have been developed, such as abdominal frames to limit thoracic excursions, gating techniques where the beam is only turned on when the tumor comes within a calculated treatment range, or internal markers that permit the guidance of the beam in real time through the breathing cycle [23]. The latter is used for robotic radiosurgery and is regarded as the most accurate body tracking method currently [24,25]. In this method, before the computed tomography (CT) scanning, usually three to four radio-opaque markers are inserted into or close to the tumor. These fiducials define a spatial reference system that can be employed to transport target coordinates from the CT to the robot's reference system. X-ray imaging is used for accurate tracking of the periodic movement connected with respiration, and to precisely correlate it with the movement of a number of external markers secured to the patient's chest. The robot is connected to optical detectors that track the external markers and anticipate the target shift and correct for it by moving the beam accordingly, and periodically to check whether the correlation model between the internal markers and the optical sources is still valid.

1.5 Current and Emerging Developments

In the last decade or so, with the growth and expanding availability of computing power, real-time image guidance has represented the driving force behind and a key factor leading to innovations in radiosurgery. Excellent results equivalent to those obtained by frame-based radiosurgical techniques have been described in the cranial radiosurgery literature. A main advantage of frameless radiosurgery is the freedom from cranial screw fixation. Exciting new applications have now become available, applicable to both benign lesions, such as meningiomas, neuromas, or AVMs; and malignant lesions, such as the primary and secondary malignant tumors of the spine [26–28].

Presently, the radiosurgical principles described above are entering the realm of body treatments in the lung, the liver, kidney, and the prostate [17, 21, 22]. It seems reasonable to estimate that the same high tumor control rates achieved in the brain for decades should also be achievable for other tumors throughout the body if exact targeting is possible. Robotic image-guided radiosurgery with its unique tracking capabilities for moving organs is ideally suited to achieve this goal. First reports on lung, liver, and prostate radiosurgery are very encouraging, and it seems obvious that the surgical disciplines need to be deeply involved in this type of treatment application similar to Leksell's view 50 years ago [2–4]. Particularly, prostate radiosurgery has become a major interest during recent years, and the first published retrospective and longitudinal studies show promising results with a comparably low toxicity profile. Large prospective trials are underway using four to five treatment sessions instead of a 6- to 8-week treatment cycle of traditional radiotherapy [29–31]. In the near future, we will learn and understand whether these new patient-friendly treatment algorithms offer real patient benefits and justify the technological investment and associated treatment costs.

Finally, in the opinion of the author, the more focused the applied radiation is, the more crucial the involvement of surgeons becomes, as the risk associated with this kind of treatment is elevated along with the promise of excellent local control. Meticulous knowledge of the treated anatomical region is needed to achieve a safe and effective treatment. This is particularly true for already operated lesions with remaining or recurrent tumors, as imaging interpretation and thus treatment planning is difficult without the surgical view. Surgeons nowadays, whether thoracic, abdominal, or urological, need to be well informed about the possibilities of radiosurgery. They should see radiosurgery as an additional tool in their surgical armamentarium to ideally direct their patients toward optimal therapy. Patient selection is ultimately the key to good overall radiosurgical results, and therefore, indications for radiosurgery should be determined in a multidisciplinary setting where the surgeon takes the lead to give the best possible treatment recommendations based on clinical and scientific results.

References

1. Leksell L (1992) Brain fragments. In: Steiner L, Forster D, Backlund E-O (eds) Radiosurgery: baseline and trends. Raven Press, New York, pp 263–292
2. Leksell L (1949) A stereotactic apparatus for intracerebral surgery. Acta Chirurg Scand 99:229–319
3. Leksell L (1951) The stereotaxic method and radiosurgery of the brain. Acta Chir Scand 102:316–319
4. Barnett GH, Linskey ME, Adler JR et al (2007) Stereotactic radiosurgery–an organized neurosurgery-sanctioned definition. J Neurosurg 106:1–5
5. Knox RCA (1915) A new therapeutic X-ray localizer. Arch Radiol Electrotherapy [Arch Roentgen Ray] 16:176–183
6. Larsson B, Leksell L, Rexed B et al (1958) The high-energy proton beam as a neurosurgical tool. Nature 182:1222–1223
7. Kjellberg RN, Koehler AM, Preston WM et al (1962) Stereotaxic instrument for use with the Bragg peak of a proton beam. Confin Neurol 22:183–189
8. Leksell L (1968) Cerebral radiosurgery. I. Gammathalanotomy in two cases of intractable pain. Acta Chir Scand 134:585–595
9. Leksell L (1971) Sterotaxic radiosurgery in trigeminal neuralgia. Acta Chir Scand 137:311–314
10. Noren GLL (1979) Stereotactic radiosurgery of acoustic tumors. In: Gabor S (ed) Stereotactic cerebral irradiation. Elsevier, Amsterdam, pp 241–244
11. Steiner L, Leksell L, Forster DM et al (1974) Stereotactic radiosurgery in intracranial arterio-venous malformations. Acta Neurochir (Wien) Suppl 21:195–209
12. Betti O, Derechinsky V (1983) Multiple-beam stereotaxic irradiation. Neurochirurgie 29:295–298
13. Colombo F, Benedetti A, Pozza F et al (1985) External stereotactic irradiation by linear accelerator. Neurosurgery 16:154–160
14. Hartmann GH, Schlegel W, Sturm V et al (1985) Cerebral radiation surgery using moving field irradiation at a linear accelerator facility. Int J Radiat Oncol Biol Phys 11: 1185–1192
15. Guthrie BL, Adler JR Jr (1992) Computer-assisted preoperative planning, interactive surgery, and frameless stereotaxy. Clin Neurosurg 38:112–131
16. Wickham LDP (1910) Radiumtherapy. Cassell, London
17. King CR, Lehmann J, Adler JR et al (2003) CyberKnife radiotherapy for localized prostate cancer: rationale and technical feasibility. Technol Cancer Res Treat 2:25–30
18. Koong AC, Le QT, Ho A et al (2004) Phase I study of stereotactic radiosurgery in patients with locally advanced pancreatic cancer. Int J Radiat Oncol Biol Phys 58:1017–1021
19. Muacevic A, Drexler C, Kufeld M et al (2009) Fiducial-free real-time image-guided robotic radiosurgery for tumors of the sacrum/pelvis. Radiother Oncol 93:37–44
20. Ryu SI, Chang SD, Kim DH et al (2001) Image-guided hypofractionated stereotactic radiosurgery to spinal lesions. Neurosurgery 49:838–846

21. Stintzing S, Hoffmann RT, Heinemann V et al (2010) Radiosurgery of liver tumors: value of robotic radiosurgical device to treat liver tumors. Ann Surg Oncol 17:2877–2883
22. Whyte RI, Crownover R, Murphy MJ et al (2003) Stereotactic radiosurgery for lung tumors: preliminary report of a phase I trial. Ann Thorac Surg 75:1097–1101
23. Adler JR Jr, Chang SD, Murphy MJ et al (1997) The Cyberknife: a frameless robotic system for radiosurgery. Stereotact Funct Neurosurg 69:124–128
24. Antypas C, Pantelis E (2008) Performance evaluation of a CyberKnife G4 image-guided robotic stereotactic radiosurgery system. Phys Med Biol 53:4697–4718
25. Chang SD, Main W, Martin DP et al (2003) An analysis of the accuracy of the CyberKnife: a robotic frameless stereotactic radiosurgical system. Neurosurgery 52:140–146; discussion 146–147
26. Furweger C, Drexler C, Kufeld M et al (2010) Patient motion and targeting accuracy in robotic spinal radiosurgery: 260 single-fraction fiducial-free cases. Int J Radiat Oncol Biol Phys 78:937–945
27. Ho AK, Fu D, Cotrutz C et al (2007) A study of the accuracy of cyberknife spinal radiosurgery using skeletal structure tracking. Neurosurgery 60:ONS147–ONS156; discussion ONS156
28. Muacevic A, Staehler M, Drexler C et al (2006) Technical description, phantom accuracy, and clinical feasibility for fiducial-free frameless real-time image-guided spinal radiosurgery. J Neurosurg Spine 5:303–312
29. Fuller DB, Naitoh J, Lee C et al (2008) Virtual HDR CyberKnife treatment for localized prostatic carcinoma: dosimetry comparison with HDR brachytherapy and preliminary clinical observations. Int J Radiat Oncol Biol Phys 70:1588–1597
30. King CR, Brooks JD, Gill H et al (2009) Stereotactic body radiotherapy for localized prostate cancer: interim results of a prospective phase II clinical trial. Int J Radiat Oncol Biol Phys 73:1043–1048
31. Xie Y, Djajaputra D, King CR et al (2008) Intrafractional motion of the prostate during hypofractionated radiotherapy. Int J Radiat Oncol Biol Phys 72:236–246

Radiosurgery as a Multidisciplinary Practice

2

Lee E. Ponsky, William Chen, and Rodney J. Ellis

CONTENTS

2.1 Abstract

The management of kidney and prostate cancer is evolving toward less-invasive treatment options, from open surgery to laparoscopic and energy-ablative techniques to stereotactic body radiotherapy (SBRT) with the aim of preserving function and minimizing side effects.

The advances of radiation therapy, including frameless stereotactic systems, image guidance and effective tumor tracking allow the application of radiosurgery principles to moving targets in the body. High doses of radiation can now be delivered safely and accurately with just a few fractions to genitourinary malignancies achieving good local control while sparing healthy organs.

A multidisciplinary team including the urologist, radiation oncologist, and physicist must work in close cooperation to establish a successful SBRT program.

2.2 Radiosurgery: A Urologist Perspective

Lee E. Ponsky

Treatments for kidney and prostate cancers have evolved significantly over the recent years. Historically, from a surgical perspective, renal tumors were only able to be treated with surgical removal. From the time of the initial description of radical nephrectomy in 1948 [1] there has been a movement toward less invasive curative intent therapy. While radical nephrectomy was a success oncologically, healthy nephrons were sacrificed and could potentially result in subsequent deterioration of renal function. The introduction of nephron-sparing surgery with partial nephrectomy met with skepticism from an oncologic standpoint. However, long-term data demonstrated relatively equivalent oncologic outcomes with improved long-term renal function. Partial nephrectomy became accepted as a standard of care for small renal masses. With the laparoscopic revolution in the 1990s, laparoscopic nephrectomy was introduced and demonstrated that patient recovery was significantly improved with this less invasive technique. Laparoscopic nephrectomy became a standard of

L.E. Ponsky et al. (eds.), *Treating Prostate Cancer and Related Genitourinary Applications*, Robotic Radiosurgery,
DOI 10.1007/978-3-642-11495-3_2,

care initially at centers of excellence and then was widely adopted as urologists learned the technique. Interestingly, because of the quicker recovery patients were experiencing, many patients who would have otherwise been ideal candidates for an open partial nephrectomy were now undergoing a laparoscopic radical nephrectomy [2, 3]. This was an unusual situation, introducing the bias of patients and their physicians to achieve the least morbidity and the quickest recovery without compromising oncologic outcomes, even at the expense of nephrons. As experts in laparoscopic surgery began to refine their skills, laparoscopic partial nephrectomy, typically offered by the advanced laparoscopic surgeon, was introduced [4]. This now began to offer patients nephron preservation with quick recovery. Interestingly, initial outcomes demonstrated a slightly increased risk of bleeding with laparoscopic partial nephrectomy compared to open partial nephrectomy. Oncologic outcomes appear to be equivalent. Patients were recovering to their baseline activities quicker after a laparoscopic partial nephrectomy [5].

It had been clearly established that patients' and physicians' priorities were on optimal oncologic outcomes, quick recovery and return to normal activities, and minimal discomfort, with nephron preservation if possible. Ablative therapies including cryoablation (destruction of tumors with freezing) and radiofrequency ablation (destruction of tumors with heat) introduced yet another option for patients, offering oncologic outcomes approaching that of surgical extirpation, yet maximal nephron preservation with minimal morbidity and recovery, where the patients achieved baseline activities within days of being treated [6, 7]. This was initially offered to patients who were considered high-risk for an extirpative surgery due to comorbidities. Our group recently demonstrated that cryoablation can in fact be offered successfully to healthy patients with small renal masses regardless of their comorbidities [8]. In the pursuit of the least invasive management of renal masses, it has been recently suggested that not all renal masses need to be treated, but in fact certain renal masses may be candidates for active surveillance [9].

The continued advancements in technology and imaging have allowed urologists to yet again evaluate the use of an ablative technology that has the potential to offer optimal oncologic outcomes with the least invasive approach. The concept of radiosurgery was initially introduced to the surgical community with Gamma Knife® (Elekta AB, Stockholm, Sweden) by neurosurgeons [10]. This clearly revolutionized the field of neurosurgery and allowed neurosurgeons to work in partnership with their radiation oncology colleagues to target brain tumors that were not ideal for surgical excision. Gamma Knife, however, was limited in application to targets within the cranium that do not move with respiration. The introduction and incorporation of advanced imaging with gating and/or tracking allowed tumors to be treated in the presence of minimal or even significant movement with respiration. CyberKnife® (Accuray Incorporated, Sunnyvale, CA) is one of the leading technologies that allow for the application of radiosurgery to a moving target [11]. Differing from the application of standard radiation therapy that works by inducing apoptosis, radiosurgery relies on highly focused and submillimeter targeting of tumors and delivering an ablative dose. This, in turn, prompts the surgeon and radiation oncologist to work in partnership to target a defined tumor and deliver a dose that can destroy a tumor with just a few fractions. Renal tumors are an example of a potential application of radiosurgery. While renal tumors have traditionally been considered to be "radioresistant," this is in fact a misnomer. Metastatic renal tumors to the brain have been treated successfully for years with Gamma Knife [12–14]. This demonstrates that the renal cell carcinoma cell line is not radio-resistant, but the dose needed to ablate the tumor is high. The dose that is likely needed to destroy a renal tumor is higher than what can be delivered by traditional external beam radiation. The dose of traditional radiation, typically delivered from a few directions around the tumor, would be so high that it would cause significant damage to the tissue in the path of the radiation beam as well as the surrounding tissue around the renal tumor. However, with the use of radiosurgery, the ablative dose of radiation can be divided into hundreds of individual low-dose beams directed from hundreds of different directions around the tumor. Each beam is a low-enough dose that it will not cause any damage to the pathway of the radiation beam, yet, at the focal point where all of the hundreds of radiation beams converge, the dose of each beam will be additive and deliver an ablative dose precisely to the tumor with minimal to no effect on the surrounding tissue. This can allow the treating team to deliver a completely noninvasive ablative treatment to a renal tumor, with no anesthesia, no pain, and no recovery time [15]. Certainly, confirmation of these possibilities requires further studies and long-term outcomes to demonstrate equivalent oncologic outcomes and the absence of long-term side effects.

This trend of moving toward less invasive approaches has also been seen among the treatment options of prostate cancer. Currently, patients have multiple options for the management of prostate cancer. Traditionally, standard external-beam radiation and surgical removal were the only options, whereas today we are able to offer patients many options, including intensity-modulated radiation therapy (IMRT), brachytherapy (low and high dose rate), radical retropubic prostatectomy, perineal prostatectomy, laparoscopic prostatectomy, robotic prostatectomy, cryoablation, high-intensity focused ultrasound (HIFU), focal therapy, and radiosurgery. With prostate cancer, patients and physicians not only demand optimal oncologic outcomes, but the side effects must also be minimized and are often the focus of the patient's decision. In the case of prostate cancer, most of the treatment options offer equivalent oncologic outcomes. This leaves the patient often weighing the side effect profiles and quality of life associated with each modality. Side effects in question include erectile dysfunction, incontinence, and rectal and bladder irritation [16]. Another aspect that is given significant consideration is time commitment required by the treatment. For example, traditional IMRT can often involve treatment 5 days a week for 6–9 weeks. This alone can be prohibitive for many patients, even if they want to avoid anesthesia that is associated with most of the other options. Radiosurgery for prostate cancer allows for treatments typically completed in 5 days [17], although it has been also reported to be completed in one treatment (Muacevic A, personal communication, 2010) To date, oncologic outcomes and side effect profiles appear equivalent to standard IMRT, however, patients can be treated in a much shorter time period [18].

Radiosurgery is a new concept for surgeons other than neurosurgeons. The adoption of radiosurgery will require surgeons to learn the concepts of radiosurgery. The anatomic knowledge is very important for successful treatments. At this point, fiducial markers are required for image guidance and urologists typically place these either transperineally or transrectally. The urologist will need to be trained on contouring and understand the terms and concepts of radiosurgery when reviewing the treatment plans. Also, the urologist must work cooperatively with their radiation oncology colleagues. It is imperative that both the urologist and radiation oncologist work together and their roles are clearly defined to be able to establish a successful program. While many urologists and radiation oncologists may feel territorial about the treatment of prostate cancer, the cooperative approach is a must. This model of cooperation has been demonstrated in many successful brachytherapy programs, which include the urologist, radiation oncologist, and physicist. If either specialty is not willing to participate in such a collaboration, ultimately they will become bypassed by patients as they seek out this technique.

2.3 Radiosurgery: A Radiation Oncologist Perspective

William Chen and Rodney J. Ellis

The management of genitourinary malignancies has evolved along technological advances. Surgical interventions have seen the progression of small and less invasive procedures, from open to laparoscopic and robotic to thermally ablative approaches.

Advances within radiation technology have broadened its utility in the treatment of genitourinary cancers as technology enables us to improve treatment effectiveness while minimizing adverse sequelae. This has enabled ablative alternatives to surgical excision in the era of stereotactic body radiation therapy (SBRT), and expanded the scope of available treatment options for adenocarcinomas of the prostate and for renal cell carcinomas (RCC).

The therapeutic use of radiation has continued to evolve since the discovery of X-rays in 1895 and the potential for radioactivity-based treatments in medicine in 1896. The basic tenets for treatment of malignant and benign diseases have remained constant, and apply not just to radiation therapy but to any treatment modality in general. The concept of the therapeutic ratio index serves as a barometer of efficacy, as we strive to maximize tumor cell death while limiting injury to the adjacent normal tissues [19].

Early after its discovery, ionizing radiation was noted to have tumoricidal properties, especially for epithelial tumors. This has become most evident as radiation doses increased and early practices delivered the dose of radiation in a few or even in single fractions. While these early efforts in hypofractionated radiation therapy resulted in appreciable tumor response, patients began to outlive their disease process, and the long-term sequelae of treatment became readily evident. Significant postradiotherapy toxicities became apparent, including fibrosis, stenosis, ulceration, and vascular injury were observed. Subsequently, these early hypofractionated schedules were soon abandoned and largely forgotten by later practitioners [20].

Compounding toxicity-related issues of radiotherapy was the imprecise nature of early radiation delivery. Without the advent of modern imaging, there was greater uncertainty in the extent of disease—both gross and microscopic. Epithelial tumors were readily visible, but internal tumors required larger treatment volumes with substantial margins to account for various inherent ambiguities and uncertainties associated with therapeutic targets within the human body. Additionally, early beam energies were available only in the lower keV range, causing the dose to healthy tissue to exceed the dose at depth.

In an effort to reduce radiotherapy-related toxicity, focus turned upon exploiting the differential effects of radiobiology between normal cells and tumor cells. Based on experiments performed in Paris in the 1920s and 1930s, it was found that a single dose of X-rays to animal testicles could not induce sterility without extensive skin damage, whereas sterilization was possible without unacceptable skin damage if the radiation was spread out over a period of time in daily fractions [19]. Subsequent experiments explained that mechanisms of sublethal damage repair, repopulation, cell cycle reassortment, and reoxygenation are the factors that allow delivery of high cumulative radiation doses by dose fractionation [21, 22]. Based on these radiobiologic principles, the overall positive differential effect in irradiation of tumor versus normal tissue provides a therapeutic index. The early experiences and promising results of giants such as Claudius Regaud and Henri Coutard in the 1920s prompted a shift toward the protracted radiotherapy fractionation method that is utilized today [23].

The advent of higher energy machines and increased popularity of cobalt-60 units in the 1950s and 1960s brought a resurgence of radiotherapy. Up to the 1950s, most external beam radiotherapy was carried out with X-rays generated at voltages up to 300 kVp. The energy profiles of these early kilovoltage units resulted in maximal dose delivery at the surface of the tissue [24]. A great limitation to treatment of deeper tumors was the skin dose. Early treatments of radiation doses began to approach maximal radiation tolerance of the skin. Megavoltage machines, such as cobalt-60 units and modern-day linear accelerators, provided skin-sparing properties of higher energy radiation and allowed protracted dose delivery over several weeks – albeit still to a large volume.

The interval improvement of diagnostic technology for radiology has improved tissue definition and tumor localization. Internal target volumes are now routinely defined utilizing computed tomography (CT) rather than fluoroscopic imaging, often in conjunction with other technologies such as magnetic resonance imaging (MRI). More recently, molecular imaging techniques, such as positron emission tomography (PET), single photon emission computed tomography (SPECT), and magnetic resonance spectroscopy imaging (MRSi), have improved delineation of tumor foci. Further improvements in the use of anatomic and molecular imaging equipment and/or fusion software now produce hybrid image sets (such as SPECT/CT, MR/MRSi, and PET/MR). Subsequently, improved delineation of tumor targeting has become routinely utilized in radiation oncology treatment planning, thus improving tumor localization, corresponding with a reduction in treatment volumes, and ultimately unnecessary radiation coverage to normal tissues [25].

Therapy has further benefited from improvements in radiation delivery. Multileaf collimation of the radiation beam and inverse treatment planning software enable IMRT, and treatment systems with imaging technologies allow verification of tumor and critical structures to provide image-guided radiation therapy (IGRT). IMRT and IGRT have been shown to improve the therapeutic ratio, allowing escalation of delivered dose while limiting toxicity. This has enabled physicians to dose-escalate in the standard fractionated treatment of prostate cancer [26].

The resurgence of hypofractionation began initially with the novel development of accurate localization systems. In 1951, a Swedish neurosurgeon named Lars Leksell employed a system for accurately navigating within the skull called "stereotaxy," which allowed precise instrumentation for biopsy, resection, and ablation [10]. Together with a radiation physicist, Borge Larsson, they developed a system in which a head frame was affixed to the skull to provide an external three-dimensional reference by which to accurately localize the intracranial target and "steer" high doses of radiation in a single session [10]. Unlike other external radiation delivery, Leksell utilized stereotaxy to avoid delivering high doses of radiation to the surrounding nontargeted radio-intolerant brain. The concept of sterotaxy and experiences with intracranial stereotactic radiosurgery (SRS) serve as a foundation for future developments of SBRT.

The ability to deliver ablative doses to the tumor was not possible with improvements in tumor localization alone. Accurate delivery of radiation is also necessary in order to limit the volume of normal tissue irradiated and prevent significant toxicities as seen in early radiotherapy. In extrapolation of the intracranial SRS into extracranial sites, Hamilton et al. presented a rigid immobilization SBRT delivery system for spinal lesions utilizing a rigid box with a clamp fixated on exposed spinous processes to establish a reference coordinate system [27]. Lax et al. developed a refined stereotactic body frame system utilizing vacuum pillow stabilization and abdominal compression to limit intrafraction diaphragmatic movement [28]. Though initially cumbersome, immobilization systems such as these are essential for accurate targeting, patient positioning, motion accounting, and delivery of dose with minimal dosimetric margins. Improvements have allowed tumor-tracking systems and frameless stereotactic systems [29].

In parallel organ systems such as the kidney, the therapeutic index for SBRT relies less upon the differential radiobiologic efficiencies of tumor and normal tissues and is more related to accurate dose delivery and rapid dose fall-off away from the targeted area. This emphasis on geography allows the delivery of ablative doses whereby only a small volume of adjacent normal tissue would be damaged.

Tumors traditionally regarded as radioresistant when utilizing conventionally fractionated radiation, such as RCC, could now be targeted with much larger doses per treatment. Large radiation doses overwhelm cell repair mechanisms, and are consequently extremely potent biologically. Early results in the metastatic setting have shown RCC to be radiosensitive to large doses per fraction [14, 30] and prompted evaluation of SBRT as a noninvasive alternative to surgical resection [31, 32].

Additionally, evidence has accumulated to show that in the special case of prostate cancer, the α/β ratio of linear and quadratic contributions to cell kill is relatively low [33–35] and more similar to late-responding normal tissues than to tumors. This characteristic suggests a hypothesis that a smaller number of larger-dose fractions should result in good local tumor control without increased normal-tissue damage [36]. Early institutional experiences have promisingly shown comparable tumor control and toxicity utilizing hypofractionated schedules, and multiinstitutional trials continue to explore long-term efficacy and safety [18].

SBRT continues to evolve as we address the fundamental limitations of tumor motion and targeting, patient positioning and motion, and dosimetric margins. Much like the origins of stereotaxy, this will require a multidisciplinary approach. Currently, the use of fiducial markers within or approximating the target may be utilized to improve tumor localization. Systems utilizing respiratory gating or tracking help account for internal tumor motion. Body-fix systems enable reproducible patient position and minimize external motion. Advanced dosimetry such as pencil beam scanning technology and Monte Carlo dose calculations enhance our understanding of where dose is delivered. The culmination of these technologies and the reproducibility of similar systems at other institutions are necessary for prospective evaluation and determination of safe fractionation regimens and delivery techniques. While still developing, molecular imaging holds a promise of intriguing advantages in SBRT. By allowing us to more precisely define the target volumes, high-dose, single- or hypofractionated courses of radiotherapy may be delivered while sparing normal tissues from the adverse late effects of radiotherapy. This may be possible through utilizing histopathology-validated hybrid molecular/anatomic image sets to more precisely guide treatment and dose modulation [25].

SBRT has provided an alternative to conventionally fractionated irradiation in the management of prostate cancer and currently is a possible alternative to resection in RCC patients with significant comorbid risks for surgery. As technology continues to advance, SBRT may continue to expand its role and utility in the management of genitourinary malignancies.

References

1. Mortensen H (1948) Transthoracic nephrectomy. J Urol 60:855–858
2. Gill IS (2000) Laparoscopic radical nephrectomy for cancer. Urol Clin North Am 27:707–719
3. Gill IS, Schweizer D, Hobart MG et al (2000) Retroperitoneal laparoscopic radical nephrectomy: the Cleveland clinic experience. J Urol 163:1665–1670
4. Rassweiler JJ, Abbou C, Janetschek G et al (2000) Laparoscopic partial nephrectomy. The European experience. Urol Clin North Am 27:721–736
5. Tierney AC (2000) Laparoscopic radical and partial nephrectomy. World J Urol 18:249–256
6. Savage SJ, Gill IS (2000) Renal tumor ablation: energy-based technologies. World J Urol 18:283–288
7. Wen CC, Nakada SY (2006) Energy ablative techniques for treatment of small renal tumors. Curr Opin Urol 16: 321–326
8. Vricella GJ, Haaga JR, Adler BL et al (2011) Percutaneous cryoablation of renal masses: impact of patient selection and treatment parameters on outcomes. Urology 77(3): 649–54
9. Derweesh IH, Novick AC (2003) Small renal tumors: natural history, observation strategies and emerging modalities of energy based tumor ablation. Can J Urol 10:1871–1879
10. Leksell L (1951) The stereotaxic method and radiosurgery of the brain. Acta Chir Scand 102:316–319
11. George R, Suh Y, Murphy M et al (2008) On the accuracy of a moving average algorithm for target tracking during radiation therapy treatment delivery. Med Phys 35:2356–2365
12. Kim DG, Chung HT, Gwak HS et al (2000) Gamma knife radiosurgery for brain metastases: prognostic factors for survival and local control. J Neurosurg 93(Suppl 3):23–29
13. Amendola BE, Wolf AL, Coy SR et al (2000) Brain metastases in renal cell carcinoma: management with gamma knife radiosurgery. Cancer J 6:372–376
14. Sheehan JP, Sun MH, Kondziolka D et al (2003) Radiosurgery in patients with renal cell carcinoma metastasis to the brain: long-term outcomes and prognostic factors influencing survival and local tumor control. J Neurosurg 98:342–349
15. Ponsky LE, Crownover RL, Rosen MJ et al (2003) Initial evaluation of Cyberknife technology for extracorporeal renal tissue ablation. Urology 61:498–501
16. Pentyala SN, Lee J, Hsieh K et al (2000) Prostate cancer: a comprehensive review. Med Oncol 17:85–105
17. King CR, Brooks JD, Gill H et al (2009) Stereotactic body radiotherapy for localized prostate cancer: interim results of a prospective phase II clinical trial. Int J Radiat Oncol Biol Phys 73:1043–1048
18. Freeman DE, King CR (2011) Stereotactic body radiotherapy for low-risk prostate cancer: five-year outcomes. Radiat Oncol 2011 Jan 10;6:3
19. Hall EJ, Giaccia AJ (2006) Radiobiology for the radiologist, 6th edn. Lippincott, Philadelphia, p 378
20. Papiez L, Timmerman R (2008) Hypofractionation in radiation therapy and its impact. Med Phys 35:112–118
21. Douglas BG, Fowler JF (1976) The effect of multiple small doses of x rays on skin reactions in the mouse and a basic interpretation. Radiat Res 66:401–426
22. Wolbarst AB, Chin LM, Svensson GK (1982) Optimization of radiation therapy: integral-response of a model biological system. Int J Radiat Oncol Biol Phys 8:1761–1769
23. Timmerman RD (2008) An overview of hypofractionation and introduction to this issue of seminars in radiation oncology. Semin Radiat Oncol 18:215–222
24. Fm K (2003) The physics of radiation therapy, 3rd edn. Lippincott, Philadelphia
25. Ellis RJ, Kaminsky DA, Zhou EH et al (2011) Ten-year outcomes: the clinical utility of single photon emission computed tomography/computed tomography ca-promab pendetide (Prostascint) in a cohort diagnosed with localized prostate cancer. Int J Radiat Oncol Biol Phys 81(1):29–34
26. Zelefsky MJ, Yamada Y, Fuks Z et al (2008) Long-term results of conformal radiotherapy for prostate cancer: impact of dose escalation on biochemical tumor control and distant metastases-free survival outcomes. Int J Radiat Oncol Biol Phys 71:1028–1033
27. Hamilton AJ, Lulu BA, Fosmire H et al (1995) Preliminary clinical experience with linear accelerator-based spinal stereotactic radiosurgery. Neurosurgery 36:311–319
28. Lax I, Blomgren H, Naslund I et al (1994) Stereotactic radiotherapy of malignancies in the abdomen. Methodological aspects. Acta Oncol 33:677–683
29. Uematsu M, Shioda A, Tahara K et al (1998) Focal, high dose, and fractionated modified stereotactic radiation therapy for lung carcinoma patients: a preliminary experience. Cancer 82:1062–1070
30. Wronski M, Maor MH, Davis BJ et al (1997) External radiation of brain metastases from renal carcinoma: a retrospective study of 119 patients from the M. D. Anderson Cancer Center. Int J Radiat Oncol Biol Phys 37:753–759
31. Beitler JJ, Makara D, Silverman P et al (2004) Definitive, high-dose-per-fraction, conformal, stereotactic external radiation for renal cell carcinoma. Am J Clin Oncol 27: 646–648
32. Wersall PJ, Blomgren H, Lax I et al (2005) Extracranial stereotactic radiotherapy for primary and metastatic renal cell carcinoma. Radiother Oncol 77:88–95
33. Wang JZ, Guerrero M, Li XA (2003) How low is the alpha/beta ratio for prostate cancer? Int J Radiat Oncol Biol Phys 55:194–203
34. Ritter M (2008) Rationale, conduct, and outcome using hypofractionated radiotherapy in prostate cancer. Semin Radiat Oncol 18:249–256
35. Macias V, Biete A (2009) Hypofractionated radiotherapy for localised prostate cancer. Review of clinical trials. Clin Transl Oncol 11:437–445
36. Fowler JF, Ritter MA, Chappell RJ et al (2003) What hypofractionated protocols should be tested for prostate cancer? Int J Radiat Oncol Biol Phys 56:1093–1104

Building a Stereotactic Radiosurgery Program for the Treatment of Prostate Cancer

3

Alan J. Katz

CONTENTS

3.1 Abstract

The focus of this chapter is to share the details of how to set up, promote, and successfully run a prostate stereotactic radiosurgery (SRS) program. Most importantly, this chapter describes what works well to promote a prostate SRS program and what does not work, so that time and money would not be wasted by those attempting to start a new prostate SRS program.

3.2 Introduction

Congratulations, you've decided to start a stereotactic radiosurgery (SRS) program for prostate cancer treatment—now what? As with any clinical program, starting an SRS prostate program presents a center with many challenges, not the least of which is getting patients at the door. I know this first hand; I launched a prostate program over 4 years ago; however, after treating over 600 patients, I have proven that it is quite feasible.

Before a program can be launched, there are several elements that need to be in place including the physical space for the center, the treatment device, and other such infrastructure, as well as the appropriate supporting staff. Existing centers will have many of these items whereas entirely new centers will not. For new centers, the issues relating to finding appropriate space and the specifics of the treatment device and other equipment depend not only on geographic location, but also center size, local regulations, and so forth. Given the regional and site-specific nature of these issues, the focus of this chapter will be to share the details of how to set up, promote, and successfully run such a prostate SRS program, assuming an office,

L.E. Ponsky et al. (eds.), *Treating Prostate Cancer and Related Genitourinary Applications*, Robotic Radiosurgery, DOI 10.1007/978-3-642-11495-3_3, © Springer-Verlag Berlin Heidelberg 2012 machine, and basic infrastructure already exist. We begin the chapter by walking through the roles of the various team members in the treatment of a prostate cancer patient to illustrate the dynamics of the program within the center and the impact of the various decisions that are made in the treatment process.

3.3 The Team

A successful program for SRS treatment of prostate cancer requires a team of professionals who embrace the treatment approach and interact well together. The primary team members should include one or more radiation oncologists, urologists, physicists, and a nurse coordinator. Each team member will have specific roles in both the setup and daily operations of prostate treatment at the center as described below. In addition, one team member should serve to spearhead the prostate program. This team member promotes and manages the program within the center to ensure smooth execution of patient treatments including patient recruitment and insurance approvals. Typically, given the nature of the prostate SRS treatment, in order for the program to grow and ensure that progress can be made, it is critical that the primary radiation oncologist be this driver of the program.

3.3.1 Radiation Oncologists' Role

In addition to serving as the prostate program team leader, the primary radiation oncologist and any additional radiation oncologists must immerse themselves in the available literature [1–4] such that they become conversant in the various methods used and outcomes reported for prostate cancer treatment. In this section, we provide an overview of the choices the radiation oncologist must consider; other chapters in this volume provide further details, and training courses provided by the device vendor can help facilitate this as well. Of course, physicists, urologists, and nurses can benefit from becoming conversant in the treatment and outcomes as well.

Prior to beginning any prostate treatment, if the radiation oncologist wishes, an Institution Review Board (IRB) approved protocol can be set up and patients can be placed on it prior to treatment. The benefits of treating on an IRB-approved protocol include providing patients with an assurance that the clinical approach is sound. Treatment on an IRB-approved protocol can also facilitate publication of outcomes, if desired. Options for an IRB-approved protocol include both a protocol developed in-house following an extensive review of currently published results, participation in an ongoing clinical study, or use of a protocol from a clinical study without formal participation in the study. Two CyberKnife®-specific (Accuray Incorporated, Sunnyvale, CA) prostate cancer clinical studies [5, 6] sponsored by Accuray are in progress, one using a homogeneous dose distribution and the other a high-dose rate (HDR) brachytherapy-like treatment approach with heterogeneous dose distribution. Details on these and other ongoing SRS clinical trials for prostate cancer can be found on the clinicaltrials.gov website, which is an online registry of clinical trials conducted in the United States and around the world. Alternatively, since a number of publications have provided treatment details and outcomes [1–3], participation in these studies could be considered optional, but it may increase the radiation oncologist's comfort level.

While patient treatment is of paramount concern, all radiation oncologists, especially the designated team-lead radiation oncologist, must tirelessly seek forums to promote, publicize, and expand the prostate program at their center. This includes giving talks about radiosurgery to potential referring physicians, including urologists and primary care physicians. These talks should highlight both the SRS approach and treatment results. For example, in my presentations, I highlight the CyberKnife technology, including the high accuracy of real-time tracking, the dose per fraction, as well as observed toxicity rates, and promising outcomes to date. The goal of such presentations is to introduce clinicians to this treatment approach and get them excited about the potentials of prostate SRS treatment. Also very useful are talks given to the general public, especially to senior groups, consisting of similar, but less technical, information. This is an effective way of educating the local public, which is especially important, as patients are rarely educated on this topic by their physicians. Since patients have a myriad of choices that can be used for their treatment, a high level of confidence and enthusiasm communicated to patients is very helpful.

3.3.2 Urologists' Role

It would be quite helpful to have a core team of urologists who have a special interest in radiosurgery that are part of the center's prostate SRS program. At this time, many centers may find this difficult to attain due to competing interests in surgery and ownership of intensity-modulated radiation therapy (IMRT) facilities by urology groups. However, if one or two urologists can be identified and educated on SRS-type prostate treatment, that would be sufficient. Not only can they be a source of patient referrals, but they can see self-referred patients and give them another point of view. As with other team members, urologists should familiarize themselves with the details of the treatments, especially the toxicity that they may be called on to manage.

While urologists can no longer be reimbursed for their participation in treatments, they can be engaged in fiducial implantation and receive reimbursement through Current Procedural Terminology (CPT) codes 55876 and 76942. Nevertheless, urologists may wish to participate in contouring and planning, but this is considered optional. Their main role is in following the patients after therapy. Specifically, they must understand when and how side effects may become manifest; understanding how PSA values respond is also of paramount importance. For instance, approximately 20–25% of patients will experience a PSA bounce up to 3 years after therapy [1, 3]; recognition of this PSA bounce by urologists is important to avoid unnecessary testing and biopsies. As such, urologists should work closely with the radiation oncologist when it comes to treatment and follow-up.

3.3.3 Physicists' Role

The role of the physicist is extremely critical in a successful prostate SRS program. The physicist must ensure the quality of the treatment plans including limiting dose to the bladder, rectum, and testes. Furthermore, the physicist must understand how to balance the treatment plan parameters with the realities of treatment. For example, while it is possible to generate an ideal treatment plan using a very large number of beams, delivery of that plan could take several hours; such an extended duration of treatment would likely result in the patient becoming fidgety and ultimately undermine the treatment. To understand these issues, physicists should be well-trained in the trade-offs between treatment plan quality and other variables such as treatment session duration. For example, with the CyberKnife System, treatment planning techniques can be discussed and familiarity with use of the new Iris® collimator (Accuray) can be obtained. As part of the program set up, the physicist and radiation oncologist also need to agree on various aspects of the treatment, including whether they wish to employ the HDR-like heterogeneous planning [6, 7] or the more common homogeneous planning [1–3], use of the IRIS collimator, and so forth, as discussed in more detail below.

3.3.4 Coordinator's Role

A nurse/insurance coordinator is a vital member of the team. A nurse who is aware of the nature of the treatments and potential side effects can interact with patients on a daily basis and increase the patient's comfort level. It is also highly desirable that a nurse be trained in the insurance approval process, though dedicated administrative staff may also fulfill this role, if the radiosurgical practice is busy enough to immerse the nurse coordinator in medical duties.

A high level of knowledge is instrumental in crafting insurance authorization requests and appeals. Furthermore, the specifics of billing policies and methodology depend greatly on whether your center is part of a hospital or a freestanding center. As such, it is highly beneficial that the nurse/insurance coordinator be well versed with billing regulations, coding, and other items specific to insurance authorization. Knowledge of the current literature is also vital in making the case for radiosurgery treatment to an insurance company. This knowledge is particularly helpful in telephone interactions with insurance companies where nurses and physicians can facilitate approval. Many of the large carriers currently do not recognize SRS as a tool for prostate cancer, but this can be overcome. One approach is for the hospital administration and/or owners of the facility to aggressively pursue contracts with the carriers. Although this may require accepting lower payments, it is well worthwhile to avoid endless battles with the carriers, which can discourage patients and end up with the patients leaving to seek other therapies. Using this approach, the lower individual payments will be made up for in the volume of patients that will be treated in a timely manner. In addition, a preapproved contract will mean less stress for prospective patients, who already are dealing with the stress of a cancer diagnosis. In either case, it is important to have the supporting documentation available for interactions with insurance carriers. Such items include references detailing the α/β ratio [8], papers supporting accelerated hypofractionation [9, 10], and published outcomes to date [1–3].

3.4 Marketing

Once the team is in place, meetings with administrative staff should focus on proper marketing of the prostate SRS program. Since many centers will not have huge urology support, direct marketing to the public is a vital component of a successful prostate SRS program. As mentioned earlier, inexpensive marketing can be done by having the radiation oncologist provide lectures to the local communities; particularly useful groups for these lectures are senior centers, retired worker groups, and other such groups with a large population of elderly members. A simple slide presentation by the radiation oncologist can stimulate interest on the part of attendees. A robust question and answer period will help bring out the elements of the therapy that will appeal to patients, such as the fact that therapy can be done in as few as 4–5 days. Evening lectures with refreshments can bring 50–100 people and often up to four patients may come in for consult as a result. It is amazing how little is known about SRS for prostate by the general public and how receptive people are once they hear the details. In the community hospital setting, these events can typically be set up by the hospital's community outreach coordinator. For freestanding clinics, as discussed below, a publicity consultant can assist with setting these activities up.

More far-reaching marketing options include internet, newspaper, radio, and TV advertising. Among these, the internet is the least expensive, but can be very useful. Your center's web site should have specific references to prostate cancer. Videos showing a treatment in action are also highly illustrative for a patient unfamiliar with radiosurgery. In addition, links to recent publications are also useful to educate a prospective patient who may be considering multiple other treatment options.

In order to effectively advertise in other media, significant funds will have to be committed, up to $500,000 per year to make a substantial impact. The greatest impact can be achieved with TV and radio advertising. Obviously, this will require a larger financial commitment, but will also return the largest dividends in terms of patients calling in for consultations. Newspaper advertisements can also be effective. My experience has shown that local newspaper ads need to be run at least weekly to have an impact. In addition, the ad must be large enough, typically a half or a full page, to catch a reader's eye. The ad should show a man, either alone or with his wife, preferably in color and a large print size should be used to emphasize key facts.

All advertisements, independent of media type, should stress the advantages of SRS therapy, including the short, 4–5 day course compared to 45 days for IMRT. An emphasis on recent data showing low toxicity and promising biochemical control rates [1–3] should also be made. Similarly, SRS potency preservation rates [2, 3, 11] should be conveyed and contrasted with IMRT or surgery [12, 13]. Furthermore, if the center has special expertise, such as a large number of cases treated, it can be placed in the ad.

Not only is the advertisement content important, but the target audience must be considered. For example, radio advertisements should be strategically placed on stations that cater to the risk group. This would include any sports stations, but also talk radio, and even "Oldies" music stations that play music from the 1950s and the 1960s.

In addition to direct-to-patient marketing, marketing to referring doctors is an option. As described earlier, this can include presentations to doctors detailing prostate SRS. Another approach is to have a person visit appropriate doctors within the community for face-to-face discussions on your center's prostate program. As with much of prostate SRS, the goal is to get the word out and inform people of the supporting literature for this treatment approach. As the above demonstrates, marketing a prostate SRS program is complex, and, if possible, professional marketing help should be sought in developing a suitable strategy.

3.5 The Patient

The patient is the lifeblood of your prostate program. The daily activities at your center revolve around your patient interactions, treatment, and follow-up; they will make or break a successful program. Every member of the prostate program team has roles in patient treatment. To highlight the dynamics associated with the daily activities of the center, the following walks through patient interaction from first contact to the decision to perform SRS treatment through to long-term patient follow-up. Each team member's roles and the impact the various decisions may have on the patient and the prostate program are illustrated. Given that my particular experience has focused on the use of the CyberKnife for prostate SRS, many of the following details will be CyberKnife-specific, but the general SRS requirements (good planning, critical structure contouring, margins, fiducial implantation, and motion management) will also apply more generally.

3.5.1 First Contact

Once the team is assembled and marketing is in place, patients will begin to call your center to learn more about your prostate program. What happens when a patient first calls your center to find out more information is extremely important. Most men who call will want more information about the treatment, rather than immediately making an appointment. During these first contact calls, men will be especially interested in how the treatment pertains to their specific situation. One thing that can quickly turn patients off is not getting a rapid response from the center, or an inadequate response from a person who cannot answer detailed questions. It is imperative that a prompt response follow an inquiry, ideally within 24 h. The team members involved in the response typically include the nurse coordinator and the radiation oncologist. The ideal person to respond to the patient is the radiation oncologist; in that way the prospective patient gets immediate feedback as to the applicability of their specific case. Patients are very impressed that a treating physician shows interest in their case at this early stage. On the other hand, when a patient can only speak to a designated triage person, who is not as well equipped in answering specific questions and concerns, they are less engaged and less likely to pursue treatment at the center. Thus, if the radiation oncologist is not the person responding to the patient, it is imperative that the nurse coordinator be well versed with the treatment and be able to provide highly relevant details to the patient. It must be remembered that men with prostate cancer have a large choice of potential therapies, and the initial experience that they have on first contact is critical in determining whether they will pursue the radiosurgery option.

3.5.2 Consultation

Patients who come for consultation are initially evaluated with history and physical exam by the radiation oncologist. In addition, they are given quality of life questionnaires such as the Expanded Prostate Cancer Index Composite (EPIC), the Sexual Health Inventory for Men (SHIM), and the American Urological Association (AUA) symptom score forms to fill out so that their urinary, bowel, and sexual function can be documented prior to treatment. These data can also be useful to monitor the overall effectiveness of your center's treatment protocol as well as for publication of results. The patients are given full discussion of all treatment options including surgery, IMRT, brachytherapy, and radiosurgery. A video to describe the procedure is a recommended tool to help educate the patients prior to their evaluation. At the time of evaluation, all data are presented, and I believe it is an excellent idea to share the most recent medical literature showing the results of radiosurgery to the patients. To make the medical literature more readily understandable to the patient, a summary sheet highlighting the results of included publications can be helpful.

The patients also should be evaluated by the center's urologist. It is particularly helpful to have an experienced urologist who can explain to the patient details about the procedure and possible side effects that may occur. Also any treatments for symptoms that may become necessary can be discussed with the patient.

3.5.3 The Decision

When the patient decides that radiosurgery makes sense for him, the next step is to obtain insurance approval. The nurse/coordinator is the team member who performs this process, as described earlier. Upon approval, the nurse/coordinator also sets up the pretreatment visit with the radiation oncologist where treatment decisions are made.

3.5.4 Treatment Decisions

Once the patient has chosen radiosurgery, and insurance approval has been obtained, the next part of the process for the radiation oncologist is decide what risk the patient has for extraprostatic extension. Generally, one can divide patients into three categories: low-, intermediate-, and high-risk patients. Low-risk patients have T1c or T2a disease, a PSA less than 10 ng/mL and a Gleason score less than 7. Intermediate-risk patients have T2B lesions with a PSA between 10 and 20 ng/mL and a Gleason score of 7 or more. High-risk patients have a PSA greater than 20 or a Gleason score of 8 or higher. In general, all patients who receive radiosurgery have organ-confined disease and therefore there are no T3 lesions.

Following the assessment of the patient's risk category, the proper treatment can be determined. Low-risk patients typically receive radiosurgery monotherapy with the treatment volume including the prostate with 5 mm margin, except 3 mm posteriorly. For intermediate-risk patients, it is recommended to also treat the proximal half of the seminal vesicles (approximately 1 cm). Based on data that has been accumulated [14], it appears that intermediate-risk patients can be well treated with SRS monotherapy and do not need external-beam radiation in addition. For high-risk patients, I believe there are two valid approaches, neither of which has been demonstrated as clearly superior. The first approach is to treat with external beam radiation to the pelvis and prostate to a dose of 45 Gy in 25 fractions followed by an SRS boost of approximately three 6.5–7 Gy fractions. Using this regimen, the patient will receive 5½ weeks of treatment, and more rectal tissue will be irradiated compared to monotherapy [15]. If these patients receive radiosurgery as a boost, this can be done with minimal margins as they already have received external-beam radiation to the periprostatic tissues. Alternatively, since no overall benefit has been shown with the use of pelvic nodal radiation [16, 17], a case can be made to deliver radiosurgery as monotherapy for these high-risk patients. High-risk patients who receive monotherapy should be treated with a wider margin on the involved side, using an 8–10 mm margin. For such patients, the treated volume would also include seminal vesicles. At the present time, there is no clear-cut difference in the two treatment outcomes, with PSA results virtually identical at 3-year follow-up [14]. The advantage of monotherapy is that there is less rectal dose, less toxicity, and a shorter duration of treatment, as monotherapy can be completed in 5 rather than 28 days.

Patients should also be counseled about hormone ablative therapy. Martinez et al. have shown that hormonal ablative therapy is of no benefit in patients receiving HDR brachytherapy with hypofractionation [18]. Therefore, we believe that patients who come to the clinic on hormone ablative therapy can discontinue it. The risks of hormone ablative therapy include fatigue, loss of libido, bone loss, increased risk of diabetes, heart disease, and cognitive dysfunction [19]. Thus, it may be possible to eliminate hormone ablative therapy provides prior to, during, and after the course of radiation to avoid these side effects without a greater risk of disease recurrence.

3.5.5 Fiducial Placement

The next step toward monotherapy treatment is fiducial seed placement. If radiosurgery will be used as a boost, seed placement can be done at the end of the course of EBRT. In general, I recommend all fiducial placements within a prostate program be performed by a small select group of doctors (radiation oncologists or urologists) to ensure a uniformity of fiducial placement. Poor seed placement makes tracking more difficult, time-consuming, and potentially less accurate. Thus, it is important that seed placement be done properly so that the patient's treatment is efficiently completed in a reasonable amount of time.

Fiducial placement can be performed transperineally, which is my preferred approach, or transrectally. Transperineal placement can easily be accomplished by using a transrectal ultrasound similar to that used for brachytherapy with a perineal template. In order to facilitate this, I have used EMLA cream, a topical anesthetic, but subcutaneous injection of lidocaine can also be used. If EMLA cream is used, it takes approximately 1 h to work. After 1 h, the patient is put in a supine position, a transrectal ultrasound is placed in the rectum and images are obtained. I use four separate needles with gold seeds embedded at the end of the needle. Using the grid, I place the first two needles into the prostate at the right and left lateral sides of the gland near the capsule. The first two seeds are placed as close to the base of the gland as possible. These two seeds should be placed at the same level, so that when orthogonal films are taken at 45° angles, the seeds do not overlap. The next two seeds are also placed with two needles toward the apex of the gland or just outside the gland. These seeds should be placed at least 2 cm apart from the adjacent seeds. The advantage of placing four seeds is that if one seed moves, the other three seeds can still be used to provide full tracking including translational, rotational, and pitch tracking. Another approach is to use stranded seeds, which eliminates the need for two of the needles. Fiducial placement can also be performed transrectally, although there is a chance of introducing bacterial infection into the prostate.

3.5.6 Treatment Planning

After waiting approximately for 1 week, the patient is scheduled for computed tomography (CT) and magnetic resonance imaging (MRI) scans that are done contemporaneously. In order to get good images with MRI, I recommend the use of gadolinium, although this is not absolutely necessary. The CT can be done without the use of any intravenous contrast. The evening before scanning, the patient gets a clean-out of two doses of bisacodyl, and then they get a Fleet® enema (Fleet Laboratories, Lynchburg, VA) on the morning of the procedure. It is very important that the patient's rectum be cleaned out prior to scanning and prior to each treatment. Occasionally, even after good clean-out, the patient still has significant air in the rectum. If this is found, the scanning is aborted and the situation can be remedied by a rectal tube or additional time to allow further evacuation. Once the scanning is done, the patient can go home.

After the scanning is complete, a physicist will perform a fusion of MRI and CT. I highly recommend the use of MRI as it shows the actual volume of the prostate much better than a computerized axial tomography (CAT) scan, especially as the apex is approached [20]. This can significantly reduce the volume of tissue treated and will reduce radiation in the periprostatic tissues including the neurovascular bundles and the penile bulb. This may also play a role in decreasing the rate of erectile dysfunction after therapy.

Planning commences once all structures have been contoured by the physician. In general, a radiation oncologist can do this, but they may work in conjunction with a urologist. The gross tumor volume (GTV) should first be contoured, including either the prostate alone or the proximal seminal vesicles also. Generally, the bladder and rectum should be contoured from well superior and to well inferior to the actual dimensions of the prostate. In order to evaluate the dose to the penile bulb, this should also be contoured. In addition, I recommend contouring the testicles so that the dose to them can be ascertained. If the dose appears to be too high, this could be remedied by eliminating some beams through the testicles. It is recommended not to allow the mean dose to the testicles to exceed 5 Gy; with this constraint there appears to be no significant loss of testicular function in terms of hypogonadism after radiosurgery [3,21,22]. Indeed, if all beams traversing the testicles can be eliminated without decreasing the PTV coverage quality this is preferable as it further reduces the mean testicular does to 2–3 Gy [22].

The next step is treatment planning which could be accomplished by the physicist. Considerations here include the number of collimators and treatment beams. With reference to our CyberKnife experience, the older G3 machine often uses three paths with two to three different collimators which have to be manually changed. The newer G4 machine combined with the use of Iris variable aperture collimator can significantly reduce treatment time by not requiring manual collimator changes. Using Iris, up to six to seven different collimators can be used, which enhances the quality of the treatment plan and reduces the D50 to the bladder and rectum by 30–40%. In general, it is recommended that treatment be delivered with approximately 130–170 beams, which can achieve a good homogenous dose plan. If the dose plan is fairly homogenous with a PTV covered by the 83–85% isodose line, then it is not necessary to contour the urethra as the urethral dose should be within tolerance.

Once the treatment planning has been completed, the treating physicians, including the radiation oncologist and urologist, will evaluate the plan and approve it. In order to approve the plan, the D50 to the rectum and bladder should ideally be at 42–45% of the total dose or lower. This is easily achievable, especially with the use of the Iris variable aperture collimator. The mean dose to the penile bulb should also be less than 40% of the maximum dose. It is advisable to do planning with shell structures and not use constraint points on the bladder, rectum, or the penile bulb.

If the radiation oncologist chooses, heterogeneous planning can be done to better emulate HDR planning, delivering a more radiobiologically potent dose to the prostate, particularly the peripheral zone of the prostate [7]. This approach will typically require more beams, more monitor units, and a longer treatment time versus homogeneous treatment plans. Also, the urethra must be identified on the CT scans by the use of a Foley catheter, as is also the case with actual HDR brachytherapy, so that the urethra may be accurately spared from areas of extreme dose intensification. The Iris platform is particularly advantageous, relative to predecessor CyberKnife models, for "HDR-like" treatments, reducing the average monitor units and beams per case by approximately 25%, and reducing the overall treatment time by up to 50%. Further follow-up is necessary to discern if there is a difference in outcomes between these two treatment approaches.

3.5.7 Treatment

After the planning has been completed and approved, the patient will come in for treatment. I have always used the daily treatment regimen from Monday to Friday to deliver five fractions. Dose has ranged from 7 to 7.25 Gy per fraction for monotherapy, or 6.5 to 7 Gy per fraction if delivered as a boost. The patients will come in having taken two bisacodyl tablets and a Fleet enema in the morning. It is also recommended that they have a light meal the night before and the morning of treatment. In the case of the CyberKnife, our experience has shown that treatment with the G3 machines should be done in approximately 45–60 min with homogenous planning assuming the fiducials are well placed and allow reasonable tracking. Using the newer G4 technology with Iris and faster machine output, the patients can be treated on the CyberKnife in approximately 30 min. My initial impression is that the dosimetry with Iris is significantly improved with regard to rectal and bladder doses. I have not found that patients need to have every other day treatment, as rectal tolerance is quite good with daily treatment especially at 7-Gy fractions [3].

All patients that I have treated also received amifostine prior to each fraction (1,500 mg mixed in approximately 40–50 cm^3 of saline advanced into the rectum 15 min before treatment). It is allowed to stay in the rectum from where it is absorbed. Amifostine is generally well tolerated; only one patient out of approximately 600 experienced an allergic reaction, and it was mild. Patients also do not become hypotensive with rectally administered amifostine as there is little to no systemic absorption [23, 24]. Nevertheless, it is not clear that amifostine is necessary to keep rectal tolerance high. Friedland et al. delivered five fractions of 7 Gy and found very low rectal toxicity with similar treatment planning in the absence of amifostine [2]. At 7.25 Gy per fraction, there was higher rectal toxicity in the Stanford experience, but it remains unknown if amifostine is necessary at that dose [1].

3.5.8 Initial Follow-Up

Patients are generally advised of the side effects they may get over the next few weeks and that they should come back for a 3-week follow-up. It is important to warn them of the 1–2 weeks of urgency, both urinary and rectal, that they are likely to encounter. Patients should be considered for alpha blockers if they develop obstructive urinary symptoms at the end of the 5 days of treatment. It is helpful to advise patients to eat one or two servings of yogurt with yeast per day, which seems to help regulate the bowels. By the third week, the majority of patients can look forward to improvement in their symptoms. When a patient returns at 3 weeks, it is advisable to have them repeat their EPIC, SHIM, and/or AUA questionnaire, which will likely show a drop in the mean scores from baseline. Very few patients should experience urinary retention requiring a catheter. This can be minimized by considering patients with severe obstructive symptoms and a large median lobe for a laser transurethral resection of the prostate (TURP) prior to undergoing radiosurgery. In so doing, patients can avoid the risk of retention and tolerate their radiosurgery treatment very well, if an interval of 4–6 weeks is allowed for healing before radiosurgery treatment.

3.5.9 Ongoing Follow-Up

Patients should be instructed to continue follow-ups with the radiation oncologist and their urologist. Monitoring of PSA at 3-month intervals for the first year, and every 6 months thereafter, is recommended and can be accomplished with alternate visits to the two physicians. EPIC, SHIM, and/or AUA scoring should also be obtained at 6-month intervals for the first 2 years. These data, along with the PSA data, can be kept easily in a Microsoft Access file or other simple database to allow examination of overall patient performance in your prostate program. A number of studies have reported prostate SRS follow-up extending to 24–36 months [1–3]. The following provides a summary of what patients can expect with ongoing follow-up based on these results and my own experience in treating over 600 prostate cancer patients using the CyberKnife.

Three months after treatment the vast majority of patients should be back to baseline with regard to urinary and rectal function. This seems to hold up on average for the first 2–3 years post-treatment. Sexual function dips on average for the first few months and tends to stay diminished with the average EPIC score down by 15–20% from the baseline [3]. This translates to roughly 15–20% of the patients reporting significant diminution in erectile function. Most of these patients, especially younger ones, can be helped effectively with medications like sildenafil. These issues are best managed by the urologist, who has more experience than the radiation oncologist in this area.

In general, regardless of dose, one can expect to see a median PSA at 1 year of 0.9–1.1 ng/mL. At 2 and 3 years, one can expect a median PSA of approximately 0.4 and 0.15 ng/mL, respectively. There is a subset of patients, mostly younger, who seem to drop their PSA more slowly. This should be recognized, as patients like this have been unnecessarily rebiopsied. As long as the trend is down, nothing but observation needs to be done. It is also very important to recognize that 20–30% of patients will experience a bounce averaging 0.2–0.5 ng/mL in their PSA in the first 3 years [1, 3]. Typically, these bounces dissipate on the next reading, as PSA should continue to dip. This pattern is similar to that seen with LDR and HDR brachytherapy [25, 26]. In my experience, overall, by 3 years, the vast majority of patients will have a PSA < 0.5 ng/mL, which may be suggestive of excellent long-term outcomes [27, 28]. PSA can still be decreasing at 4 years after treatment, which is near the extent of data to date; thus, it is difficult to describe the average time to nadir. At this point, however, it appears that the average time to nadir will be at least 30–36 months and maybe longer.

In the patients I have treated, late bowel and bladder side effects have typically taken an average of 12–15 months to develop. Few patients seem to experience any late side effects beyond 24 months, although a small percentage of patients (1–3%) can be expected to develop late rectal bleeding [3]. Thus far this seems to be true whether amifostine is administered or not [2, 29]. This bleeding is generally mild and tends to resolve on its own after a few months. A few of these patients may benefit from laser cauterization if symptoms do not abate on their own. Urinary side effects usually are related to prostatic urethritis, rather than cystitis, and up to 10% of patients can experience dysuria and urge incontinence from this. Most of these patients can be treated with a medication such as solifenacin or tolterodine and obtain relief. Over a period of a few months, this tends to resolve. Patients who develop mild necrosis at the superior urethra have benefited from hyperbaric oxygen treatments, with complete healing noted on cystoscopy. Less than 1% of patients have developed severe urinary symptoms, such as frank incontinence or severe urethral stricture [3]. Most patients who develop such late symptoms should be treated with medication and cystoscopy; biopsy should be avoided, as this may exacerbate the problem.

3.6 Summary

This chapter describes the roles and interactions of the various team members within a prostate SRS program. Successful development of a prostate SRS program requires a devotion to the treatment approach, communication between team members, and a forward-looking marketing campaign that is able to get patients in the door. Patients are the most important aspect of the program and it is important to remember that prostate cancer patients know they have a choice in treatment. A well-designed and executed SRS program that considers all aspects of patient interactions and treatment will go a long way in itself to help promote your program through patient referral.

References

1. King CR, Brooks JD, Gill H et al (2009) Stereotactic body radiotherapy for localized prostate cancer: interim results of a prospective phase II clinical trial. Int J Radiat Oncol Biol Phys 73:1043–1048
2. Friedland JL, Freeman DE, Masterson-McGary ME et al (2009) Stereotactic body radiotherapy: an emerging treatment approach for localized prostate cancer. Technol Cancer Res Treat 8:387–392
3. Katz AJ, Santoro M, Ashley R et al (2010) Stereotactic body radiotherapy for organ-confined prostate cancer. BMC Urol 10:1
4. Katz A (2010) CyberKnife radiosurgery for prostate cancer. Technol Cancer Res Treat 9(5):463–472
5. Meier R. CyberKnife radiosurgery for organ-confined prostate cancer: homogenous dose distribution; 2008
6. Fuller DB. CyberKnife radiosurgery for low & intermediate risk prostate cancer: emulating HDR brachytherapy dosimetry; 2008
7. Fuller DB, Naitoh J, Lee C et al (2008) Virtual HDR CyberKnife treatment for localized prostatic carcinoma: dosimetry com-parison with HDR brachytherapy and preliminary clinical observations. Int J Radiat Oncol Biol Phys 70:1588–1597
8. Fowler JF (2005) The radiobiology of prostate cancer including new aspects of fractionated radiotherapy. Acta Oncol 44:265–276
9. Martinez AA, Gustafson G, Gonzalez J et al (2002) Dose escalation using conformal high-dose-rate brachytherapy improves outcome in unfavorable prostate cancer. Int J Radiat Oncol Biol Phys 53:316–327
10. Collins CD, Lloyd-Davies RW, Swan AV (1991) Radical external beam radiotherapy for localised carcinoma of the prostate using a hypofractionation technique. Clin Oncol (R Coll Radiol) 3:127–132
11. Wiegner EA, King CR (2010) Sexual function after stereotactic body radiotherapy for prostate cancer: results of a prospective clinical trial. Int J Radiat Oncol Biol Phys 78(2):442–448
12. Zelefsky MJ, Chan H, Hunt M et al (2006) Long-term outcome of high dose intensity modulated radiation therapy for patients with clinically localized prostate cancer. J Urol 176:1415–1419
13. Dubbelman YD, Dohle GR, Schroder FH (2006) Sexual function before and after radical retropubic prostatectomy: a systematic review of prognostic indicators for a successful outcome. Eur Urol 50:711–718; discussion 718–720
14. Katz A, Santoro M, Ashley R et al (in press) Stereotactic body radiotherapy with and without external beam radiation therapy in treatment of organ confined prostate cancer. European Society for Therapeutic Radiology and Oncology Annual Meeting
15. Katz A, Santoro M, Ashley R et al (2010) Stereotactic body radiotherapy as boost for organ-confined prostate cancer. Technol Cancer Res Treat 9(6):575–582
16. Pommier P, Chabaud S, Lagrange JL et al (2007) Is there a role for pelvic irradiation in localized prostate adenocarcinoma? Preliminary results of GETUG-01. J Clin Oncol 25: 5366–5373
17. Lawton CA, DeSilvio M, Lee WR et al (2007) Results of a phase II trial of transrectal ultrasound-guided permanent radioactive implantation of the prostate for definitive management of localized adenocarcinoma of the prostate (radiation therapy oncology group 98–05). Int J Radiat Oncol Biol Phys 67:39–47
18. Martinez AA, Demanes DJ, Galalae R et al (2005) Lack of benefit from a short course of androgen deprivation for unfavorable prostate cancer patients treated with an accelerated hypofractionated regime. Int J Radiat Oncol Biol Phys 62:1322–1331
19. Bagrodia A, Diblasio CJ, Wake RW et al (2009) Adverse effects of androgen deprivation therapy in prostate cancer: current management issues. Indian J Urol 25:169–176
20. Sannazzari GL, Ragona R, Ruo Redda MG et al (2002) CT-MRI image fusion for delineation of volumes in three-dimensional conformal radiation therapy in the treatment of localized prostate cancer. Br J Radiol 75:603–607
21. King CR, Lo A, Kapp DS (2009) Testicular dose from prostate cyberknife: a cautionary note. Int J Radiat Oncol Biol Phys 73:636–637; author reply 637
22. Fuller DB (2009) Testicular dose from prostate cyberknife: a cautionary note in regard to King et al. Int J Radiat Oncol Biol Phys 73:637

23. Athanassiou H, Antonadou D, Coliarakis N et al (2003) Protective effect of amifostine during fractionated radiotherapy in pa-tients with pelvic carcinomas: results of a randomized trial. Int J Radiat Oncol Biol Phys 56:1154–1160
24. Simone NL, Menard C, Soule BP et al (2008) Intrarectal amifostine during external beam radiation therapy for prostate cancer produces significant improvements in Quality of Life measured by EPIC score. Int J Radiat Oncol Biol Phys 70:90–95
25. Toledano A, Chauveinc L, Flam T et al (2006) PSA bounce after permanent implant prostate brachytherapy may mimic a biochemical failure: a study of 295 patients with a minimum 3-year followup. Brachytherapy 5:122–126
26. Pinkawa M, Piroth MD, Holy R et al (2010) Prostate-specific antigen kinetics following external-beam radiotherapy and tem-porary (Ir-192) or permanent (I-125) brachytherapy for prostate cancer. Radiother Oncol 96(1): 25–29
27. Zelefsky MJ, Shi W, Yamada Y et al (2009) Postradiotherapy 2-year prostate-specific antigen nadir as a predictor of long-term prostate cancer mortality. Int J Radiat Oncol Biol Phys 75:1350–1356
28. Stock RG, Klein TJ, Cesaretti JA et al (2009) Prognostic significance of 5-year PSA value for predicting prostate cancer recurrence after brachytherapy alone and combined with hormonal therapy and/or external beam radiotherapy. Int J Radiat Oncol Biol Phys 74:753–758
29. Freeman DE, Friedland JL, Masterson-McGary ME (2010) Stereotactic radiosurgery for low-intermediate risk prostate cancer: an emerging treatment approach. Am J Clin Oncol 33:208

Part II

Historical and Current Prostate Cancer Issues

Prostate Anatomy and Prostate Cancer Screening, Diagnosis, Staging, and Prevention

4

Eric Umbreit, Mark Shimko, and Matthew Gettman

CONTENTS

4.1 Abstract

The prostate is located between the bladder and the external sphincter and normally is 4 cm in length and 4–5 cm in width.

Prostate cancer is the third leading cause of cancer-related death in men. Prostate serum antigen (PSA) is used for the screening, diagnosis, treatment, and monitoring of prostate cancer. PSA screening alone has a higher detection rate than digital rectal examination alone, but detection rates are highest when the two exams are combined. The diagnosis of prostate cancer is made histologically by prostate needle biopsy in the majority of cases. The most widely accepted grading system is the Gleason grading system, which is based on the architectural pattern of the prostate glands. Based on current evidence, 5α-reductase inhibitors have been shown to reduce the relative incidence of prostate cancer compared to placebo.

4.2 Prostate Anatomy

4.2.1 General

The prostate is located between the bladder and the external sphincter (Fig. 4.1). The normal adult prostate is approximately 4 cm in length and 4–5 cm in width [1]. It is traversed throughout its length by the posterior urethra and is fixed to the pelvic floor by fascial investments [2]. The endopelvic fascia is a continuation of the endoabdominal fascia and two dense condensations of the endopelvic fascia on the anterior prostate affix it to the pubis as the puboprostatic/pubovesical ligament. These ligaments contain detrusor (bladder) muscle fibers and stabilize the prostate, urethra, and bladder to the pubic bone [3, 4]. Anteriorly, the prostate is covered by a rich plexus of veins known as the deep venous complex, or Santorini's

L.E. Ponsky et al. (eds.), *Treating Prostate Cancer and Related Genitourinary Applications*, Robotic Radiosurgery, DOI 10.1007/978-3-642-11495-3_4,

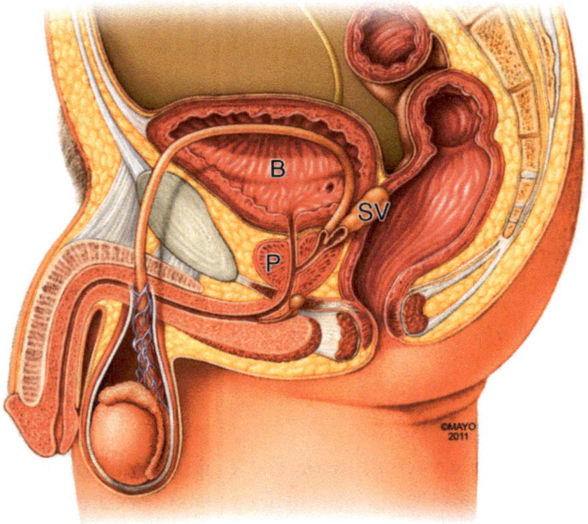

Fig. 4.1 3-D Sagittal representation of the prostate and its anatomic relationships within the pelvis

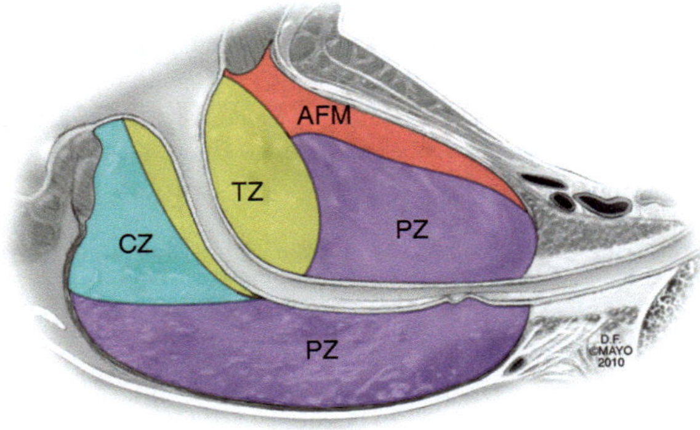

Fig. 4.2 Anatomical zones of the prostate gland as depicted by McNeal [7]. AFM = Anterior fibromuscular zone, TZ = Transition zone, CZ = Central zone, PZ = Peripheral zone

plexus [5]. Posteriorly, the prostate is separated from the rectum by Denonvilliers' fascia (or rectoprostatic fascia), which embryologically is derived from the peritoneum [6].

4.2.2 Gross Anatomy

The prostate is covered by a fibrous capsule and consists of four glandular regions or zones that can be distinguished by ultrasonic examination of the prostate (Fig. 4.2) [7]. They include the peripheral, central, and transitional zones. There is also an anterior fibromuscular stroma. Anatomically, no true lobar anatomy exists and the bulk of the gland is composed of the peripheral zone, which makes up 75% of the volume, whereas the central zone generally constitutes 25%. The posterior aspect of the prostate is traversed by the ampullae of the vas deferens, which exit in the ejaculatory ducts of the posterior urethra. The posterior urethra has a small mound on its dorsal aspect, termed the verumontanum. In the middle of the verumontanum is a small pit called the utricle, a Mullerian (paramesonephric) remnant. The ejaculatory ducts exit on the verumontanum.

4.2.3 Microscopic Anatomy

A glandular structure, the prostate is made up of mucosal, submucosal, and main prostatic glands arranged concentrically around the prostatic urethra [8]. The glands are surrounded by fibromuscular stroma (Fig. 4.3) and distributed into external and periurethral glands. The external glands comprise the majority of the glandular tissue within the prostate. The main ducts consist of tubuloalveolar elements, with simple or pseudostratified epithelium.

The prostatic secretion is colorless, watery, and makes up one-third of the ejaculate volume. It is rich in zinc, citric acid, acid phosphatase, fibrolysin, PSA, and other proteases involved with liquefaction of semen. The prostate gland is an androgen-dependent organ and the conversion of testosterone into dihydrotestosterone within the prostate stimulates its growth.

4.2.4 Blood Supply, Lymphatics, and Innervation

The primary blood supply to the prostate is via the bilateral prostatic arteries, which derive from the inferior vesical artery. Two main groups of arteries occur: capsular and urethral. Some accessory vessels to the prostate are supplied from the middle hemorrhoidal and internal pudendal arteries as well. The venous drainage of the prostate is through a prostatic plexus, which joins in Santorini's plexus and then

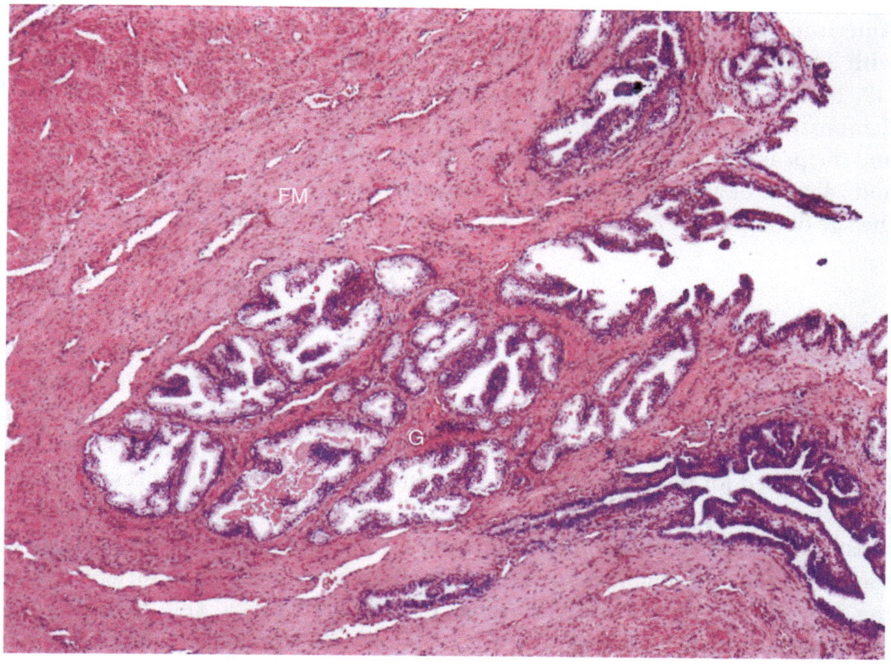

Fig. 4.3 Microscopic representation of benign prostate gland. Central glands (*G*) are surrounded by fibromuscular stroma (*FM*)

drains into the internal iliac (hypogastric) veins [5]. The prostatic plexus also joins with the prevertebral veins (Batson's plexus). This prevertebral plexus has been implicated in the spread of prostate cancer to the vertebral bodies [9].

Prostatic lymphatic drainage is highly variable and dependent on location within the gland. The main prostatic lymphatics drain into the periprostatic network, which is composed of three groups: the superior gland drains into the external iliac lymph nodes, the lateral gland usually drains into the hypogastric and obturator lymph nodes and the posterior prostatic gland drains to the presacral area [10]. Lymphatic spread of prostate cancer most frequently involves the hypogastric, external iliac, and obturator lymph nodes [11].

Innervation of the prostate is via the pelvis plexus, made up of parasympathetic input from the pelvic splanchnic nerves and sympathetic input from the hypogastric plexus and nerve [12, 13]. The past 25 years have emphasized a "nerve sparing" approach to radical prostatectomy and cystectomy [14]. In reality this operation is a neurovascular sparing technique that separates the neurovascular bundle from the prostate. The bundle contains fibers that innervate the corpora cavernosa, prostate, and urethral sphincter [13, 15]. The neurovascular bundle is located along the posterior lateral prostate at the base. More distally, the neurovascular bundle closes in on the apex of the prostate and dives into the pelvic floor lateral to urethral sphincter [15, 16].

4.3 Prostate Cancer

Prostate cancer is the most common internal tumor and the third leading cause of cancer death in men [17]. Prostate cancer accounts for approximately 180,000 new cases annually, 29,000 cancer-related deaths annually, and corresponds to a lifetime risk of 17.6% for whites and 20.6% for African Americans [18]. Most prostate cancers do not cause death and less than 5% of those with prostate cancer will die from prostate cancer [19]. Only 25% of prostate cancers are thought to be clinically significant. Prostate cancer incidence is age and race dependent, as 75% of cases occur at or after the age of 65 and African

American men have a 40% increased risk of disease with 2.4 times the risk of cancer-specific mortality [17, 19, 20]. The most recent SEER cancer statistics demonstrate prostate cancer risk increases with age and the peak incidence occurs between the ages of 70 and 74 years of age, with almost 85% diagnosed after the age of 65 years [17].

4.3.1 Prostate Cancer Screening

The combination of digital rectal exam (DRE), serum PSA, and transrectal ultrasound-guided prostatic biopsy is used for the early detection of prostate cancer. While DRE and serum PSA testing remain the most useful initial assessment for prostate cancer, their use in asymptomatic men as a means of screening for prostate cancer with the goal of reduced prostate cancer mortality by earlier detection and treatment has remained controversial [21–23]. The advent of PSA testing and screening has resulted in a significant downward stage migration, and the number of patients receiving treatment for localized disease has dramatically increased [20]. However, early detection has not conclusively improved health outcomes [22]. Although the value of PSA screening remains an issue of debate, men presenting for annual health examinations should be made aware of the availability, benefits, and consequences of PSA testing. It is important for men to make an informed decision regarding routine PSA screening.

PSA screening alone has a higher detection rate than DRE alone, but detection rates are highest when the two exams are combined [24, 25]. The pathologic features of prostate cancer detected by DRE tend to be more aggressive than those revealed by PSA testing [24]. Therefore, the two exams often detect distinct cancer types and are complementary to one another. They are recommended in combination.

4.3.1.1 Digital Rectal Examination

An abnormal digital rectal examination (DRE), or prostate nodule, raises concerns for prostate cancer and is an indication for prostate biopsy [26]. The consistency of a nodule is variable and often described as rubbery, firm, or hard. The nodule itself may range from well circumscribed to irregular and diffuse. The presence of a prostate nodule as an isolated finding with normal PSA is uncommon.

Carcinoma on DRE is palpable as firm, indurated nodules or regions within the prostate gland often characterized by having a woody consistency. They usually arise in the posterior peripheral region. As the prostatic carcinomas progress, the entire gland can become firm. With more advanced disease, the medial and lateral sulci of the prostate may become obliterated. Eventually, these tumors may progress beyond the capsule of the prostate, extending superiorly into the seminal vesicles and laterally toward the pelvic side wall causing fixation of the gland.

Benign prostatic hyperplasia on DRE typically consists of variable enlargement with rubber consistency and findings are generally limited to the prostate. Sometimes adenomas are palpably soft, well-circumscribed nodules. Infectious etiologies of an abnormal DRE include prostatitis and abscess. DRE during prostatitis may demonstrate a warm, tender prostate that can be fluctuant or boggy in consistency. A prostatic abscess is evident by localized fluctuant, tender region within the prostate and suggestive clinical symptomology. A calculus may be evident by a hard, firm, and small nodule.

4.3.1.2 Prostate-Specific Antigen

PSA is a serine protease produced by prostatic epithelium and periurethral glands with a half-life of 2–3 days [27]. It liquefies the seminal coagulum. PSA is a commonly used laboratory test for the screening, diagnosis, treatment, and monitoring of prostate cancer. It is thought to become elevated in the serum when prostatic architecture is disrupted and the basal layer or basement membrane has compromised integrity.

Other etiologies of an elevated PSA include advanced age, benign enlargement of the prostate, infection, prostatic biopsy, aggressive DRE, prostatic infarction, recent transurethral instrumentation, or recent catheterization. PSA should not be evaluated in the setting of untreated bacterial prostatitis or within 3–4 weeks of prostate instrumentation or biopsy due to risk of false elevation.

A clear definition of a normal serum PSA value remains controversial. Based on the Baltimore Longitudinal Study of Aging, elevated PSA traditionally begins with >4.0 ng/mL. Median PSA is 0.7 ng/mL during the fourth decade and rises to a median of 1.7 ng/mL by the seventh decade [28]. Across all races at ages greater than 50 years, 7.9% of men randomly screened have PSA > 4.0 ng/mL and, according to the Prostate Cancer Prevention Trial (PCPT), approximately 25% of men with PSA > 4.0 ng/mL harbor prostate cancer [28, 29]. However, PSA 2.1–3.0 and 3.1–4.0 corresponded to a 24% and 27% rate of prostate cancer, respectively. Beginning with the PCPT trial, it has become clear that PSA level represents a continuum of risk that is affected by family history and ethnicity. Clearly there is no absolute lower cutoff or normal PSA to indicate absence of prostate cancer and some have advocated for a cutoff of 2.5 ng/mL, especially for African Americans and men with a family history [30].

PSA, Age, and Race-Adjusted

An age-specific scale of normal PSA values has been proposed, based on the observation that PSA rises with age, in an effort to reduce unnecessary prostate biopsies [31] (Table 4.1). Based on the observation that African American males have higher average PSA values when adjusted for age, some authors have proposed PSA adjusted for race as well as age. Use of race-adjusted PSA is controversial [32].

PSA, Free, and Total

PSA is found either free in serum or bound to serum proteins. It has been postulated that prostate cancer cells produce more binding protein with PSA [33]. Thus, patients with prostate cancer tend to have lower free PSA levels in proportion to total PSA.

Table 4.1 Proposed age-specific reference range for PSA [31]

Age (year)	Age-specific reference range (ng/mL)
40–49	0.0–2.5
50–59	0.0–3.5
60–69	0.0–4.5
70–79	0.0–6.5

Table 4.2 Probability of prostate cancer by percent-free PSA in men with a total PSA between 4.0 and 10.0 ng/mL [36]

% Free PSA	Prostate cancer probability (%)
0–10	56
10–15	28
15–20	20
20–25	16
>25	8

Measurement of the free PSA percentage can improve the specificity of PSA as a cancer screening test [33, 34]. Percent-free PSA is most useful for patients with mildly elevated PSA (4.0–10.0 ng/mL) [35]. A specific threshold for biopsy is controversial for free PSA percentage, which ranges from <15% to <25% (Table 4.2). A higher threshold will have improved sensitivity with lower specificity [36].

PSA Kinetics and PSA Velocity (PSAV)

PSAV and PSA doubling time (PSADT) are two parameters of PSA kinetics used by urologists. PSAV is the change of PSA over the course of 1 year measured by three separate values over a period of at least 18 months (Fig. 4.4). Early studies suggested a diagnostic value of a PSAV of >0.75 ng/mL/year; however, the use of PSAV has become more controversial in recent studies [37, 38]. Regardless, a high pretreatment PSAV (>2.0 ng/mL/year) has been shown to correlate with a worse prognosis after radiotherapy or radical prostatectomy [38].

PSA Density

PSA density may be useful with PSA levels 4–10 ng/mL and a previous negative biopsy. This is calculated by dividing PSA by the transrectal ultrasound prostate volume (Fig. 4.5). This calculation is useful in distinguishing benign prostatic hyperplasia from

$$\mathrm{PSAV} = 0.5\left(\frac{\mathrm{PSA}_2 - \mathrm{PSA}_1}{\mathrm{Time}_1} + \frac{\mathrm{PSA}_3 - \mathrm{PSA}_2}{\mathrm{Time}_2}\right)$$

Fig. 4.4 PSA velocity equation. PSA_1 = 1st PSA measurement (ng/mL), PSA_2 = 2nd PSA measurement (ng/mL), PSA_3 = 3rd PSA measurement (ng/mL), $Time_1$ = interval between PSA_1 and PSA_2 (year), $Time_2$ = interval between PSA_2 and PSA_3 (year)

$$\text{PSAD} = \frac{\text{PSA(ng/mL)}}{\text{Prostate Volume (cc)}}$$

Fig. 4.5 PSA density equation. Prostate volume is usually acquired via transrectal ultrasound

prostate cancer [21]. Using a cutoff of 0.1 ng/mL/cm^3, PSA specificity is improved, avoiding 31% of repeat biopsies but misses 10% of cancers [39]. There is currently no consensus on a cutoff value for PSA density.

PCLO Trial and ERSPC Study

Recently, two large, multicenter prostate cancer screening trials – the Prostate, Lung, Colorectal, and Ovarian Cancer Screening (PLCO) study from the United States and the European Randomized Study of Screening in Prostate Cancer (ERSPC) study from Europe – described their 10-year results. The PLCO found a higher risk of cancer diagnosis in the screening cohort but no cancer-specific survival advantage for the group [22]. In contrast, the ERSPC demonstrated a cancer-specific survival benefit for the screening arm by 7–8 years [23].

The PLCO trial [22] included 76,000 men between the ages of 55 and 74 in the screening and control groups from 1993 to 2001. Patients in the screening arm had annual PSA and DRE and men in the control arm were not screened. Biopsy in the screening arm was based on abnormal DRE or PSA > 4 ng/mL. Specific treatment for prostate cancer was not directed by the study. After a median follow-up of 11.5 years, screening was associated with an increased risk of prostate cancer diagnosis (HR 1.17) but no significant difference in prostate cancer mortality was demonstrated (0.24% vs. 0.21%). However, one the most important aspects of the PLCO trial interfered with its ability to answer whether or not screening reduced prostate cancer mortality; unfortunately, the control arm was contaminated by widespread prostate cancer screening. During the first 6 years of the study, at least 52% of men in the control arm had undergone PSA screening and 46% underwent DRE.

The ERSPC study [23] recruited 162,243 men between the ages of 55 and 69 and randomized them to the screening or control arms from 1991 to 2003. The screening arm was followed less aggressively with PSA and an average of 2.1 PSA tests were drawn over the course of the study. DRE was used sporadically and often only in cases of equivocal PSA values. Most centers used an abnormal DRE or PSA > 3.0 ng/mL as indications for biopsy. Specific treatment of prostate cancer was not designated by the study. With a median follow-up of 9 years, the risk ratio of cancer specific mortality for the screened arm was 0.80 ($p = 0.01$). On secondary analysis of those who adhered to the screening protocol, the risk ratio was closer to 0.70 [40]. This mortality benefit with screening became evident between 7 and 8 years. The authors also concluded that the number needed to screen to prevent one death was 1,410 and the number needed to treat was 48. Data on contamination of the control arm with screening demonstrates a rate of 15% at the most [26].

Based on these studies, it is safe to conclude that there is a survival benefit to screening, but it may not extend to all men of all ages, especially those over 75 years old. Optimal screening intervals and indications for biopsy were touched on indirectly in these studies as well. It appears less frequent testing can still provide a survival benefit. However, the screened arm in the European trial had a higher rate of cancer-specific death than the PLCO, which could be secondary to the longer intervals between screening examinations. Long-term reporting of these trials should improve our understanding of the utility of prostate cancer screening.

4.3.2 Prostate Cancer Diagnosis

The diagnosis of prostate cancer is made histologically by prostate needle biopsy in the majority of cases. Prostate cancer rarely causes symptoms early in the course of the disease because the majority of adenocarcinomas arise in the periphery of the gland, which is distant from the urethra. The presence of systemic symptoms suggests locally advanced or metastatic disease. Thus, suspicion of prostate cancer resulting in a recommendation for prostate biopsy is most often raised by abnormalities of serum PSA or findings on DRE.

Prior to widespread PSA testing, clinicians relied on DRE and performed finger-guided nodule biopsies. However, with an increased number of men coming to biopsy for an elevated PSA and normal DRE, transrectal ultrasound-guided (TRUS) biopsy has become more routinely template-based.

4.3.2.1
Transrectal Biopsy

During TRUS biopsy, the prostate volume can be assessed and any noted lesions may be characterized. Traditionally, an 18-gauge spring-loaded needle core biopsy gun can be used in conjunction with the ultrasound probe. Most probes are made with attachments that allow the biopsy gun to pass directly through it. Suspicious lesions within the prostate include hypoechoic nodules; however, most hypoechoic lesions are not cancer [41]. Flanigan et al. noted that only 18% of hypoechoic nodules seen on transrectal ultrasound were found to have prostate cancer [41]. Additionally, 50% of prostate cancers larger than 1 cm cannot be detected by TRUS [42]. Despite the limitations of TRUS to detect prostate cancer, any palpable or visual nodule must be biopsied. Most providers will then proceed to a template biopsy.

Sextant Biopsy
The first routinely used template was the sextant biopsy. This method retrieved one core from each the left and right base, mid, and apex of the gland. This demonstrated a remarkable improvement in prostate cancer detection compared to digitally directed biopsies [43]. Over time this template has been replaced with even more sensitive biopsy designs (Fig. 4.6).

Extended Biopsy Templates
Many modifications have been proposed to the traditional six-core sextant biopsy and most of these recommendations have integrated the importance of targeting the peripheral gland [44–46]. Apical, base, and laterally directed biopsies yield an approximate 25% increase in prostate cancer detection [46, 47]. Most studies conclude that extended biopsy techniques demonstrate superior prostate cancer detection without increasing patient discomfort or morbidity [48].

More recently, researchers have argued for much more aggressive biopsy schemes than the traditional 10–12 core biopsy. One study of over 300 patients compared patients undergoing 6-, 12-, 18-, and 21-core templates [47]. The authors concluded a 21-core template improved cancer detection and reported a 25% and 11% improvement for 12- versus 6- and 21- versus 12-core techniques, respectively. However, it has also been demonstrated that these "saturation" biopsy techniques do improve cancer detection as an initial biopsy strategy [49]. In a meta-analysis of published literature, there was no significant benefit gained by taking more than 12 cores [50]. Additionally, the authors found patients undergoing 18 or more needle samples experienced increased discomfort and morbidity.

In conclusion, most urologists consider it standard to do an initial prostate biopsy with 10–12 cores, including apically and laterally directed biopsies. If a patient requires additional biopsies for diagnosis or confirmation of extent of disease, it is reasonable to consider "saturation" biopsy techniques of 18 or more cores, especially for larger prostates.

4.3.3
Prostate Cancer Grade and Staging

4.3.3.1
Gleason Score

The most widely accepted grading system is the Gleason grading system, which is based on the

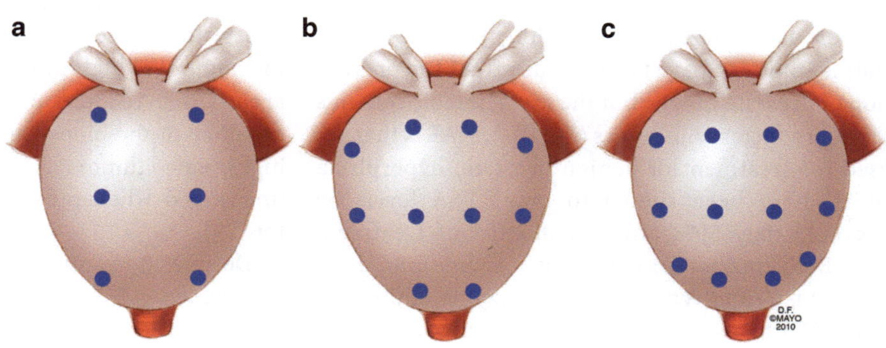

Fig. 4.6 Transrectal ultrasound-guided prostate biopsy templates
(a) 6-core biopsy template
(b) 10-core biopsy template
(c) 12-core biopsy template

architectural pattern of the prostate glands [51]. Cellular characteristics are not used to determine Gleason grade. The two most representative areas of the tumor are graded from 1 to 5. These two grades are added to obtain the Gleason score or sum. This score is reported as the most prevalent grade plus the second most prevalent grade (i.e., 4+3>2). Generally, the higher scores correspond to worse cancer-specific prognosis [52].

4.3.3.2 TNM Stage (AJCC 2010)

The tumor, node, metastases (TNM) classification and Anatomic Stage/Prognostic Groups are the most commonly utilized clinical staging systems today. First adopted in 1975 by the American Joint Committee for Cancer (AJCC), the system has undergone multiple revisions. The most recent modification occurred in 2010. In the modern PSA era, approximately 90% of newly diagnosed prostate cancer will be localized [20]. Patients with high Gleason scores and/or elevated PSA levels have a high risk of extraprostatic disease [53], but are categorized as localized disease when there is no clinical or radiographic evidence of extraprostatic disease. The AJCC 2010 TNM staging for prostate cancer is presented in Table 4.3 and Anatomic Stage/Prognostic Groups are presented in Table 4.4.

4.3.4 Prostate Cancer Prevention

4.3.4.1 The Role of 5a-Reductase Inhibitors in Prostate Cancer Prevention: PCPT and REDUCE Trial

Numerous medications, including selenium, zinc, statins, and teas, have been evaluated for the prevention of prostate cancer, but the most notable remains the 5α-reductase inhibitors (5-ARIs). 5-ARIs that are used for treatment of benign prostatic hyperplasia (BPH) have been shown to lower PSA levels by approximately 50% after 12 months of treatment [29]. Both finasteride (type 2 isoenzyme inhibitor) and dutasteride (type 1 and 2 isoenzyme inhibitors) lower PSA to a similar degree [54]. Men should have a pretreatment PSA recorded for future reference and then be followed with at least annual PSA measurements.

The Prostate Cancer Prevention Trial (PCPT) examined finasteride for prevention of prostate cancer. Over 18,000 men with age ≥55 years, normal prostate exam and PSA ≤3.0 ng/mL were randomized to finasteride 5 mg daily or to placebo and followed for 7 years [55]. Finasteride decreased the risk of developing prostate cancer by 25% but men taking finasteride were more likely to have high-grade cancers and sexual side effects. Multiple authors have identified several biases that may account for the increase in high-grade cancer in the finasteride arm [56–58]. Biases that have been identified include increased sensitivity of DRE and PSA as diagnostic tools, the impact of smaller prostate volume at time of biopsy in the finasteride arm and the use of extended biopsy techniques. Based on these publications, the American Urological Associations and the American Society of Clinical Oncology released a statement suggesting the development of high-grade cancers is not a problem and that clinicians should discuss the risks and benefits of 5-ARI therapy regarding a decreased risk of prostate cancer, decreased urinary symptoms, and increased sexual side effects [59].

The REDUCE study group recently published their results using dutasteride for prostate cancer prevention [54]. In this 4-year, international, multicenter, placebo-controlled, randomized trial, dutasteride was associated with a 5.1% absolute reduction and 23% relative reduction in the incidence of prostate cancer detected on biopsy at the end of the study. These men were biopsied at the 4-year mark regardless of an indication for biopsy (abnormal DRE or elevated PSA). When only evaluating biopsies performed for cause, the rate of prostate cancer detected was relatively the same in the dutasteride group versus placebo (16.6% vs. 16.7%, respectively). Additionally, like finasteride in the PCPT, dutasteride failed to reduce the number of high-grade tumors. Some authors have argued that reduced prostate volumes increase the accuracy of the biopsy and cause easier detection of high-grade tumors. However, these results were unchanged when prostate volumes were accounted for [29].

Despite the continued controversy, based on current evidence, 5-ARIs reduce the relative incidence of prostate cancer by 25% compared to placebo. These

Table 4.3 TNM prostate cancer staging systems

Primary tumor (T)			
Clinical			
	TX		Primary tumor cannot be assessed
	T0		No evidence of primary tumor
	T1		Clinically inapparent tumor neither palpable nor visible by imaging
		T1a	Tumor incidental histologic finding in 5% or less of tissue resected
		T1b	Tumor incidental histologic finding in more than 5% of tissue resected
		T1c	Tumor identified by needle biopsy
	T2		Tumor confined to the prostate
		T2a	Tumor involves one-half of one lobe or less
		T2b	Tumor involves more than one-half of one lobe but not both lobes
		T2c	Tumor involves both lobes
	T3		Tumor extends through the prostate capsule
		T3a	Extracapsular extension (unilateral or bilateral)
		T3b	Tumor invades seminal vesicle
	T4		Tumor is fixed or invades adjacent structures other than seminal vesicles such as external sphincter, rectum, bladder, levator muscles and/or pelvic sidewall
Pathologic (pT) – following prostatectomy			
	pT2		Organ confined
		pT2a	Unilateral, one-half of one side or less
		pT2b	Unilateral, involving more than one-half of side but not both sides
		pT2c	Bilateral disease
	pT3		Extraprostatic extension
		pT3a	Extraprostatic extension or microscopic invasion of bladder neck
		pT3b	Seminal vesicle invasion
	pT4		Invasion of rectum, levator muscles and/or pelvic wall
Regional lymph nodes (N)			
Clinical			
	NX		Regional lymph nodes were not assessed
	N0		No regional lymph node metastasis
	N1		Metastasis in regional lymph node(s)
Pathologic			
	pNX		Regional nodes not sampled
	pN0		No positive regional nodes
	pN1		Metastases in regional node(s)
Distant metastasis (M)			
	M0		No distant metastasis
	M1		Distant metastasis
	M1a		Nonregional lymph node(s)
	M1b		Bone(s)
	M1c		Other site(s) with or without bone disease

medications may not prevent high-grade tumor progression but they offer the possibility of fewer patients with indolent cancer receiving unnecessary biopsy and treatment morbidities. Following a discussion of the risks and benefits of this therapy, patients should be offered 5-ARIs as possible chemoprevention agents.

4.3.4.2 Chemoprevention Using Dietary Modification or Nutritional Supplements

Many patients are interested in "natural" chemoprevention and modifications to prevent the development of prostate cancer. However, dietary

Table 4.4 Anatomic stage/prognostic groups

Group	T	N	M	PSA	Gleason
I	T1a–c	N0	M0	PSA < 10	Gleason ≤ 6
	T2a	N0	M0	PSA < 10	Gleason ≤ 6
	T1–T2a	N0	M0	PSA X	Gleason X
II	T1a–c	N0	M0	PSA < 20	Gleason 7
	T1a–c	N0	M0	PSA ≥ 10 < 20	Gleason ≤ 6
	T2a	N0	M0	PSA < 20	Gleason ≤ 7
	T2b	N0	M0	PSA < 20	Gleason ≤ 7
	T2b	N0	M0	PSA X	Gleason X
IIB	T2c	N0	M0	Any PSA	Any Gleason
	T1–2	N0	M0	PSA ≥ 20	Any Gleason
	T1–2	N0	M0	Any PSA	Gleason ≥ 8
III	T3a–b	N0	M0	Any PSA	Any Gleason
IV	T4	N0	M0	Any PSA	Any Gleason
	Any T	N1	M0	Any PSA	Any Gleason
	Any T	Any N	M1	Any PSA	Any Gleason

modification and nutritional supplementation have never demonstrated benefit in randomized trials. In 2009, three trials evaluating nutritional supplements in the prevention of prostate cancer were published.

Selenium and Vitamin E Cancer Prevention Trial (SELECT)

The SELECT trial randomized over 35,000 men to supplementation with selenium, vitamin E, or both versus placebo [60]. Patients were accrued over a 7-year period and the trial was terminated secondary to lack of efficacy. No statistical difference in prostate cancer rates were demonstrated among the four groups. Based on this trial, neither selenium nor vitamin E should be advocated for the prevention of prostate cancer.

Vitamin E and Vitamin C (Physician's Health Study II)

In the Physician's Health Study II, nearly 15,000 men were randomized to vitamin E, vitamin C, multivitamin, or betacarotene in a number of combinations versus placebo [61]. Despite 8 years of follow-up, the authors did not report a significant difference between any of the combinations of supplements and placebo. Additionally, analyses of only adherent patients did not change the outcome. At this time, none of these supplementations should be promoted for protection from prostate cancer.

Folate and Aspirin (Aspirin/Folate Polyp Prevention Study)

This trial was designed to determine the possible preventive properties of aspirin and folate for colon cancer. In a secondary analysis, folate was associated with an increased risk of prostate cancer [62]. The probability of a prostate cancer diagnosis was 9.7% in the folic acid group compared to 3.3% in the placebo group (HR 2.63; 95% CI 1.23–5.65). Overall, there were a small number of prostate cancer events and final recommendations about folic acid and prostate cancer are difficult to generate.

References

1. Crafts R (1979) Textbook of human anatomy, 2nd edn. Wiley, New York
2. Takenaka A, Hara R, Soga H et al (2005) A novel technique for approaching the endopelvic fascia in retropubic radical prostatectomy, based on an anatomical study of fixed and fresh cadavers. BJU Int 95:766–771
3. Myers RP (2002) Detrusor apron, associated vascular plexus, and avascular plane: relevance to radical retropubic prostatectomy – anatomic and surgical commentary. Urology 59:472–479
4. Steiner MS (1994) The puboprostatic ligament and the male urethral suspensory mechanism: an anatomic study. Urology 44:530–534
5. Santorini G (1724) De virorum naturalibus [Concerning the male genitalia]. In: Observationes Anatomicae. G. Baptista Recurti, Venice, p p. 202
6. Myers RP (2001) Practical surgical anatomy for radical prostatectomy. Urol Clin North Am 28:473–490
7. McNeal JE (1981) The zonal anatomy of the prostate. Prostate 2:35–49
8. Kerr J (2000) Atlas of functional histology, 1st edn. Mosby, Barcelona
9. Onuigbo WI (1975) Batson's theory of vertebral venous metastasis: a review. Oncology 32:145–150
10. Cellini N, Luzi S, Mantini G et al (2003) Lymphatic drainage and CTV in carcinoma of the prostate. Rays 28:337–341
11. Heidenreich A, Ohlmann CH, Polyakov S (2007) Anatomical extent of pelvic lymphadenectomy in patients undergoing radical prostatectomy. Eur Urol 52:29–37
12. Mauroy B, Demondion X, Drizenko A et al (2003) The inferior hypogastric plexus (pelvic plexus): its importance

in neural preservation techniques. Surg Radiol Anat 25: 6–15

13. Baader B, Herrmann M (2003) Topography of the pelvic autonomic nervous system and its potential impact on surgical intervention in the pelvis. Clin Anat 16:119–130
14. Walsh PC, Donker PJ (2002) Impotence following radical prostatectomy: insight into etiology and prevention. 1982. J Urol 167:1005–1010
15. Lunacek A, Schwentner C, Fritsch H et al (2005) Anatomical radical retropubic prostatectomy: 'curtain dissection' of the neurovascular bundle. BJU Int 95:1226–1231
16. Costello AJ, Brooks M, Cole OJ (2004) Anatomical studies of the neurovascular bundle and cavernosal nerves. BJU Int 94:1071–1076
17. Damber J-E, Aus G (2008) Prostate cancer. Lancet 371: 1710–1721
18. Jemal A, Tiwari RC, Murray T et al (2004) Cancer statistics, 2004. CA Cancer J Clin 54:8–29
19. American Cancer Society (2005) Cancer facts and figures 2005. American Cancer Society, Atlanta
20. Walsh PC, DeWeese TL, Eisenberger MA (2007) Clinical practice. Localized prostate cancer. N Engl J Med 357: 2696–2705
21. Benson MC, Whang IS, Pantuck A et al (1992) Prostate specific antigen density: a means of distinguishing benign prostatic hypertrophy and prostate cancer. J Urol 147: 815–816
22. Andriole GL, Crawford ED, Grubb RL 3rd et al (2009) Mortality results from a randomized prostate-cancer screening trial. N Engl J Med 360:1310–1319 [Erratum appears in N Engl J Med. 2009;360(17):1797]
23. Schroder FH, Hugosson J, Roobol MJ et al (2009) Screening and prostate-cancer mortality in a randomized European study. N Engl J Med 360:1320–1328
24. Catalona WJ, Hudson MA, Scardino PT et al (1994) Selection of optimal prostate specific antigen cutoffs for early detection of prostate cancer: receiver operating characteristic curves. J Urol 152:2037–2042
25. Littrup PJ, Kane RA, Mettlin CJ et al (1994) Cost-effective prostate cancer detection. Reduction of low-yield biopsies. Investigators of the American Cancer Society National Prostate Cancer Detection Project. Cancer 74: 3146–3158
26. Ciatto S, Zappa M, Villers A et al (2003) Contamination by opportunistic screening in the European Randomized Study of Prostate Cancer Screening. BJU Int 92(Suppl 2):97–100
27. Lilja H (1985) A kallikrein-like serine protease in prostatic fluid cleaves the predominant seminal vesicle protein. J Clin Invest 76:1899–1903
28. Catalona WJ, Beiser JA, Smith DS (1997) Serum free prostate specific antigen and prostate specific antigen density measurements for predicting cancer in men with prior negative prostatic biopsies. J Urol 158:2162–2167
29. Thompson IM, Tangen CM, Goodman PJ et al (2009) Chemoprevention of prostate cancer. J Urol 182:499–507; discussion 508
30. Catalona WJ, Ramos CG, Carvalhal GF et al (2000) Lowering PSA cutoffs to enhance detection of curable prostate cancer. Urology 55:791–795
31. Oesterling JE, Jacobsen SJ, Chute CG et al (1993) Serum prostate-specific antigen in a community-based population of healthy men. Establishment of age-specific reference ranges. JAMA 270:860–864
32. Morgan TO, Jacobsen SJ, McCarthy WF et al (1996) Age-specific reference ranges for prostate-specific antigen in black men. N Engl J Med 335:304–310
33. Christensson A, Bjork T, Nilsson O et al (1993) Serum prostate specific antigen complexed to alpha 1-antichymotrypsin as an indicator of prostate cancer. J Urol 150:100–105
34. Lilja H (1993) Significance of different molecular forms of serum PSA. The free, noncomplexed form of PSA versus that complexed to alpha 1-antichymotrypsin. Urol Clin North Am 20:681–686
35. Catalona WJ, Southwick PC, Slawin KM et al (2000) Comparison of percent free PSA, PSA density, and age-specific PSA cutoffs for prostate cancer detection and staging. Urology 56:255–260
36. Catalona WJ, Partin AW, Slawin KM et al (1998) Use of the percentage of free prostate-specific antigen to enhance differentiation of prostate cancer from benign prostatic disease: a prospective multicenter clinical trial. JAMA 279: 1542–1547
37. Carter HB, Pearson JD, Metter EJ et al (1992) Longitudinal evaluation of prostate-specific antigen levels in men with and without prostate disease. JAMA 267:2215–2220
38. O'Brien MF, Cronin AM, Fearn PA et al (2009) Pretreatment prostate-specific antigen (PSA) velocity and doubling time are associated with outcome but neither improves prediction of outcome beyond pretreatment PSA alone in patients treated with radical prostatectomy. J Clin Oncol 27: 3591–3597
39. Babaian RJ, Kojima M, Ramirez EI et al (1996) Comparative analysis of prostate specific antigen and its indexes in the detection of prostate cancer. J Urol 156:432–437
40. Roobol MJ, Kerkhof M, Schröder FH et al (2009) Prostate cancer mortality reduction by prostate-specific antigen-based screening adjusted for nonattendance and contamination in the European Randomised Study of Screening for Prostate Cancer (ERSPC). Eur Urol 56:584–591
41. Flanigan RC, Catalona WJ, Richie JP et al (1994) Accuracy of digital rectal examination and transrectal ultrasonography in localizing prostate cancer. J Urol 152:1506–1509
42. Sedelaar JP, Vijverberg PL, De Reijke TM et al (2001) Transrectal ultrasound in the diagnosis of prostate cancer: state of the art and perspectives. Eur Urol 40:275–284
43. Hodge KK, McNeal JE, Terris MK et al (1989) Random systematic versus directed ultrasound guided transrectal core biopsies of the prostate. J Urol 142:71–74; discussion 74–75
44. Terris MK, McNeal JE, Stamey TA (1992) Detection of clinically significant prostate cancer by transrectal ultrasound-guided systematic biopsies. J Urol 148:829–832
45. Presti JC Jr, Chang JJ, Bhargava V et al (2000) The optimal systematic prostate biopsy scheme should include 8 rather than 6 biopsies: results of a prospective clinical trial. J Urol 163:163–166; discussion 166–167
46. Eskew LA, Bare RL, McCullough DL (1997) Systematic 5 region prostate biopsy is superior to sextant method for

diagnosing carcinoma of the prostate. J Urol 157:199–202; discussion 202–193
47. de la Taille A, Antiphon P, Salomon L et al (2003) Prospective evaluation of a 21-sample needle biopsy procedure designed to improve the prostate cancer detection rate. Urology 61:1181–1186
48. Scattoni V, Zlotta A, Montironi R et al (2007) Extended and saturation prostatic biopsy in the diagnosis and characterisation of prostate cancer: a critical analysis of the literature. Eur Urol 52:1309–1322
49. Jones JS, Patel A, Schoenfield L et al (2006) Saturation technique does not improve cancer detection as an initial prostate biopsy strategy. J Urol 175:485–488
50. Eichler K, Hempel S, Wilby J et al (2006) Diagnostic value of systematic biopsy methods in the investigation of prostate cancer: a systematic review. J Urol 175:1605–1612
51. Gleason DF, Mellinger GT (1974) Prediction of prognosis for prostatic adenocarcinoma by combined histological grading and clinical staging. J Urol 111:58–64
52. Gleason DF, Mellinger GT, Veterans Administration Cooperative Urological Research Group (2002) Prediction of prognosis for prostatic adenocarcinoma by combined histological grading and clinical staging. 1974. J Urol 167:953–958; discussion 959
53. Partin AW, Mangold LA, Lamm DM et al (2001) Contemporary update of prostate cancer staging nomograms (Partin Tables) for the new millennium. Urology 58:843–848
54. Andriole GL, Bostwick DG, Brawley OW et al (2010) Effect of dutasteride on the risk of prostate cancer. N Engl J Med 362:1192–1202
55. Thompson IM, Goodman PJ, Tangen CM et al (2003) The influence of finasteride on the development of prostate cancer. N Engl J Med 349:215–224
56. Cohen YC, Liu KS, Heyden NL et al (2007) Detection bias due to the effect of finasteride on prostate volume: a modeling approach for analysis of the Prostate Cancer Prevention Trial. J Natl Cancer Inst 99:1366–1374
57. Pinsky P, Parnes H, Ford L (2008) Estimating rates of true high-grade disease in the prostate cancer prevention trial. Cancer Prev Res 1:182–186
58. Kaplan SA, Roehrborn CG, Meehan AG et al (2009) PCPT: evidence that finasteride reduces risk of most frequently detected intermediate- and high-grade (Gleason score 6 and 7) cancer. Urology 73:935–939
59. Kramer BS, Hagerty KL, Justman S et al (2009) Use of 5-alpha-reductase inhibitors for prostate cancer chemoprevention: American Society of Clinical Oncology/American Urological Association 2008 Clinical Practice Guideline. J Clin Oncol 27:1502–1516
60. Lippman SM, Klein EA, Goodman PJ et al (2009) Effect of selenium and vitamin E on risk of prostate cancer and other cancers: the Selenium and Vitamin E Cancer Prevention Trial (SELECT). JAMA 301:39–51
61. Gaziano JM, Glynn RJ, Christen WG et al (2009) Vitamins E and C in the prevention of prostate and total cancer in men: the Physicians' Health Study II randomized controlled trial. JAMA 301:52–62
62. Figueiredo JC, Grau MV, Haile RW et al (2009) Folic acid and risk of prostate cancer: results from a randomized clinical trial. J Natl Cancer Inst 101:432–435

Prostate Surgery and the Evolution to Minimally Invasive Therapies

5

Lee E. Ponsky and Gino Vricella

CONTENTS

5.1 Abstract

Like many therapies, the treatment of prostate cancer has evolved over the years. While the radical prostatectomy began as the initial curative treatment, it was associated with significant co-morbidities that greatly affected a patient's quality of life. The improvement in surgical technique and improved description of the anatomy has led to significant improvements in the outcomes. Advances in irradiation techniques have also added to the options a patient has to consider when deciding on a treatment for his prostate cancer. Treatments have continued to improve to become less invasive and less impactful on a patient's quality of life. However, to date, the options all have very similar outcomes in regard to cancer control, potency and urinary control, which have been described as the "trifecta" goal of prostate cancer treatment.

5.2 Open Radical Prostatectomy

The initial description of radical prostatectomy for prostate cancer was by Hugh Hampton Young in 1905, which was performed via the perineal approach [1]. Millin subsequently described the radical retropubic approach in 1945; however, the procedure was not widely adopted because of significant incontinence and impotence issues [2]. Patrick Walsh's description and development of anatomic radical retropubic prostatectomy allowed for the dissection to be performed with better visualization and preservation of the cavernous nerves and external sphincter muscle [3, 4]. This led to a significant reduction in the two most common surgical complications, incontinence and impotence, at rates of 3% and 30%, respectively [5].

L.E. Ponsky et al. (eds.), *Treating Prostate Cancer and Related Genitourinary Applications*, Robotic Radiosurgery,
DOI 10.1007/978-3-642-11495-3_5, © Springer-Verlag Berlin Heidelberg 2012

5.3 External Beam Radiotherapy

Pasteau and Degrais were the first to describe the use of radiation with curative intent of prostate cancer in 1914 [6]. Since then, a number of technological advances in planning and delivery systems have occurred to offer radiotherapy as one of the main treatment modalities in the armamentarium against prostate cancer.

External beam radiotherapy (EBRT) uses beams of gamma radiation or X-rays directed at the prostate through multiple fields. The mechanism of action is primarily through the induction of unrepairable double-strand breaks in DNA. The expression of radiation damage does not occur until the target cells enter mitosis in their cell cycle. In addition, radiation also induces programmed cell death, or apoptosis [7].

Over the past 20 years, there has been an evolution in radiation technologies, from conventional radiation therapy to three-dimensional conformal radiotherapy (3D-CRT) to intensity-modulated radiation therapy (IMRT). All of these techniques use the same high-energy X-rays delivered to the target, however, difference exist in the method of planning the radiation delivery. Conventional radiotherapy planning relies on two-dimensional (2D) fluoroscopic images to determine the radiation fields, which are now considered outdated for prostate radiation therapy. The incorporation of computed tomography (CT) into radiotherapy was a major development, which allowed the pelvic anatomy to be outlined and reformatted into a 3D volumetric image. These 3D images could then be utilized to create multiple customized fields that conform to the target while minimizing the dose to the surrounding tissues (i.e. bladder and rectum). The introduction of IMRT was another major technological advancement for radiation therapy of prostate cancer. While similar to 3D-CRT in using a 3-D image set by CT, IMRT is capable of localizing the radiation dose to geometrically complex fields.

5.4 Brachytherapy

Permanent interstitial prostate brachytherapy as a curative-intent treatment for prostate cancer has been performed since the 1960s. Initial descriptions involved open lymphadenectomy, at which time patients underwent placement of radioactive seeds inserted directly into the prostate gland via a retropubic approach with "finger-guidance" [8]. Given the relatively unfavorable results, the procedure was largely abandoned until the late 1980s, when ultrasound image guidance was developed and used in conjunction with transperineal placement of the radioactive seeds, as a definitive treatment for localized prostate cancer [9]. Modern prostate brachytherapy uses a transrectal ultrasound probe with a template that overlies the perineum. Prior to initiating therapy, a transrectal ultrasound-based volume study is typically performed to assess prostate volume and to determine the number of needles and corresponding radioactive seeds, the isotope, and the isotope strength required for the procedure. With the patient under general or local anesthesia, needles are inserted through the perineum via a perineal template and radioactive seeds (the most common permanent implants are iodine-125 or palladium-103) are placed into the prostate to achieve a planned conformal dose distribution. After the implant has been completed, a CT scan or an X-ray image is obtained to check the postimplant dosimetry.

5.5 Laparoscopic Radical Prostatectomy

Laparoscopic radical prostatectomy via the transperitoneal approach was initially described by Schuessler 1992, with the first series of nine cases being reported 5 years later by the same group [10, 11]. They concluded that "laparoscopic radical prostatectomy is not an efficacious alternative to open radical prostatectomy as a curative treatment of clinically localized prostate cancer," citing excessive operative times and multiple technical difficulties [11]. Renewed interest in laparoscopic prostatectomy occurred in 1998 and 1999, when two separate groups from France (Montsouris and Creteil) reported successful adaptations of the technique with competitive operative times [12, 13]. Rassweiler described an ascending laparoscopic technique similar to the classic anatomic radical prostatectomy in a series of 100 patients [14]. This evolution of a standardized laparoscopic technique, with initial outcomes being similar to the classic open procedures led to widespread interest in the laparoscopic approach to radical prostatectomy. In 2001 Bollens and colleagues modified their initial experience with the transperitoneal approach and described a technique for an extraperitoneal laparoscopic radical prostatectomy [15]. They maintained that the extraperitoneal approach was analogous to the classic open retropubic technique. While the extraperitoneal technique does offer theoretic advantages, this approach can be much more challenging because of the smaller working space [16]. In 2001, there was yet another major modification to the laparoscopic radical prostatectomy technique with the introduction of the robotic technology using the da Vinci® surgical system (Intuitive Surgical, Sunnyvale, CA). There are many who attribute the increase in the application of minimally invasive techniques of radical prostatectomy to surgical robotics [17]. Selected advantages cited by proponents of the robotic system include three-dimensional stereoscopic visualization, flexibility in performing complex movements, minimal fatigue due to ergonomic design, and, most notably, the ease of intracorporeal suturing. Robotic prostatectomy may also have a shorter learning curve than standard laparoscopy, potentially allowing novice laparoscopists to complete these procedures [17, 18]. Some criticisms, however, include the loss of tissue resistance or tactile feedback, and cost [19]. The surgical robot system requires a tremendous capital investment, the laparoscopic instruments have a finite number of procedures before they must be replaced, and the annual maintenance and per-case disposable instrument costs make this technology prohibitive to many centers, limiting the widespread implementation of such a device worldwide.

5.6 Cryoablation

Cryoablation destroys tissue using extremely cold temperatures. Cryoablation can be considered therapeutically directed frostbite. The technique of cryotherapy was initially described by Cooper and Lee in the 1960s. At that time, the technique made use of a small-caliber vacuum-insulated liquid nitrogen cryoprobe, which allowed for organ targeting [20]. Although there are various theories explaining the mechanism of tissue injury via cryoablation, the most accepted hypothesis is that freezing of the tissue directly results in cellular death [21–23]. This occurs through two mechanisms: (1) direct cellular damage from disruption of the cellular membrane by ice crystals and (2) vascular compromise from thrombosis and ischemia [22].

The initial introduction of cryoablation for the treatment of prostate cancer was fraught with numerous complications, commonly including urethral sloughing, urinary incontinence, and urethrorectal fistula. These complications were thought to be due to a lack of accurate monitoring of the freezing process. With the advent of transrectal ultrasound (TRUS) in the 1980s, there were significant improvements in prostate cryosurgery in terms of enabling real-time imaging of the prostate and using ultrasonography for precise placement of multiple cryoprobes. The introduction of a urethral warming catheter significantly reduced urethral sloughing and subsequent strictures [23]. Although these adjustments improved cryoablative surgery, the continued incidence of rectourethral fistula as well as continued substandard oncologic outcomes prevented cryotherapy from being accepted. It was not until late 1990s that cryoablation was reintroduced as a technique for prostate cancer treatment. The new gas-driven probes were smaller and utilized a brachytherapy template to achieve precise placement of probes transperineally. Temperature sensors were utilized for improved control of the freeze zone and a urethral warming catheter was always employed to protect the urethra [24].

With the introduction of the third generation cryotherapy technology, there has been a significant decrease in morbidity compared to those reported with the first generation cryosurgery. Currently, rectal and bladder complications are reported to be approximately <0.5% in patients undergoing primary cryoablation [25–27]. Third generation cryosurgery is associated with an incontinence rate of up to 5.5%, urethral sloughing rates up to 6.7%, and up to 5.5% of the patients require transurethral resection of the prostate (TURP) due to bladder outlet obstruction following cryotherapy [26, 28]. Impotence remains a significant problem after cryosurgery. In most series, even with the third generation techniques, nearly all patients develop impotence [29, 30]. Although in a study by Robinson et al., 13% of patients regained potency and an additional 34% remained sexually active with the assistance of erectile aides 3 years after cryoablation [31].

5.7 High-Intensity Focused Ultrasound

High-intensity focused ultrasound (HIFU) is a minimally invasive approach that uses targeted ultrasound waves to treat prostate cancer. To deliver this ablative therapy, a probe is inserted transrectally and a high-energy ultrasound wave is targeted at a specific point in the prostate. Acoustic energy, precisely directed at the prostate, is absorbed by the prostate tissue and converted into thermal energy with intraprostatic temperatures reaching upwards of 100°C [32]. This results in coagulating heat, high pressure, cavitation bubbles, and chemically active free radicals, resulting in a focal area of tissue destruction due to coagulative necrosis [33]. HIFU of the prostate can be performed under either spinal or general anesthesia with the patient lying on his side or in the dorsal lithotomy position. With both the imaging and the treatment probe placed transrectally, the prostate is imaged and a therapeutic plan is created. A series of adjacent target zones are mapped to each cross-sectional level of the prostate gland. Once the treatment is ready to commence, the machine automatically cycles through the outlined treatment plan. The treating physician must monitor the ultrasound changes of the tissue to ensure no characteristics of overheating are evident. A monitoring device automatically deactivates the machine if the patient moves, and cooling fluid is circulated around the treatment probe to protect the rectal wall. Up to 3 months are required for necrosis to occur and, because the energy is nonionizing, treatment can be repeated if necessary.

HIFU is widely available in Europe and Canada; however, at the current time, it is only available in the USA via clinical trials. During a large, open-label, multicenter study in Europe, just over 400 patients underwent HIFU for prostate cancer between 1995 and 1999. Of the 288 patients that were rebiopsied after treatment, 87% were negative for carcinoma. Complications included urinary incontinence in 13.1% and rectourethral fistulas in 1.3%. Follow-up was relatively short, at just over 13 months and the treatment protocol evolved during the trial, making the interpretation of these results somewhat difficult [34]. In a more recent study, Uchida and colleagues treated 503 patients between 1999 and 2006 with HIFU for T1–3N0M0 prostate cancer. The biochemical disease-free survival (BDFS) at 5 years for all patients was 63.5%, with actuarial BDFS in low-, intermediate-, and high-risk groups being 86.3%, 64.8%, and 31.3%, respectively. Negative prostate biopsy results were found in 80.2%. Complications included urethral stricture, impotence, epididymitis, and urinary incontinence in 16%, 14%, 4%, and 0.8%, respectively [35].

5.8 Stereotactic Radiosurgery

The ultimate goals of radiation therapy would be precise tumor targeting and safe delivery of higher doses of radiation, while reducing the amount of normal tissue toxicity associated with these higher doses of radiation.

Hypofractionation refers to the use of larger-than-conventional doses of radiation per fraction. Several investigators have determined that the α/β ratio for prostate cancer is much lower than previously thought, which implies a high sensitivity to dose-per-fraction size [36, 37]. Therefore, a hypofractionated regimen would deliver higher tumor control rates while maintaining a biologically equivalent dose to normal tissues (i.e., bladder and rectum) for late toxicity and reduce the acute toxicity seen with the common current treatments, permanent-seed brachytherapy, or IMRT. In addition, a shortened course of radiotherapy would be a much more appealing option than conventional radiotherapy in terms of logistics (1-week versus a 6- to 9-week course of daily treatments) with a significant cost differential.

A precise delivery of large-dose fractions demands a system that is capable of overcoming daily target position variations and potential organ motion to a degree of unprecedented precision in order to not inflict debilitating damage. The CyberKnife® (Accuray Incorporated, Sunnyvale, CA) is a 6-MV linear accelerator mounted on a computer-controlled robotic arm. Real-time correction for target organ daily position changes or motion during radiation delivery is accomplished via an orthogonal pair of digital X-ray imaging devices monitoring the position of fiducial markers previously placed within the target organ. These fiducial markers consist of several gold "seeds" placed throughout the prostate via transrectal ultrasound guidance. Since the planning CT scan is obtained with these seeds in place, it is the relative position of the seeds with respect to the contoured organ that serves as reference points. This allows radiation delivery with a precision of <0.5 mm and a tracking error of <1 mm [38].

Results are limited as few centers in the USA have adopted this technology, which was originally described for use on intracranial tumors, to treat carcinoma of the prostate. In a recent Phase I/II trial, 40 patients were prospectively enrolled to evaluate the feasibility and toxicity of stereotactic hypofractionated radiotherapy to the prostate for localized, low-risk prostate cancer [39]. The median follow-up was 41 months, with five patients dying of nonprostate-related causes. Acute and late genitourinary (GU) and gastrointestinal (GI) toxicities were evaluated and PSA values and self-reported sexual function responses were recorded at specific intervals. Acute Grade 2 or less GU and GI toxicities were 48.5% and 39%, respectively; only one patient had an acute Grade 3 GU toxicity, which required catheterization, but resolved with ibuprofen and tamsulosin. Late Grade 2 or less GU and GI toxicities were 45% and 37%, respectively, with no late Grade 3 toxicities reported. This study is promising, in that it demonstrates the feasibility of delivering hypofractionated radiotherapy to the prostate, acceptable GU and GI toxicity rates and appropriate biochemical response. Multiple other studies are currently underway to assess acute and chronic morbidities of the CyberKnife treatment for prostate cancer as well as to confirm the long-term BDFS [40, 41].

5.9 Conservative Management

In patients with localized prostate cancer, the small, well-differentiated prostate cancers have repeatedly been shown to be associated with slow growth rates and an uncertainty as to the absolute need to treat all low-risk tumors. These findings have influenced a number of researchers, clinicians, and patients to consider *active surveillance* for highly selected patients with prostate cancer. Active surveillance is completely different from watchful waiting, which refers to monitoring of the patient until the development of metastatic disease that would require palliative therapy. Active surveillance allows for delayed primary treatment when there is evidence of cancer progression, such as a rising PSA level or biopsy findings consistent with an increase in volume or histological grade. The rationale for this approach stems from the fact that increasing numbers of older men are being diagnosed with prostate cancer as the result of PSA screening. Given the fact the treatment of older men who have low-grade disease is unlikely to affect their life span, these patients are managed expectantly until the first sign of disease progression, at which point active therapy is instituted [42]. The differentiating factor between active surveillance and watchful waiting is that, with active surveillance, there is still the goal to treat with curative intent.

Traditionally, this deferred treatment has been reserved for men with a life expectancy of less than 10 years [43]. Early data demonstrate that this approach may be a reasonable alternative to definitive treatment in older men who have low-volume, low-grade prostate cancer [44, 45]. In one case series that involved almost 300 men who were followed with an active surveillance protocol, one-third had evidence of disease progression, but overall, at 8 years follow-up, less than 1% had died from cancer [46]. It has also been shown that surveillance offers 10-year survival rates and quality-adjusted life years similar to those achieved with radical prostatectomy or radiotherapy [47]. This may not be the case, however, for patients with high-risk disease and Gleason scores >7. According to a population-based study by Lu-Yao and Yao, these patients have a better 5-year overall and disease-specific survival with active intervention than with observation [48]. These findings were echoed by a prospective, randomized clinical trial of almost 700 men with localized prostate cancer who were assigned to a watchful waiting protocol versus radical prostatectomy. In this study, Bill-Axelson and colleagues found that radical prostatectomy reduced disease-specific mortality, overall mortality, and the risks of metastasis, and local progression [49].

The potential downfalls of active monitoring for men with clinically localized disease would include multiple biopsies, which could complicate subsequent attempts at nerve-sparing surgery, or worse, delay definitive treatment for which the window of opportunity for cure may have been missed. A more recent study by Warlick and colleagues, however, found that delayed prostate cancer surgery for patients with small, lower-grade prostate cancers did not appear to compromise curability, although longer follow-up will be necessary to confirm these findings [50]. A universal regimen for active surveillance has not been defined, but most reports describe a clinical strategy that includes regular PSA level measurement and DRE with a periodic repeat prostate biopsy along with an option of more active therapy if biochemical (increasing PSA) or histopathologic (increased tumor grade or volume) progression occurs [41].

5.10 Future Trends

There are multiple techniques for treating prostate cancer that will likely become more developed in the coming years. The incorporation of imaging, i.e., transrectal ultrasound and MRI, may serve a role in assisting the physician to identify the neurovascular bundles and precise margins of the prostate dissection and/or focused treatment. There will certainly be more incorporation of ablative therapies in the treatment of prostate cancer, such as cryotherapy and HIFU. The utilization of these techniques for patients who have failed standard initial radiation therapy will likely provide a potentially curative option for patients with possibly decreased morbidity compared to a salvage prostate removal. Yet another area of great interest currently is the concept of focal therapy. This concept goes against all of the conventional teachings of prostate cancer and its respective therapies; prostate cancer is traditionally considered a multifocal disease. However, with the advance of ablative therapies, improvements in imaging and additional testing that can help reliably identify appropriate candidates treating only part of the prostate (only where the cancer exists) may have a role in the future.

It is only so much smaller that we can make our incisions and only so much better that we can improve our instruments, however, computers and imaging technologies will continue to evolve and progress at astronomical rates. It is with these developments and the appropriate incorporation into the clinical practice of treating patients with prostate cancer that true advancements will be made in the future.

References

1. Young HH (1905) The early diagnosis and radical cure of carcinoma of the prostate. Johns Hopkins Hosp Bull 16:315–321
2. Millin T (1945) Retropubic prostatectomy; a new extravesical technique; report of 20 cases. Lancet 2:693–696
3. Walsh PC, Donker PJ (1982) Impotence following radical prostatectomy: insight into etiology and prevention. J Urol 128:492–497
4. Walsh PC (2007) The discovery of the cavernous nerves and development of nerve sparing radical retropubic prostatectomy. J Urol 177:1632–1635
5. Kundu SD, Roehl KA, Eggener SE et al (2004) Potency, continence and complications in 3,477 consecutive radical retropubic prostatectomies. J Urol 172:2227–2231
6. Pasteau O, Degrais P (1914) The radium treatment of cancer of the prostate. Arch Roentgen Ray 18:396
7. Sklar GN, Eddy HA, Jacobs SC et al (1993) Combined antitumor effect of suramin plus irradiation in human prostate cancer cells: the role of apoptosis. J Urol 150:1526–1532
8. Sogani PC, Whitmore WF Jr, Hilaris BS et al (1980) Experience with interstitial implantation of iodine 125 in the treatment of prostatic carcinoma. Scand J Urol Nephrol Suppl 55:205–211
9. Blasko JC, Ragde H, Grimm PD (1991) Transperineal ultrasound-guided implantation of the prostate: morbidity and complications. Scand J Urol Nephrol Suppl 137:113–118
10. Schuessler WW, Kavoussi L, Clayman RV (1992) Laparoscopic radical prostatectomy: initial case report [abstr 130]. J Urol Suppl 147:246A

11. Schuessler WW, Schulam PG, Clayman RV et al (1997) Laparoscopic radical prostatectomy: initial short-term experience. Urology 50:854–857
12. Abbou CC, Salomon L, Hoznek A et al (2000) Laparoscopic radical prostatectomy: preliminary results. Urology 55: 630–634
13. Guillonneau B, Cathelineau X, Barret E et al (1999) Laparoscopic radical prostatectomy: technical and early oncological assessment of 40 operations. Eur Urol 36: 14–20
14. Rassweiler J, Sentker L, Seemann O et al (2001) Heilbronn laparoscopic radical prostatectomy. Technique and results after 100 cases. Eur Urol 40:54–64
15. Bollens R, Van den Bossche M, Roumeguere T et al (2001) Extraperitoneal laparoscopic radical prostatectomy. Results after 50 cases. Eur Urol 40:65–69
16. Trabulsi EJ, Guillonneau B (2005) Laparoscopic radical prostatectomy. J Urol 173:1072–1079
17. Menon M, Shrivastava A, Tewari A et al (2002) Laparoscopic and robot assisted radical prostatectomy: establishment of a structured program and preliminary analysis of outcomes. J Urol 168:945–949
18. Ahlering TE, Skarecky D, Lee D et al (2003) Successful transfer of open surgical skills to a laparoscopic environment using a robotic interface: initial experience with laparoscopic radical prostatectomy. J Urol 170:1738–1741
19. Guillonneau B (2003) What robotics in urology? A current point of view. Eur Urol 43:103–105
20. Cooper IS, Lee AS (1961) Cryostatic congelation: a system for producing a limited, controlled region of cooling or freezing of biologic tissues. J Nerv Ment Dis 133:259–263
21. Baust JG, Gage AA (2005) The molecular basis of cryosurgery. BJU Int 95:1187–1191
22. Gage AA, Baust J (1998) Mechanisms of tissue injury in cryosurgery. Cryobiology 37:171–186
23. Hoffmann NE, Bischof JC (2002) The cryobiology of cryosurgical injury. Urology 60:40–49
24. Onik GM, Cohen JK, Reyes GD et al (1993) Transrectal ultrasound-guided percutaneous radical cryosurgical ablation of the prostate. Cancer 72:1291–1299
25. Saliken JC, Donnelly BJ, Rewcastle JC (2002) The evolution and state of modern technology for prostate cryosurgery. Urology 60:26–33
26. Bahn DK, Lee F, Badalament R et al (2002) Targeted cryoablation of the prostate: 7-year outcomes in the primary treatment of prostate cancer. Urology 60:3–11
27. Donnelly BJ, Saliken JC, Ernst DS et al (2002) Prospective trial of cryosurgical ablation of the prostate: five-year results. Urology 60:645–649
28. Ellis DS (2002) Cryosurgery as primary treatment for localized prostate cancer: a community hospital experience. Urology 60:34–39
29. Han KR, Cohen JK, Miller RJ et al (2003) Treatment of organ confined prostate cancer with third generation cryosurgery: preliminary multicenter experience. J Urol 170: 1126–1130
30. Shinohara K (2003) Prostate cancer: cryotherapy. Urol Clin North Am 30:725–736, viii
31. Robinson JW, Donnelly BJ, Saliken JC et al (2002) Quality of life and sexuality of men with prostate cancer 3 years after cryosurgery. Urology 60:12–18
32. Madersbacher S, Pedevilla M, Vingers L et al (1995) Effect of high-intensity focused ultrasound on human prostate cancer in vivo. Cancer Res 55:3346–3351
33. Chapelon JY, Ribault M, Vernier F et al (1999) Treatment of localised prostate cancer with transrectal high intensity focused ultrasound. Eur J Ultrasound 9:31–38
34. Thuroff S, Chaussy C, Vallancien G et al (2003) High-intensity focused ultrasound and localized prostate cancer: efficacy results from the European multicentric study. J Endourol 17:673–677
35. Uchida T, Nitta M, Hongo S et al (2007) High-intensity focused ultrasound for the treatment in 503 patients with localized prostate cancer. Urology 70:2
36. Bentzen SM, Ritter MA (2005) The alpha/beta ratio for prostate cancer: what is it, really? Radiother Oncol 76: 1–3
37. King CR, Fowler JF (2001) A simple analytic derivation suggests that prostate cancer alpha/beta ratio is low. Int J Radiat Oncol Biol Phys 51:213–214
38. King CR, Lehmann J, Adler JR et al (2003) CyberKnife radiotherapy for localized prostate cancer: rationale and technical feasibility. Technol Cancer Res Treat 2:25–30
39. Madsen BL, Hsi RA, Pham HT et al (2007) Stereotactic hypofractionated accurate radiotherapy of the prostate (SHARP), 33.5 Gy in five fractions for localized disease: first clinical trial results. Int J Radiat Oncol Biol Phys 67:1099–1105
40. Freeman DE, King CR (2011) Stereotactic body radiotherapy for low-risk prostate cancer: five-year outcomes. Radiat Oncol 6:3
41. King CR, Brooks JD, Gill H et al (2011) Long-term outcomes from a prospective trial of stereotactic body radiotherapy for low-risk prostate cancer. Int J Radiat Oncol Biol Phys 2011 Feb. 5 (Epub Ahead of print)
42. Allaf ME, Carter H (2005) The results of watchful waiting for prostate cancer. AUA Update Series 24:1–7
43. Fowler FJ Jr, McNaughton Collins M, Albertsen PC et al (2000) Comparison of recommendations by urologists and radiation oncologists for treatment of clinically localized prostate cancer. JAMA 283:3217–3222
44. Carter HB, Walsh PC, Landis P et al (2002) Expectant management of nonpalpable prostate cancer with curative intent: preliminary results. J Urol 167:1231–1234
45. Johansson JE (1994) Expectant management of early stage prostatic cancer: Swedish experience. J Urol 152: 1753–1756
46. Klotz L (2005) Active surveillance for prostate cancer: for whom? J Clin Oncol 23:8165–8169
47. Choo R, Klotz L, Danjoux C et al (2002) Feasibility study: watchful waiting for localized low to intermediate grade prostate carcinoma with selective delayed intervention based on prostate specific antigen, histological and/or clinical progression. J Urol 167:1664–1669
48. Lu-Yao GL, Yao SL (1997) Population-based study of long-term survival in patients with clinically localised prostate cancer. Lancet 349:906–910
49. Bill-Axelson A, Holmberg L, Ruutu M et al (2005) Radical prostatectomy versus watchful waiting in early prostate cancer. N Engl J Med 352:1977–1984
50. Warlick C, Trock BJ, Landis P et al (2006) Delayed versus immediate surgical intervention and prostate cancer outcome. J Natl Cancer Inst 98:355–357

Part III

Prostate Motion

Prostate Motion: Implications and Management Strategies

Alison Tree, Vincent Khoo, and Nick van As

CONTENTS

6.1 Abstract

Further developments in precision and high-dose radiotherapy for patients with prostate cancer demand a greater understanding of prostate motion and the ways it can be managed. Prostate movement can occur unpredictably both between fractions and during fractions of radiotherapy. Nearly 14% of conventional radiotherapy treatments are given when the prostate displacement exceeds the CTV-PTV margin [1]. This chapter discusses the three mechanisms of prostate motion: translational movements, rotational movements, and prostate deformation. We discuss the factors that induce or affect prostate motion, such as rectal movement, as well as ways of detecting and characterizing movement of the prostate with various imaging techniques. Imaging modalities that can detect prostate position prior to radiotherapy are reviewed including CT on rails, TomoTherapy®, fiducials with kV imaging using CyberKnife®, and electromagnetic transponders (Calypso®). Methods of adapting treatment to mitigate these effects are discussed. These include

L.E. Ponsky et al. (eds.), *Treating Prostate Cancer and Related Genitourinary Applications*, Robotic Radiosurgery,
DOI 10.1007/978-3-642-11495-3_6, © Springer-Verlag Berlin Heidelberg 2012

off-line corrections after imaging, online imaging, and correction and adaptive replanning. Conclusions regarding the standard of care for prostate cancer patients are presented, along with avenues for future research.

6.2 Introduction

While we develop ever more precise ways of delivering radiotherapy to patients with prostate cancer, these must be accompanied by a greater understanding of prostate motion, its implications and ways in which this motion can be reduced or accommodated. Prostate movement can be unpredictable and occurs both between fractions and during fractions of radiotherapy [1–3]. It is known that radiotherapy dose escalation increases biochemical disease-free control [4, 5], and there are theoretically robust reasons why hypofractionation may improve the therapeutic ratio of prostate radiotherapy [6, 7]. However, without greater compensation for prostate motion, dose escalation and hypofractionation are not likely to improve tumor control without increasing toxicity [4, 8].

Radiotherapy planning involves the definition of a gross tumor volume (GTV), clinical tumor volume (CTV) and planning tumor volume (PTV). In contrast to other tumor sites, for prostate cancer a GTV is rarely used, as the entire prostate is used as a surrogate for the CTV, i.e. the region that has the potential to harbor microscopic disease [9]. In order to accommodate the uncertainties of treatment, a margin is put around the CTV to ensure that the inconsistencies of treatment setup are unlikely to compromise the irradiation of the CTV. With conventional linear accelerator (linac)-based radiotherapy, typically 8–10 mm is added to the CTV, with a smaller margin (e.g., 6–8 mm) posteriorly. This margin accounts for inaccuracies in the setup, both random and systematic, and also allows for prostate motion within the pelvis.

This chapter will focus on the body of knowledge regarding prostate movement and will discuss possible ways of compensating for this.

6.3 Normal Prostate Movement

Prostate movement can occur in six ways: anterior-posterior (AP), superior-inferior (SI), left-right (LR), pitch, roll, and yaw. Translational movements (AP, SI, LR) can be corrected by movement of the treatment couch. Rotational movements (pitch, roll, and yaw) are more difficult to mitigate. This type of motion is illustrated in Fig. 6.1.

6.3.1 Translational Movements

Prostate movement has been extensively studied and this subject was reviewed by Langen and Jones in 2001 [10]. They reviewed the literature on translational movements, but did not include a discussion of rotational movements which were less well studied at that point. It is clear from their review that prostate movement is greatest in the AP and SI directions and least in the LR direction [10, 11]. While the mean prostate displacement in most of these studies was less than 1 mm overall, the standard deviations in the studies reviewed ranged from 1.5 to 4.1 mm AP, from 0.7 to 1.9 mm LR, and for SI motion from 1.7 to 4.5 mm, indicating a larger variation than the mean position would suggest. Most of these studies involved a series of CT scans at intervals over the course of radiotherapy and none used real-time prostate tracking.

There are good anatomical reasons why certain directions have a greater magnitude of movement than others. The prostate is held inferiorly by the superior fascia of the urogenital diaphragm, which limits movement, and infero-laterally by the levator ani muscle, which also reduces movement in the lateral plane. In contrast, the prostate sits adjacent to the rectum posteriorly, which causes rather than restricts prostate motion.

Studies have also shown extensive movement of the prostate over the course of a few minutes, and this can be as much as 9.1 mm AP, 8.6 mm SI, and 4.8 mm LR over the course of 8–16 min [12].

More recently, many studies have investigated prostate movement with the use of daily portal imaging,

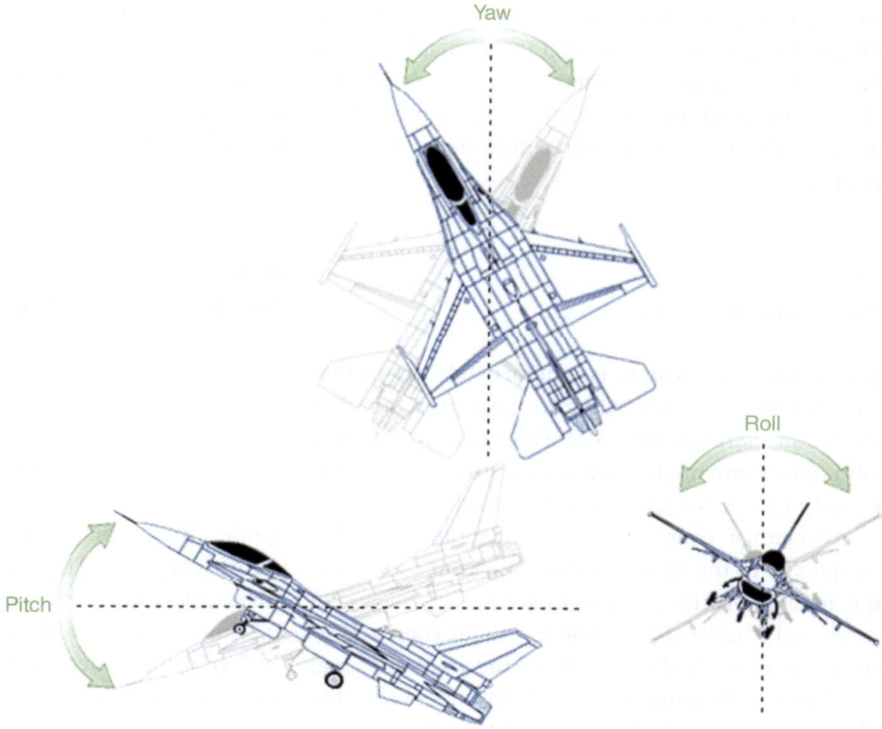

Fig. 6.1 Rotational movements (Acme Worldwide Enterprises, Inc.)

often using metal fiducials implanted in the prostate. Adamson et al. used kV portal imaging, as well as pre- and post-treatment CT imaging to assess movement of the prostate in 30 patients, totaling 571 fractions of radiotherapy [13]. He found that patients had maximum vector displacements of ≥3 and ≥5 mm in 46% and 19% of cases, respectively, which was similar to that found by Kupelian et al. [14]. The clinical significance of prostate movement is brought home by studies showing that 13.9% of daily treatments are displaced by more than the conventional CTV-PTV margin [1] hence part of the prostate will be "missed" on that day.

Continuous tracking with the Calypso® system (discussed later) has enabled more detailed analysis of the characteristics of prostate movement. Movement of the prostate in the SI and AP planes has been found to be linked, presumably due to the effects of bowel peristalsis pushing the prostate in the anterior-superior direction [11]. Motion in the LR plane is thought to be mostly due to pelvic rotation [11].

Interestingly two patterns of motion have been distinguished. The first of these is the "slow drift," usually in the posterior–inferior direction, thought to be the effect of either slow-moving rectal peristalsis or the gradual relaxation of the pelvic musculature as the patient lies on the couch [11]. This movement is usually small in magnitude, but is persistent and cumulative so that over prolonged periods of time, the effect can be enhanced. With conventional margins this is insignificant for most patients, but in order to reduce margins and hence toxicity, image guidance would be needed in order to avoid a geographical miss during longer fractions.

The second type of prostate movement is the short-lived and seemingly random movement, usually in the anterior and superior directions, hypothesized to be related to sudden bowel peristalsis [11]. These movements can be large (>10 mm) but due to their unpredictability and brevity may be difficult to compensate for.

6.3.2 Prostate Rotation

Rotation of the prostate has been less well studied. The predominant direction of rotation is described as the "nodding of the prostate in the sagittal plane" and this is found to have a mean value of 3.1° and standard deviations of 4.9 degrees (systematic component) and 4.7 degrees (random component) [15]. Some systems are now able to assess and correct for rotational movements [16, 17].

6.3.3 Prostate Deformation

In addition, the prostate is a deformable organ that can alter its shape according to local pressure. It is important therefore not to consider the prostate as a solid object moving in three dimensions, but instead a partly pliable structure whose outline can significantly change over time. This introduces further complexity to the ideal of conforming our radiotherapy delivery precisely to the prostate.

Several studies have monitored prostate movement using cine MRI which tracks the prostate in real time [18, 19]. Imaging the prostate in this way has the advantage of being able to detect more complex deformatory prostate movements such as focal compression by the rectum. Kerkof et al. pictorially represent the changes in prostate outline seen in MRI with variations in rectal filling, which were found to be 2.9-fold over five to six MRI sessions [20]. They found that the AP dimension of the prostate varies by 10% and 18% with a 2.6- and 5.1-fold increase in rectal volume [20], which can affect the dose to the rectum, although with margins of 4 mm they found this to be of negligible clinical significance.

It has been reported elsewhere that significant prostate deformation is usually unrelated to rectal filling, but a reduction in prostate size of 0.5% per fraction during the course of radiotherapy was noted. This small study also suggested that prostate deformation is more likely in patients who have undergone a transurethral resection of the prostate [21].

6.3.4 Seminal Vesicle Movement

Seminal vesicle (SV) movement has also been investigated in some studies. It is acknowledged that seminal vesicle movement has a greater mean amplitude than that of the prostate [10, 22], with anterior displacements of over 10 mm in 7% of cases (median 3 mm, maximum 22 mm) [22]. Factors affecting seminal vesicle movement are similar to those causing prostate movement and will be discussed below as a single entity.

6.4 Factors Affecting Prostate Movement

6.4.1 Breathing

Perhaps surprisingly, the effect of breathing on prostate motion can be detected. Although some early studies found this to be significant [23], when digital fluoroscopy is used to monitor the position of fiducials, mean prostate movements of 0.04 mm LR, 0.47 SI, and 0.2 mm AP can be detected [24]. In the context of higher displacements due to other causes, these are unlikely to be significant. Accordingly, the use of abdominal compression to limit the effect of respiration has not been found to be useful in reducing prostate motion [25].

6.4.2 Bladder Filling

Bladder filling has a minor contribution to prostate movement despite evidence that bladder volume has been found to change by an average of 14% over the course of 18 min [26]. The filling of the bladder which occurs during a fraction of radiotherapy can induce a posterior shift in the position of the prostate. However this only occurs if the rectum is relatively empty and the bladder volume would need to increase by at least 60% during the fraction to move the prostate back 1 mm.

6.4.3 Patient Position

The standard for prostate patients is for the patients to be treated supine. As well as being preferred by patients, there is a suggestion that the prostate moves less in the supine position [27] (see Table 6.1).

Table 6.1 Prostate movement in the prone and supine positions [27]

	Prone (mean displacement in mm ± SD)	Supine (mean displacement in mm ± SD)
AP ($p=0.47$)	2.1 ± 1.2	1.7 ± 1.44
SI ($p=0.16$)	2.2 ± 2.0	1.6 ± 1.8
LR ($p=0.03$)	1.0 ± 1.2	0.6 ± 0.9

6.4.4 Time

When we perform a planning CT scan, we hope that the position of the prostate at that moment will be representative of its position over the forthcoming weeks. However all prostates have a range of movement, and some patients will be scanned with their prostate in an "extreme" position for them. This will introduce a systematic error as for most days the prostate position will differ from its position during the CT scan. Even if the planning CT was performed while the prostate was in an "average" position, there will be oscillation around this point, causing interfraction movement.

In addition, the position of the prostate varies during the daily radiation treatment, called intrafraction prostate movement. It has been found that the chance of a patient's prostate moving 2, 3, or 4 mm increases during 6 min on the treatment couch, hence there seems to be a "drift" in prostate movement the longer the patient lies on the bed [2, 3]. This movement occurred in all directions but was most significant in the AP and SI directions where by 6 min over 10% of patients had drifts of >2 mm. Larger movements seem less time-dependent [2, 3].

6.4.5 Rectal Filling

It is well recognized that rectal filling has the most significant physiological effect on prostate position [10]. Rectal filling can be due to fecal matter or rectal gas. Solid fecal matter can cause persistent displacement of the prostate or may induce peristaltic movement causing prostate motion. Rectal gas may cause prostate displacement of shorter duration, but the effect of solid versus gaseous rectal distension on prostate motion has been less well studied.

The chance of having a 3-mm displacement of the prostate is 10% within 1 min if the rectum is full. However, with an empty rectum, it takes 20 min to have a 10% risk of a 3-mm displacement [18]. Rectal wall motion is greatest at the prostate's base and hence the chance of geographical miss is greatest here [28].

In addition, the larger the rectum, the higher the chance of a rectal peristaltic movement [19], hence the larger the chance of a significant movement of the prostate. This is corroborated by the documented increase in biochemical failure for patients with larger rectums at planning [29].

During a course of radiotherapy the average rectal filling decreases, consistent with radiotherapy's known effect on bowel function [28].

6.5 Imaging Systems for Treatment Guidance

Historically patients have been set up to permanent marks on the skin and imaged infrequently with portal films showing only bony anatomy, which corresponds only moderately to the position of the prostate [30]. Innovative use of imaging technologies has enabled accurate visualization of the prostate and these methods are outlined below. Three-dimensional image guidance has recently been the subject of an ESTRO review [31] and readers are directed here for a more in-depth discussion of the topic. The prostate can be imaged before and after delivery of radiotherapy, or it can be tracked during radiation delivery itself.

6.5.1 CT on Rails

The patient is set up on the linac and then the couch is moved to an imaging position where the CT on rails slides over the treatment couch and obtains diagnostic quality kV CT images, which are coregistered with the planning CT (Fig. 6.2). The method provides high-quality imaging but no intrafraction information is available [31–34].

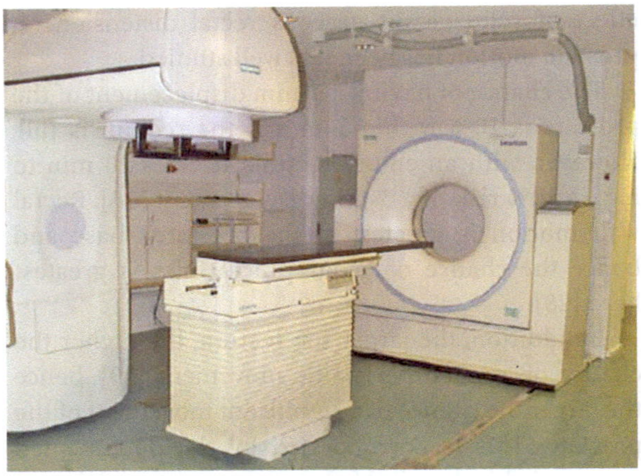

Fig. 6.2 Siemens CT on rails system [31]

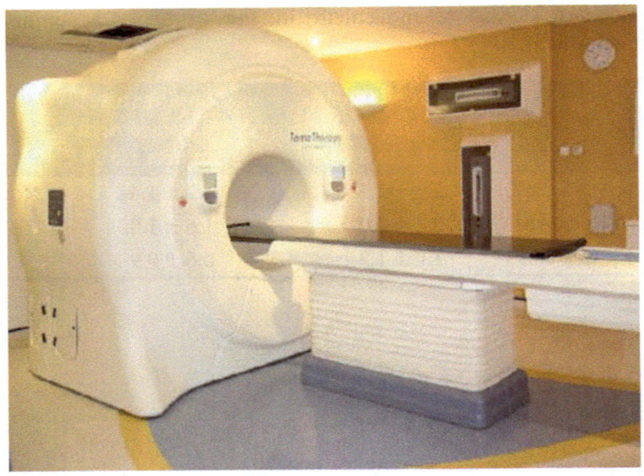

Fig. 6.3 TomoTherapy® (From [31])

6.5.2 Kilovoltage Cone-Beam CT

Cone beam CT is achieved using a diagnostic X-ray source and a flat panel detector integrated with a linac [35]. One major advantage of this system compared to "CT on rails" is that the patient is not moved between treatment setup and scan. The image quality is inferior to CT on rails for soft tissue delineation and definition of the prostate margins can be difficult.

6.5.3 Megavoltage Cone-Beam CT

Megavoltage (MV) cone-beam systems were initially developed in the 1980s and were based on a single-slice tomogram generated through one gantry rotation. The MV quality of images is poorer than kV CT, but there are fewer artifacts produced by prostheses, and it allows accurate identification of fiducial markers. Alignment of the target is simple as the treatment beam is used to acquire the image. A problem with MV CT is the relatively high dose, typically 1–3 cGy per exposure (see supplementary materials for reference [31]) received by the target while acquiring an image. This compares to around 17 mGy for a kV cone-beam CT [36]. However, as with all CT methods, the seminal vesicles can be visualized, which is an advantage over fiducial-based methods.

6.5.4 TomoTherapy® (Using MVCT)

Tomotherapy® (Tomotherapy Inc., Madison, WI) is a technique whereby radiation is delivered by a beam rotating around a patient (Fig. 6.3). Basically it is a CT scanner where the diagnostic X-ray tube has been replaced with a linac and the collimating jaws replaced with a binary collimator consisting of small high-density metal leaves. CT-image acquisition, using a lower energy than for treatment, is acquired with all leaves open prior to treatment [35]. The system incorporates a rapid auto-matching system, which enables daily online positional correction prior to treatment and correction of both random and systematic errors [37]. The couch moves through the cone as the gantry rotates delivering radiation in a helical manner [38–40].

6.5.5 Ultrasound

BAT ultrasound has been used to measure displacement relative to the planning scan and suggest shifts prior to treatment [41]. Some studies indicated that this technique may reduce toxicity [41].

Further analysis of this technique, compared to implanted fiducials, has shown that transabdominal ultrasound to be less accurate in guiding image-guided radiotherapy [42–44].

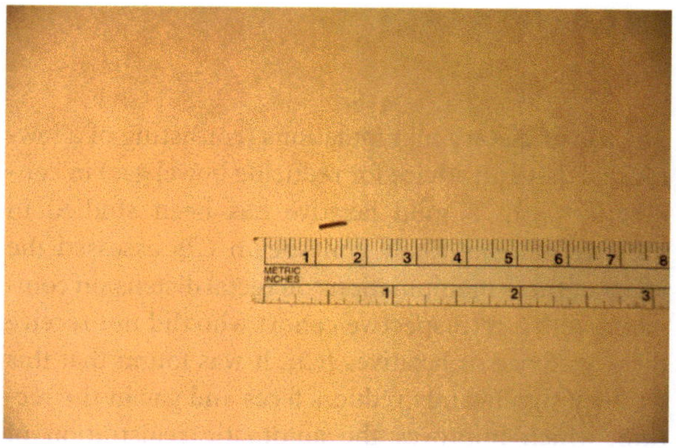

Fig. 6.4 Gold fiducial

6.5.6 Fiducials with kV Imaging

Transrectal ultrasound is usually used to implant gold markers, approximately 1 mm long, into the prostate (Fig. 6.4). These can also be implanted by the transperineal route. Typically three are used, although more are employed for some studies. Most users allow 1 week between marker placement and planning CT to allow for settling of marker position [17]. The fiducials are easily seen with kV portal imaging, which is usually set up to record two orthogonal images to localize the seeds. Interobserver variation in fiducial localization was found to be small, with only 3–5% of recordings having a discrepancy in excess of 2 mm [45].

The gold seeds appear to be stable within the prostate and intraprostate migration is small [46–48]. The average absolute marker positional variation was 1.01 mm, with only 1% of markers showing a significant change in their position over a course of radiotherapy, mostly due to prostate deformation [49]. The procedure appears safe and well tolerated by patients [50]. One disadvantage of prostate fiducials is that they cannot directly determine seminal vesicle position. However some centers are now investigating the feasibility of seminal vesicle fiducial implantation [51].

The CyberKnife® (Accuray Incorporated, Sunnyvale, CA) uses fiducials located with kV imaging to locate the prostate prior to delivering each beam of radiotherapy [52]. The use of fiducials to improve accuracy of radiotherapy delivery is discussed further in the section below titled "Online Corrective Strategies."

Fiducial imaging using kV portal images has been compared with cone beam CT [53]. The two modalities suggested shifts that were discordant by more than 5 mm in 28% of cases, which leaves us wondering which modality was "right." The authors suggest reasons why the two may not agree including the additional time taken to perform the cone beam CT, the poor image quality that could compromise accurate localization, and prostate deformation that may distort fiducial positioning. The authors conclude that they feel kV fiducial imaging is the best use of their resources due to its accuracy and efficiency. Another similar study found that using cone beam CT localization of fiducials was concordant with their localization on portal kV imaging, but that soft-tissue localization was less concordant, supporting the hypothesis that the soft-tissue definition is the crucial step in this process [54]. These studies underline the point that the accuracy of determining the prostate position for each system must be known and accounted for.

6.5.7 Calypso®

The Calypso® system (Calypso® Medical Inc., Seattle, WA) uses electromagnetic transponders, which are also inserted under transrectal ultrasound guidance. When put into an electromagnetic field, these transponders are able to be precisely localized and track the prostate movement in real time. Each transponder has a unique resonant frequency and hence each one can be tracked independently.

The transponder position remains within 2 mm of its reference position in >80% of measurements, and it should be remembered that the transponder position can be displaced by rectal filling, as with the prostate itself [12]. The Calypso® system is attractive because prostate movement can be tracked without extra radiation exposure. The prostate position can be tracked continuously during treatment, and the beam interrupted when a predefined tolerance is exceeded. The patient can then be set up to the updated prostate position. Studies using Calypso® have shown that pre- and post-treatment imaging is not sensitive for predicting prostate motion during the fraction, and that frequent intermittent sampling is inferior to continuous monitoring [55]. Real-time motion monitoring with Calypso® would facilitate significant reductions in the margins needed for treatment [56]. Integration of the Calypso® system with closed-loop motion management strategies is being investigated [57].

6.5.8 MR-Linac

Several centers have published on prototypes of a system consisting of a linear accelerator guided by an on-board MRI [58, 59]. This system appears to have excellent geometric accuracy and low distortion [60] and clearly is an important avenue for future research.

6.6 Strategies to Reduce Prostate Movement

6.6.1 Endorectal Balloon

The insertion of an endorectal balloon is believed to stabilize the position of the prostate for the purpose of radiotherapy delivery (Fig. 6.5). The balloon is usually inflated with 100 mL of water and has the added advantage of displacing the dorsal rectal wall away from the radiotherapy field and hence could reduce toxicity. Some studies have shown this to reduce intrafraction prostate movement [61], while this has not been reproduced in some studies [62].

6.6.2 Pharmaceutical

Some centers have used bowel relaxants (e.g., buscopan) to reduce bowel movement during radiotherapy. It has been noted that these reduce the incidence of clinically visible bowel movements from 58% to 42% [19].

6.6.3 Dietary

The use of dietary manipulations (consisting of a low-residue diet and advice for reducing bowel gas) in conjunction with a mild laxative has been studied in prostate patients. Daily cone beam CTs assessed the effect of these manipulations on rectal distension compared with a retrospective cohort who did not receive dietary advice or laxatives [63]. It was found that this strategy significantly reduces feces and gas in the rectum, which improves the automatic registration of daily CTs with the planning CT, thereby facilitating daily online corrections. There was also a nonsignificant trend for dietary manipulations to reduce prostate movement [63]. However, others have found that an antiflatulence diet and milk of magnesia has no significant effect on rectal size or intrafraction prostate movement [21]. Despite this many centers use mild laxatives for prostate patients undergoing radiotherapy.

6.7 Strategies to Accommodate Prostate Movement in Radiotherapy: Interfraction Movement

Methods for accommodating prostate motion distinguish between interfraction prostate movement (i.e., day-to-day) and intrafraction (movement during the delivery of radiotherapy). Interfraction movement is generally of a larger amplitude than intrafraction movement, as might be intuitively expected [64]. Strategies to accommodate movement can involve moving the couch, altering the MLC configuration, or moving the beam relative to the patient.

6.7.1 Online vs. Offline

There are two general strategies for accommodating interfraction prostate movement. One involves daily monitoring of the position of the prostate, either via soft tissue imaging, or the position of fiducials, then an online correction can be made, thus reducing both the systematic and random error of the setup. While this may be

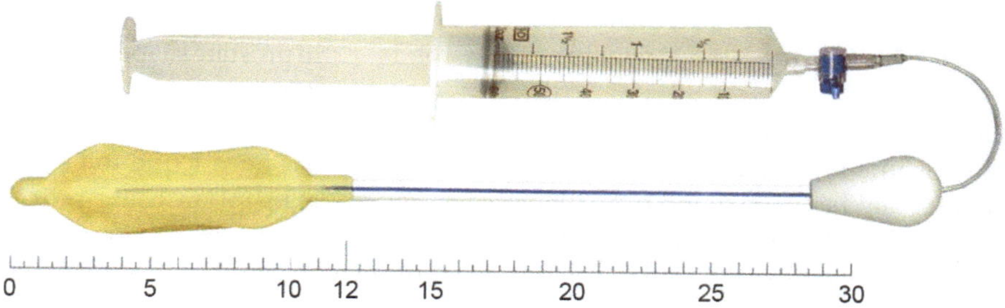

Fig. 6.5 Endorectal balloon (From [61])

labour-intensive if radiographer input is needed, many "closed loop" systems have now been developed where the correction is applied remotely, making record, correct, and verify systems quick and simple to use.

The second way of adjusting for prostate motion is to monitor the position over several fractions at the start of a course of treatment, and then average the data collected, to reduce the systematic error associated with the treatment. This is called offline correction and can be less labor-intensive for the medical staff on the radiotherapy unit but does not account for most of the random error in prostate motion. This can also facilitate adaptive replanning offline.

6.7.2 Offline Corrective Strategies for Interfraction Movement

6.7.2.1 Average Shifts

Attempts have been made to monitor prostate movement in individual patients for the first few fractions and then average the shifts needed for these days. This has been found to slightly reduce the chance of geographical miss, but overall it was concluded that daily imaging is needed to ensure the prostate is covered each day [1]. This has been corroborated in a second study, which investigated a range of offline correction protocols and found that due to variation in the systematic and random errors during a course of radiotherapy, offline corrective models are less accurate than would be desirable [46].

6.7.2.2 Individualized Margins

It is known that prostate movement exhibits a high degree of individual variation [11]. Therefore there has been some interest in individualizing planning margins to better reflect the movement of the prostate in each patient. This prevents those with a relatively stable prostate position being penalized with a larger planning target volume than is necessary.

6.7.2.3 Individualized Planning

Daily cone beam CTs over the first few fractions of radiotherapy have been used to generate an average prostate contour and an average rectal contour [52, 65]. An adaptive plan was then generated and the adequacy of this was assessed with weekly scans. This method facilitated the coverage of the prostate within the PTV on 96% of treatments, with the other 4% mostly missing by only 1 mm. This was achieved with a reduction of the CT V to PTV margin to 7 mm, resulting in a 29% reduction in the PTV volume and a 19% reduction in the volume of rectum receiving >65 Gy [52].

The benefit of adaptive radiotherapy (i.e., replanning after monitoring patient position) in terms of margin reduction has been studied. Lei et al. noticed systematic and patient-specific rotational displacements of the prostate, and suggest that these persist throughout a treatment course. By performing adaptive replanning after imaging the first five fractions, they found that a margin reduction of 1.4–2.0 mm was possible, translating into a reduction in PTV volume of 19–27% [66].

6.7.3 Online Corrective Strategies for Interfraction Movement

The use of daily gold fiducial imaging with resulting couch shifts improves the accuracy of radiotherapy delivery and has been found to facilitate reduction in margins from 8 mm (and 6 mm posteriorly) to 4 mm (and 3 mm posteriorly) without significant loss in PTV coverage [67]. Other studies have found similar reductions in the margins necessary from 5.7 mm LR, 7.9 mm SI, and 7.7 mm AP to 3.6 mm LR and 3.7 mm SI and AP [56] [68]. Much work has been done by many centers to quantify the potential margin reductions with fiducial imaging but a more in-depth discussion is beyond the scope of this chapter [69–71]. Reductions in margins such as this can only be safely achieved with image guidance. It is worthwhile considering that while we aim to reduce margins and hence toxicity, this must be monitored in terms of clinical outcomes. Engels et al. [72] noted an increase in biochemical failure in a small cohort of patients who had implanted fiducials and reduced margins using a daily X-Ray image registration procedure.

Fiducials can be combined with advanced correction protocols to achieve a high level of precision. Graf et al. used kV imaging to assess fiducial position relative to digitally reconstructed radiographs (DRRs) from the planning CT scan. Their algorithm then corrects for translational and all three rotational movements using the Robotics Tilt Module device® (BrainLAB AG, Feldkirchen, Germany). A second image of the fiducials was taken after the shift and a second correction was made if necessary. Using this second correction, margins could be reduced to 1.8–2.1 mm [22].

As discussed above, even with excellent localization of the prostate prior to each fraction, intrafraction movement can cause errors large enough to compromise treatment. Some centers are therefore exploring the feasibility of real-time fiducial detection on a linac [46, 73]. While it appears to be technically feasible, more clinical trials need to be published detailing the success of this technology in treating patients.

Using daily CT images, it has been found that even when using couch shifts to account for daily prostate movement, the resulting dose distributions are suboptimal. In 5% of fractions the prostate volume receiving 100% of the planned dose is 15–20% less than on the planning scan [74]. Movement of the couch can account for setup error and interfraction movement, but has no mechanism for compensating for a change in prostate shape or intrafraction movement. However, it is now possible to account for rotation in one plane by rotation of the gantry on the lateral fields and this has been found to be feasible in practice [16]. Image registration using helical CT images prior to treatment, and adjustment of the couch position and gantry angles allowed reduction of CTV-PTV margins from 8 to 5 mm without compromising on dosimetric coverage [16]. A technique of recontouring the prostate on the daily CT and performing image registration to this contour would further reduce margins to 3 mm, but the time needed was not thought to be practical for daily treatments with this schedule [16].

The next step for improving techniques in adaptive radiotherapy using conventional linacs is to perform a fast replan on a daily basis. This involves recontouring the prostate on the daily MVCT image, performing a modified replan by adjusting MLC positions and adjusting beam weightings, and then treating the patient on that day's plan. Despite the seeming complexity of this, the authors report the replan can be achieved in 6–10 min and that the resulting increased risk of prostate motion with the extended treatment time is more than compensated for by the increase in plan conformality [75].

They compared this method to standard online correction (i.e., performing couch shifts relative to the prostate position) and found that their method improved rectal dose-volume histograms (DVHs) without compromising on PTV coverage, despite using only a 2-mm margin around the CTV (compared to 5 and 3 mm posteriorly for their online couch adjustment method) [75]. Other groups have corroborated these findings [76] and clearly this is an area where there is need for further investigation.

6.8 Strategies to Accommodate Prostate Movement in Radiotherapy: Intrafraction Movement

Traditionally patients were set up to tattoos and lasers but we now have the technology to quantify the accuracy of this strategy. Quigley et al. determined the accuracy of a traditional setup compared to the location of electromagnetic transponders using the Calypso® system. They found that in over 75% of treatment sessions the prostate was more than 5 mm removed from the location suggested by the traditional setup methods [30]. Over 10% had an initial positioning misalignment of more than 15 mm, which would mean that the prostate would not be covered adequately by the radiotherapy field. The comparison between traditional setup margins and those possible with the Calypso® system has also been investigated. It was found that when using Calypso® to monitor prostate position in real time, significant margin reductions were possible, which would result in a significant reduction in PTV volume and hence late toxicity to surrounding structures (see Table 6.2) [3].

Litzenberg found remarkably similar results using Calypso®, also confirming that accuracy improves with frequency of assessment [56]. However it should also be borne in mind that even for early prostate cancers, there is a risk of undiscovered extracapsular extension [77, 78], which needs to be incorporated into the CTV. The margins in Table 6.3 are simply for the CTV to PTV margin.

Without real-time imaging, it is estimated that intrafraction movement necessitates an additional 2–3 mm margin [3, 79] in addition to the margin needed to account for other errors in the treatment delivery system.

When prostate position is assessed daily before and after radiation delivery, this is as a surrogate for the position of the prostate during radiotherapy delivery. Some have suggested that performing pre- and post-radiotherapy scans is a poor indicator of the prostate position in between. The sensitivity of these scans predicting displacements of between 3 and 7 mm during treatment was found to be less than 60% in one study [55] but 75–81% in another study [26], which equates to an accuracy of 95% within 3.1-mm displacement.

The dosimetric impact of prostate motion and the potential gains of online image guidance have been studied. Intensity-modulated arc therapy in combination with the Calypso® system to monitor prostate position has been found to significantly improve dose distributions to the PTV in comparison to arc therapy without tracking. This can be achieved by adjustment of the multileaf collimator configuration to accommodate the position of the prostate [80].

It is important to note, however, that the Calypso® transponders are not currently suitable for use in conjunction with MRI, as they induce significant artifact [81]. This is an issue for treatment planning and would also be an issue if MR-Linacs become commercially available (see Sect. 6.5.8).

The CyberKnife® system uses a robotically mounted linear accelerator to deliver a large number of small conformal beams and has a treatment delivery accuracy of <1 mm [17, 82–84]. The system incorporates two orthogonal kV imagers that detect the location of implanted fiducials and then corrects the beam position prior to delivery. Corrections can be made remotely both translationally and rotationally, which represents a significant improvement on conventional techniques.

The frequency of fiducial imaging, usually every 30–60 s, determines the accuracy of prostate localization, and the frequency can be individualized for each patient to reflect the stability of their prostate position during treatment [85]. Using the InTempo system® (Accuray, Sunnyvale, CA), if the prostate position is found to have moved in excess of predetermined limits between successive beams, then the time

Table 6.2 CTV to PTV margin reductions allowable using Calypso®-guided online correction and a 5-mm action threshold [3]

	Skin set-up margins (mm)	Margins using Calypso® (mm)
Left-right	8.4	1.3
Superior-inferior	10.8	2.3
Anterior-posterior	14.7	2.8

Table 6.3 CTV to PTV margin reductions suggested in [56]

	Skin set-up margins (mm)	Margins using Calypso® to set up prior to treatment only (mm)	Margins using Calypso® to set up prior to each beam (mm)	Margins using Calypso® to continuously monitor (mm)
Left-right	8.2	1.8	1.4	1.3
Superior-inferior	10.2	5.8	2.3	1.5
Anterior-posterior	12.5	7.1	1.8	1.5

between imaging and beam delivery ("image age") is set to a maximum of 15 s, thereby increasing the frequency of imaging [17]. In general an imaging frequency of 40 s has been found to be adequate [52] but for some patients their prostate movement is such that systems such as InTempo® would enable greater accuracy.

CyberKnife® is usually used for hypofractionated prostate treatments, for example five fractions of 7.25 Gy. Because of the high dose per fraction, low number of fractions and the rapidity of prostate motion described above, it is essential that image guidance is used [86]. Although the system has a technical accuracy of <1 mm, most centers that have published use margins of 5 mm in all directions except 3 mm posteriorly [83, 87] for prostate in order to adequately treat any extracapsular spread. Thin-cut planning CTs (e.g., slice thickness 1.25 mm) along with CT-MRI fusion are used to improve accuracy of target definition.

6.9 Summary

The characteristics of prostate movement have been extensively studied over the last 20 years. Prostate movement has the potential to compromise cure of prostate cancer and increase toxicity of the surrounding normal structures. Traditionally geometric margins have been used to account for prostate movement at the expense of increasing dose to the rectum.

With the advent of daily prostate localization, treatment accuracy can be improved by adapting for interfraction and even intrafraction prostate motion. Treatment delivery techniques specific to an individual's prostate motion characteristics can further improve the accuracy of treatment and reduce margins for uncertainty.

Interfraction and intrafraction movement are clearly both important, but strategies to accommodate the latter will clearly address the former as well, assuming one image is acquired before the initiation of treatment. Prostate deformation is harder to quantify but likely to be significant, particularly if margins are reduced. More work is needed to develop adaptive planning solutions, which can cope with a deformable organ.

Image-guided radiotherapy should now be the standard of care and the gold standard should include assessment and correction for movement during each fraction. This will enable margin reduction and the possibility of hypofractionation for prostate cancer. Further work is needed to determine optimal margins to establish the feasibility of MRI-guided radiotherapy and further explore the possibilities for daily adaptive replanning.

References

1. Perks J, Turnbull H, Liu T et al (2011) Vector analysis of prostate patient setup with image-guided radiation therapy via kV cone beam computed tomography. Int J Radiat Oncol Biol Phys 79(3):915–919
2. Both S, Wang KK, Plastaras JP et al (2010) Real-time study of prostate intrafraction motion during external beam radiotherapy with daily endorectal balloon. Int J Radiat Oncol Biol Phys
3. Su Z, Zhang L, Murphy M, et al (2010) Analysis of prostate patient setup and tracking data: potential intervention strategies. Int J Radiat Oncol Biol Phys
4. Khoo VS, Dearnaley DP (2008) Question of dose, fractionation and technique: ingredients for testing hypofractionation in prostate cancer–the CHHiP trial. Clin Oncol (R Coll Radiol) 20:12–14
5. Tree A, Khoo VS (2009) Treatment of early prostate cancer: radiotherapy including brachytherapy. Trends Urol Gynaecol Sex Health 14:18–23
6. Dasu A (2007) Is the alpha/beta value for prostate tumors low enough to be safely used in clinical trials? Clin Oncol (R Coll Radiol) 19:289–301
7. Hoskin PJ, Dearnaley DP (2007) Hypofractionation in clinical trials for prostate cancer. Clin Oncol (R Coll Radiol) 19:287–288
8. Khoo VS (2005) Radiotherapeutic techniques for prostate cancer, dose escalation and brachytherapy. Clin Oncol (R Coll Radiol) 17:560–571
9. Khoo VS (2010) Imaging for radiotherapy treatment planning, Chapter 52. In: Husband J, Reznek R (eds) Imaging in oncology, 3rd edn. Informa UK Ltd, London
10. Langen KM, Jones DT (2001) Organ motion and its management. Int J Radiat Oncol Biol Phys 50:265–278
11. Langen KM, Willoughby TR, Meeks SL et al (2008) Observations on real-time prostate gland motion using electromagnetic tracking. Int J Radiat Oncol Biol Phys 71:1084–1090
12. Tanyi JA, He T, Summers PA et al (2010) Assessment of planning target volume margins for intensity-modulated radiotherapy of the prostate gland: role of daily inter- and intrafraction motion. Int J Radiat Oncol Biol Phys 78:1579–1585
13. Adamson J, Wu Q (2010) Prostate intrafraction motion assessed by simultaneous kilovoltage fluoroscopy at

megavoltage delivery I: clinical observations and pattern analysis. Int J Radiat Oncol Biol Phys 78:1563–1570
14. Kupelian P, Willoughby T, Mahadevan A et al (2007) Multi-institutional clinical experience with the Calypso® System in localization and continuous, real-time monitoring of the prostate gland during external radiotherapy. Int J Radiat Oncol Biol Phys 67:1088–1098
15. de Boer HC, van Os MJ, Jansen PP et al (2005) Application of the No Action Level (NAL) protocol to correct for prostate motion based on electronic portal imaging of implanted markers. Int J Radiat Oncol Biol Phys 61:969–983
16. Wu Q, Ivaldi G, Liang J et al (2006) Geometric and dosimetric evaluations of an online image-guidance strategy for 3D-CRT of prostate cancer. Int J Radiat Oncol Biol Phys 64:1596–1609
17. Kilby W, Dooley JR, Kuduvalli G et al (2010) The cyberKnife robotic radiosurgery system in 2010. Technol Cancer Res Treat 9:433–452
18. Ghilezan MJ, Jaffray DA, Siewerdsen JH et al (2005) Prostate gland motion assessed with cine-magnetic resonance imaging (cine-MRI). Int J Radiat Oncol Biol Phys 62:406–417
19. Padhani AR, Khoo VS, Suckling J et al (1999) Evaluating the effect of rectal distension and rectal movement on prostate gland position using cine MRI. Int J Radiat Oncol Biol Phys 44:525–533
20. Kerkhof EM, van der Put RW, Raaymakers BW et al (2008) Variation in target and rectum dose due to prostate deformation: an assessment by repeated MR imaging and treatment planning. Phys Med Biol 53:5623–5634
21. Nichol AM, Warde PR, Lockwood GA et al (2010) A cinematic magnetic resonance imaging study of milk of magnesia laxative and an antiflatulent diet to reduce intrafraction prostate motion. Int J Radiat Oncol Biol Phys 77:1072–1078
22. Beard CJ, Kijewski P, Bussiere M et al (1996) Analysis of prostate and seminal vesicle motion: implications for treatment planning. Int J Radiat Oncol Biol Phys 34:451–458
23. Dawson LA, Litzenberg DW, Brock KK et al (2000) A comparison of ventilatory prostate movement in four treatment positions. Int J Radiat Oncol Biol Phys 48:319–323
24. Cheung P, Sixel K, Morton G et al (2005) Individualized planning target volumes for intrafraction motion during hypofractionated intensity-modulated radiotherapy boost for prostate cancer. Int J Radiat Oncol Biol Phys 62:418–425
25. Rosewall T, Chung P, Bayley A et al (2008) A randomized comparison of interfraction and intrafraction prostate motion with and without abdominal compression. Radiother Oncol 88:88–94
26. Adamson J, Wu Q (2009) Inferences about prostate intrafraction motion from pre- and posttreatment volumetric imaging. Int J Radiat Oncol Biol Phys 75:260–267
27. Wilder RB, Chittenden L, Mesa AV et al (2010) A prospective study of intrafraction prostate motion in the prone vs. supine position. Int J Radiat Oncol Biol Phys 77:165–170
28. Sripadam R, Stratford J, Henry AM et al (2009) Rectal motion can reduce CTV coverage and increase rectal dose during prostate radiotherapy: a daily cone-beam CT study. Radiother Oncol 90:312–317
29. Heemsbergen WD, Hoogeman MS, Witte MG et al (2007) Increased risk of biochemical and clinical failure for prostate patients with a large rectum at radiotherapy planning: results from the Dutch trial of 68 GY versus 78 Gy. Int J Radiat Oncol Biol Phys 67:1418–1424
30. Quigley MM, Mate TP, Sylvester JE (2009) Prostate tumor alignment and continuous, real-time adaptive radiation therapy using electromagnetic fiducials: clinical and cost-utility analyses. Urol Oncol 27:473–482
31. Korreman S, Rasch C, McNair H et al (2010) The European Society of Therapeutic Radiology and Oncology-European Institute of Radiotherapy (ESTRO-EIR) report on 3D CT-based in-room image guidance systems: a practical and technical review and guide. Radiother Oncol 94:129–144
32. Stutzel J, Oelfke U, Nill S (2008) A quantitative image quality comparison of four different image guided radiotherapy devices. Radiother Oncol 86:20–24
33. Owen R, Kron T, Foroudi F et al (2009) Comparison of CT on rails with electronic portal imaging for positioning of prostate cancer patients with implanted fiducial markers. Int J Radiat Oncol Biol Phys 74:906–912
34. Wong JR, Gao Z, Uematsu M et al (2008) Interfractional prostate shifts: review of 1870 computed tomography (CT) scans obtained during image-guided radiotherapy using CT-on-rails for the treatment of prostate cancer. Int J Radiat Oncol Biol Phys 72:1396–1401
35. Verellen D, Ridder MD, Linthout N et al (2007) Innovations in image-guided radiotherapy. Nat Rev Cancer 7:949–960
36. Walter C, Boda-Heggemann J, Wertz H et al (2007) Phantom and in-vivo measurements of dose exposure by image-guided radiotherapy (IGRT): MV portal images vs. kV portal images vs. cone-beam CT. Radiother Oncol 85:418–423
37. Burnet NG, Adams EJ, Fairfoul J et al (2010) Practical aspects of implementation of helical tomotherapy for intensity-modulated and image-guided radiotherapy. Clin Oncol (R Coll Radiol) 22:294–312
38. Boswell S, Tome W, Jeraj R et al (2006) Automatic registration of megavoltage to kilovoltage CT images in helical tomotherapy: an evaluation of the setup verification process for the special case of a rigid head phantom. Med Phys 33:4395–4404
39. Welsh JS, Lock M, Harari PM et al (2006) Clinical implementation of adaptive helical tomotherapy: a unique approach to image-guided intensity modulated radiotherapy. Technol Cancer Res Treat 5:465–479
40. Mackie TR (2006) History of tomotherapy. Phys Med Biol 51:R427–R453
41. Pinkawa M, Pursch-Lee M, Asadpour B et al (2008) Image-guided radiotherapy for prostate cancer. Implementation of ultrasound-based prostate localization for the analysis of inter- and intrafraction organ motion. Strahlenther Onkol 184:679–685
42. Scarbrough TJ, Golden NM, Ting JY et al (2006) Comparison of ultrasound and implanted seed marker prostate localization methods: Implications for image-guided radiotherapy. Int J Radiat Oncol Biol Phys 65:378–387
43. McNair HA, Mangar SA, Coffey J et al (2006) A comparison of CT- and ultrasound-based imaging to localize the prostate for external beam radiotherapy. Int J Radiat Oncol Biol Phys 65:678–687
44. Langen KM, Pouliot J, Anezinos C et al (2003) Evaluation of ultrasound-based prostate localization for image-guided radiotherapy. Int J Radiat Oncol Biol Phys 57:635–644

45. Kong V, Lockwood G, Yan J et al (2010) The effect of registration surrogate and patient factors on the interobserver variability of electronic portal image guidance during prostate radiotherapy. Med Dosim
46. Litzenberg DW, Balter JM, Lam KL et al (2005) Retrospective analysis of prostate cancer patients with implanted gold markers using off-line and adaptive therapy protocols. Int J Radiat Oncol Biol Phys 63:123–133
47. Nichol AM, Brock KK, Lockwood GA et al (2007) A magnetic resonance imaging study of prostate deformation relative to implanted gold fiducial markers. Int J Radiat Oncol Biol Phys 67:48–56
48. van der Heide UA, Kotte AN, Dehnad H et al (2007) Analysis of fiducial marker-based position verification in the external beam radiotherapy of patients with prostate cancer. Radiother Oncol 82:38–45
49. Kupelian PA, Willoughby TR, Meeks SL et al (2005) Intraprostatic fiducials for localization of the prostate gland: monitoring intermarker distances during radiation therapy to test for marker stability. Int J Radiat Oncol Biol Phys 62:1291–1296
50. Moman MR, van der Heide UA, Kotte AN et al (2010) Long-term experience with transrectal and transperineal implantations of fiducial gold markers in the prostate for position verification in external beam radiotherapy; feasibility, toxicity and quality of life. Radiother Oncol 96:38–42
51. Mercuri AL, Lim Joon D, Khoo V et al (2008) The impact of prostate and seminal vesicle motion during prostate cancer radiotherapy on planning margins. Int J Radiat Oncol Biol Phys 72:312
52. Nijkamp J, Pos FJ, Nuver TT et al (2008) Adaptive radiotherapy for prostate cancer using kilovoltage cone-beam computed tomography: first clinical results. Int J Radiat Oncol Biol Phys 70:75–82
53. Barney BM, Lee RJ, Handrahan D et al (2011) Image-Guided Radiotherapy (IGRT) for prostate cancer comparing kV imaging of fiducial markers with Cone Beam Computed Tomography (CBCT). Int J Radiat Oncol Biol Phys 80(1): 301–305
54. Moseley DJ, White EA, Wiltshire KL et al (2007) Comparison of localization performance with implanted fiducial markers and cone-beam computed tomography for on-line image-guided radiotherapy of the prostate. Int J Radiat Oncol Biol Phys 67:942–953
55. Noel C, Parikh PJ, Roy M et al (2009) Prediction of intrafraction prostate motion: accuracy of pre- and post-treatment imaging and intermittent imaging. Int J Radiat Oncol Biol Phys 73:692–698
56. Litzenberg DW, Balter JM, Hadley SW et al (2006) Influence of intrafraction motion on margins for prostate radiotherapy. Int J Radiat Oncol Biol Phys 65:548–553
57. Sawant A, Smith RL, Venkat RB et al (2009) Toward submillimeter accuracy in the management of intrafraction motion: the integration of real-time internal position monitoring and multileaf collimator target tracking. Int J Radiat Oncol Biol Phys 74:575–582
58. Fallone BG, Murray B, Rathee S et al (2009) First MR images obtained during megavoltage photon irradiation from a prototype integrated linac-MR system. Med Phys 36: 2084–2088
59. Lagendijk JJ, Raaymakers BW, Raaijmakers AJ et al (2008) MRI/linac integration. Radiother Oncol 86:25–29
60. Wachowicz K, Stanescu T, Thomas SD et al (2010) Implications of tissue magnetic susceptibility-related distortion on the rotating magnet in an MR-linac design. Med Phys 37:1714–1721
61. D'Amico AV, Manola J, Loffredo M et al (2001) A practical method to achieve prostate gland immobilization and target verification for daily treatment. Int J Radiat Oncol Biol Phys 51:1431–1436
62. van Lin EN, van der Vight LP, Witjes JA et al (2005) The effect of an endorectal balloon and off-line correction on the interfraction systematic and random prostate position variations: a comparative study. Int J Radiat Oncol Biol Phys 61:278–288
63. Smitsmans MH, Pos FJ, de Bois J et al (2008) The influence of a dietary protocol on cone beam CT-guided radiotherapy for prostate cancer patients. Int J Radiat Oncol Biol Phys 71:1279–1286
64. Aubry JF, Beaulieu L, Girouard LM et al (2004) Measurements of intrafraction motion and interfraction and intrafraction rotation of prostate by three-dimensional analysis of daily portal imaging with radiopaque markers. Int J Radiat Oncol Biol Phys 60:30–39
65. Nuver TT, Hoogeman MS, Remeijer P et al (2007) An adaptive off-line procedure for radiotherapy of prostate cancer. Int J Radiat Oncol Biol Phys 67:1559–1567
66. Lei Y, Wu Q (2010) A hybrid strategy of offline adaptive planning and online image guidance for prostate cancer radiotherapy. Phys Med Biol 55:2221–2234
67. Pawlowski JM, Yang ES, Malcolm AW et al (2010) Reduction of dose delivered to organs at risk in prostate cancer patients via image-guided radiation therapy. Int J Radiat Oncol Biol Phys 76:924–934
68. Skarsgard D, Cadman P, El-Gayed A et al (2010) Planning target volume margins for prostate radiotherapy using daily electronic portal imaging and implanted fiducial markers. Radiat Oncol 5:52
69. Graf R, Wust P, Budach V et al (2009) Potentials of on-line repositioning based on implanted fiducial markers and electronic portal imaging in prostate cancer radiotherapy. Radiat Oncol 4:13
70. McNair HA, Hansen VN, Parker CC et al (2008) A comparison of the use of bony anatomy and internal markers for offline verification and an evaluation of the potential benefit of online and offline verification protocols for prostate radiotherapy. Int J Radiat Oncol Biol Phys 71:41–50
71. Meijer GJ, de Klerk J, Bzdusek K et al (2008) What CTV-to-PTV margins should be applied for prostate irradiation? Four-dimensional quantitative assessment using model-based deformable image registration techniques. Int J Radiat Oncol Biol Phys 72:1416–1425
72. Engels B, Soete G, Verellen D et al (2009) Conformal arc radiotherapy for prostate cancer: increased biochemical failure in patients with distended rectum on the planning computed tomogram despite image guidance by implanted markers. Int J Radiat Oncol Biol Phys 74:388–391
73. Court LE, Dong L, Lee AK et al (2005) An automatic CT-guided adaptive radiation therapy technique by online modification of multileaf collimator leaf positions

for prostate cancer. Int J Radiat Oncol Biol Phys 62: 154–163
74. Peng C, Ahunbay E, Chen G et al (2010) Characterizing interfraction variations and their dosimetric effects in prostate cancer radiotherapy. Int J Radiat Oncol Biol Phys 79(3):909–914
75. Ahunbay EE, Peng C, Holmes S et al (2010) Online adaptive replanning method for prostate radiotherapy. Int J Radiat Oncol Biol Phys 77:1561–1572
76. Thongphiew D, Wu QJ, Lee WR et al (2009) Comparison of online IGRT techniques for prostate IMRT treatment: adaptive vs repositioning correction. Med Phys 36:1651–1662
77. Davis BJ, Pisansky TM, Wilson TM et al (1999) The radial distance of extraprostatic extension of prostate carcinoma: implications for prostate brachytherapy. Cancer 85: 2630–2637
78. Chao KK, Goldstein NS, Yan D et al (2006) Clinicopathologic analysis of extracapsular extension in prostate cancer: should the clinical target volume be expanded posterolaterally to account for microscopic extension? Int J Radiat Oncol Biol Phys 65:999–1007
79. Beltran C, Herman MG, Davis BJ (2008) Planning target margin calculations for prostate radiotherapy based on intrafraction and interfraction motion using four localization methods. Int J Radiat Oncol Biol Phys 70:289–295
80. Keall PJ, Sawant A, Cho B et al (2011) Electromagnetic-guided dynamic multileaf collimator tracking enables motion management for intensity-modulated arc therapy. Int J Radiat Oncol Biol Phys 79:312–320
81. Zhu X, Bourland JD, Yuan Y et al (2009) Tradeoffs of integrating real-time tracking into IGRT for prostate cancer treatment. Phys Med Biol 54:N393–N401
82. Antypas C, Pantelis E (2008) Performance evaluation of a CyberKnife G4 image-guided robotic stereotactic radiosurgery system. Phys Med Biol 53:4697–4718
83. King CR, Lehmann J, Adler JR et al (2003) CyberKnife radiotherapy for localized prostate cancer: rationale and technical feasibility. Technol Cancer Res Treat 2:25–30
84. Coste-Maniere E, Olender D, Kilby W et al (2005) Robotic whole body stereotactic radiosurgery: clinical advantages of the Cyberknife integrated system. Int J Med Robot 1: 28–39
85. Xie Y, Djajaputra D, King CR et al (2008) Intrafractional motion of the prostate during hypofractionated radiotherapy. Int J Radiat Oncol Biol Phys 72:236–246
86. Hossain S, Xia P, Chuang C et al (2008) Simulated real time image guided intrafraction tracking-delivery for hypofractionated prostate IMRT. Med Phys 35:4041–4048
87. Oermann EK, Slack RS, Hanscom HN et al (2010) A pilot study of intensity modulated radiation therapy with hypofractionated stereotactic body radiation therapy (SBRT) boost in the treatment of intermediate- to high-risk prostate cancer. Technol Cancer Res Treat 9: 453–462

The Evolution of Conventionally Fractionated External-Beam Radiotherapy: Contemporary Techniques (3D-CRT/IMRT/IGRT)

7

Donald B. Fuller

CONTENTS

7.1 Abstract

This chapter will focus on the technological and clinical evolution of conventionally fractionated external-beam radiotherapy against prostate cancer. Advances in imaging and radiotherapy techniques during treatment planning and delivery, such as 3D conformal radiotherapy (3D-CRT), intensity-modulated radiotherapy (IMRT), and image-guided radiotherapy (IGRT) resulted in a more accurate definition of the prostate target volume and reduced complications due to better sparing of adjacent normal tissues. In consequence, an increased therapeutic dose can now be delivered more safely with a significant superiority of biochemical disease-free survival.

Robotic IMRT represents the next generation of conventional extended-fractionation delivery options, with the benefits of continual intrafraction tracking and beam correction, normally associated with robotic radiosurgery.

7.2 Introduction

Although external-beam radiotherapy (EBRT) has a decade's long history of clinical use and long-term follow-up data in the treatment of prostate cancer, its absolute efficacy in the cure of this disease has still not been definitively established. It has become obvious that doses such as 60–66 Gy over 30–37 fractions that were once thought to be adequate are in fact wholly inadequate and progressively worse over increasing follow-up periods when subjected to long-term prostate-specific antigen (PSA)-based follow-up evaluation [1–3].

Further exacerbating the basic dose adequacy problem, targeting inaccuracies due to technological limitations of older radiotherapy-targeting methodology have also contributed to the insufficient treatment of

L.E. Ponsky et al. (eds.), *Treating Prostate Cancer and Related Genitourinary Applications*, Robotic Radiosurgery,
DOI 10.1007/978-3-642-11495-3_7, © Springer-Verlag Berlin Heidelberg 2012

even early-stage prostate cancer lesions, with early demonstration of a vastly higher biochemical relapse rate in "conventionally" treated patients, relative to those treated with CT-based 3D conformal technique (3D-CRT), in spite of similar total doses being delivered with either method [4]. This strongly implies "geographic miss" as an explanation for the higher failure rate in the non-CT-planned group.

Patients that may have otherwise been considered "controlled" according to the normalization of their follow-up digital rectal exam (DRE) following radiotherapy, in fact often have a "biochemical relapse" of their disease, as PSA-based evaluation is far more sensitive to a treatment failure than "clinical" endpoints such as DRE or positive radiologic study. In other words, since the advent of routine PSA-based follow-up, there has been a fundamental reassessment of the dose–response curve required to cure a typical case of prostate cancer with a course of external-beam radiotherapy.

This PSA-driven reappraisal has led to a radiotherapy dose escalation trend over the last two decades, as clinicians have sought to increase the effectiveness of conventionally fractionated external-beam radiotherapy [2, 5–7]. In parallel with dose escalation, there has been an evolution of "image guidance" methods to more accurately direct the treatment and compensate for changes in the location of the prostate from day to day as the treatment course progresses [8–10].

The topics of hypofractionation radiobiology and image-guided robotic hypofractionated stereotactic body radiotherapy (SBRT) for prostate cancer are amply addressed elsewhere within this textbook, and as such, will not be covered in any significant detail in this chapter, which instead, will focus on the evolution of *conventionally* fractionated external beam radiotherapy against prostate cancer.

7.3 Evolution of Treatment Planning Technique and Radiotherapy Delivery Process

Prior to 1980, virtually all external-beam radiotherapy treatment planning for prostate cancer was accomplished with the use of plain X-ray-based simulation techniques, with radio-opaque contrast in the bladder, urethra and the rectum, used to visualize the base of the bladder, the "beak" of the urethra, and the anterior wall of the rectum, respectively. During that era, this simulation methodology was felt sufficient to accurately define the limits of the prostate; essentially giving its location by "subtraction" by defining the configuration of its surrounding organs, and surrounding pelvic bony constraints. The prostate itself was not directly visualized by this technique.

In 1982, the Mallinckrodt Institute group from St. Louis reported the use of CT-based planning in 100 consecutive patients with prostate cancer, describing a disturbing discordance in the actual location of the prostate and seminal vesicles as defined by CT imaging, versus where they were presumed to be based on contrast-enhanced plain film simulation, with the non-CT-based simulation method judged as leading to inadequate target volume coverage in 7% of "seminal vesicle negative" cases and 53% of "seminal vesicle positive" cases [11].

Although this early emergence of CT-based prostate and seminal vesicle target volume evaluation began to shed light on the problem of accurately covering the prostate target volume, it underestimated the true magnitude of the problem, as this and other reports of the era assumed constant prostate and seminal vesicle location throughout the treatment course – the phenomenon of interfraction and intrafraction prostate/seminal vesicle motion having not yet been defined in the literature. Nonetheless, CT-based planning represented the first major step of our era toward more accurate definition of the prostate target volume. The process of importing CT images directly into the radiotherapy treatment-planning computer, to be contoured for tumor targeting and normal tissue dose limitation purposes, became known as "three-dimensional conformal radiotherapy" (3D-CRT) and became the standard of care by the year 2000 [3].

The next paradigm-shifting stage of treatment planning development was the advent of intensity-modulated radiotherapy (IMRT). IMRT derives its source treatment planning data from the same CT-based images as basic 3D-CRT treatment planning, but also often takes advantage of co-registered MR images for better prostate anatomic definition. It also uses a different planning algorithm to calculate the best dose distribution. IMRT for prostate cancer makes use of an inverse-planning process, to vary the fluence of the radiation distribution across a beam's-eye profile, in addition to conforming the beam around the edges of the CT-defined target volume. This feature introduces the capability to create a concave isodose line against a convex encroaching structure, leading to a far more conformal three dimensional dose-sculpting capability in the process. This property allows the exclusion of greater amounts of surrounding tissues, specifically, the rectum, enabling a larger dose of therapeutic radiation to be directed toward the prostate planning target volume for a given volume of rectal dose exposure, fundamentally improving the therapeutic ratio [2, 12].

7.4 Image Guidance

Beyond IMRT, the next technologic advance was image-guided targeting, using ultrasound, X-ray, or CT imaging to localize the prostate and correct for intrafractional motion and daily errors in patient positioning [8–10]. Collectively these imaging-based methods are known as "image-guided radiotherapy" (IGRT) and represent a significant improvement in targeting quality, enabling a more accurate delivery of the highly conformal IMRT dose pattern, relative to simple skin mark reference-based targeting strategies [13, 14].

7.5 Dose Response

There has been a clear demonstration of dose–response curve for the local control of prostate cancer, with improved biochemical relapse-free survival rates observed with higher radiotherapeutic doses [2, 5–7]. Unfortunately, due to the concomitant exposure of adjacent normal tissues beyond prostate, there is also a similar dose–response curve for normal tissue complications [5].

The MD Anderson Hospital (MDAH) 3D-CRT dose escalation trial showed a statistically significant superiority of biochemical disease-free survival for the patients randomized for the higher-dose arm (78 Gy versus 70 Gy), with subset analysis demonstrating the most significant benefit in the "high-risk" and "PSA > 10 ng/mL" groups [15]. A significantly higher risk of clinical relapse, distant metastases, and prostate cancer induced death was also observed in the lower-dose arm "high-risk" and "PSA > 10 ng/ml" subsets, strongly suggesting, as have others, that local failure serves as a reservoir for subsequent dissemination, ultimately increasing the risk of suffering and dying from the disease, further increasing the clinical importance of local control. Concomitantly, there was also a statistically significant increased incidence of grade 2 and higher rectal complications observed in the dose-escalated group, with a secondary observation that the rectal complication rate was reduced if the volume of rectum receiving >70 Gy was less than 25% [5].

The Memorial Sloan Kettering (MSKCC) group demonstrated a clear dose–response curve for all prostate cancer prognostic groups, including favorable-risk, intermediate-risk, and high-risk groups, over an escalating dose range from 64.8 to 86.4 Gy, at 1.8 Gy per fraction, evaluated in 5.4-Gy total dose increments. Unlike the MDAH series, the MSKCC series did not demonstrate an increased complication rate in the dose escalation arm. In fact, a lower incidence of rectal complication was observed in the dose escalation arms, and the postulated reason for this reduced complication rate was the significantly greater prevalence of the IMRT delivery technique with better rectal sparing from the high-dose region, in the high dose-study arms [2]. In subsequent updated reporting from the MSKCC dose progression, even "ultrahigh-dose" IMRT (86.4 Gy) appears to have a lower rectal toxicity rate than lower doses delivered by "conventional" 3D-CRT [6]. There appears to be no significant dose–response relationship for urinary tract toxicity in either of the MDAH or the MSKCC series [2, 5, 6].

Another convincing demonstration of an outcome advantage with conventional fractionation dose escalation has been provided by the updated Proton Radiation Oncology Group (PROG) trial report [7]. This is not specifically a proton study, as both arms received mixed proton-photon treatment plans, but rather is a randomized *dose escalation* study (70.2 GyE versus 79.2 GyE). This trial has demonstrated a greater than 50% reduction in biochemical relapse rates in the high- versus low-dose arms, with 8.9 years of median follow-up; 16.7% versus 32.4%, respectively, with a highly significant benefit in the low-risk group (7.1% versus 28.2%; $p<0.0001$) and a borderline significant benefit in the smaller intermediate-risk group (30.4% versus 42.1%; $p=0.06$). There was a modestly increased incidence of ≥grade 2 late GI and GU complications in the dose escalation arm, borderline significant for GI ($p=0.0895$), but no significant difference in the incidence of ≥grade 3 complications, and no difference in patient-reported GI or GU quality of life outcomes.

A subsequent evaluation of delayed patient-reported rectal toxicity in the PROG study indicated that the more important predictor of delayed rectal toxicity was the *volume* of rectum exposed to a given dose of radiation, with borderline statistically significant increased patient-reported GI dysfunction with higher V60, V65, V70, and V75 levels [14]. There was no difference seen by prescribed total prostate dose (70.2 GyE versus 79.2 GyE). This led the authors to conclude that further prostate dose escalation should be possible as long as GI dose volume limitation constraints are met. This study appears to reinforce the rectal toxicity observation from the MSKCC study, each independently suggesting that the volume of rectum exposed to moderate–high dose radiation is probably more significant in the development of subsequent toxicity than the absolute maximum dose received by the rectum [2, 6, 16].

7.6 Next-Generation Treatment

Although ultrasound-based prostate targeting has been one of the prototypical IGRT approaches, its accuracy is degraded by a variability of interobserver image interpretation, leading to subjective differences in set-up correction magnitude, which may be of similar or larger magnitude than the prostate motion itself [17, 18]. Additionally, this method has systematic measurement differences from CT-based and fiducial-based methods, leading to an impression that its accuracy is limited compared particularly with fiducial-based methods, perhaps with the greatest utility in adjusting the AP dimension and the greatest potential inaccuracy in the superior-inferior dimension [18]. As such ultrasound would represent an incremental rather than a final image guidance development. Daily CT image-based guidance may offer a higher quality image to interpret, but in the absence of implanted fiducial markers to three dimensionally co-register, this method also potentially suffers from at least some degree of interobserver image interpretation variation, potentially reducing the overall accuracy of that process relative to fiducial-based set up [18].

To reduce interobserver and patient-to-patient variability, more objective IGRT processes are desirable. Electromagnetic tracking tools such as Calypso® (Calypso Medical Technologies, Inc., Seattle, WA) and CyberKnife® (Accuray Incorporated, Sunnyvale, CA) represent promising next-generation advances. Each of these systems addresses initial target volume localization efficiently and with precision using electromagnetic and image-guided principles, respectively. They also create the capability to update the prostate location throughout each treatment fraction, thus tracking the intrafraction motion in addition to the interfraction setup adjustment [18–21].

Carrying the IGRT-based targeting logic to the next step, "4D" radiotherapy has ensued, with the "fourth dimension" representing the updating of the target acquisition and beam-aiming data after the initial IGRT step, over the entire life of each individual fraction, to continuously adjust beam-aiming to compensate for the sometimes dynamic processes of continued prostate motion that may occur over the period of a fraction [22–24]. Several methods have been devised to accomplish continuously updated target tracking, including real-time electromagnetic tracking, fluoroscopy-based tracking, and the image-guided fiducial-based robotic CyberKnife platform [19, 20].

The reduced set-up uncertainty provided by electromagnetic tracking allows enough of a CTV-to-PTV margin reduction relative to other set-up methods to facilitate the delivery of dose-escalated IMRT with reduced patient-reported GI toxicity, representing a promising next generation development [25]. Practically applied though, the electromagnetic tracking method still requires a definition of quantitative transponder motion tolerance boundaries, with interruption and repositioning of the patient when these limits are violated, retaining a "manual" correction step in the process that may slightly reduce the speed and accuracy compared with the fully evolved result that would be available with a fully automated detection and correction approach. Furthermore, the electromagnetic tracking method, although theoretically capable of providing sub-millimeter X-Y-Z tracking capability, does not allow for the dynamic correction of beam-aiming due to targeting errors created by rotational prostate motion.

The CyberKnife system represents a fully automated feedback-loop detection and correction system, capable of end-to-end sub-millimeter prostate targeting accuracy, including a capability to fully correct for rotational as well as translational forms of prostate motion, as long as the target is imaged frequently enough (≤40-second imaging frequency for a typical patient) [21]. Thus, at this time, the CyberKnife system appears to represent the most fully evolved, automated, and accurate external-beam radiotherapeutic prostate-targeting system currently available.

7.7 Robotic IMRT Using the CyberKnife System

Although IMRT represents a new dimension of beam manipulation capability, its quality and ability to maximize the reduction of normal tissue dose exposure is even further improved by the optimization of gantry angles ("better gantry angles make better IMRT plans") [26]. The inherent non-coplanar geometry of the CyberKnife platform applies a far larger number of beam-targeting angles than standard coplanar IMRT to a given target volume, theoretically improving dose-molding, thereby reducing the dose to the normal tissues. Further supporting this theory, there is a published comparison of prostate CyberKnife stereotactic body radiotherapy (SBRT) versus standard coplanar gantry-based SBRT treatment plans, indicating a superior normal tissue-sparing outcome with the CyberKnife-delivered technique [20].

In clinical practice, the CyberKnife Robotic Radiosurgery System has been almost exclusively used as a radiosurgical or robotic SBRT device, engineered to deliver conformal, ablative radiation treatments in one to five fractions to a wide variety of malignant lesions in the CNS, head and neck, lung, liver, pancreas, prostate, and other sites [27–35]. Although there is no medical reason, this device has not been used to deliver conventionally fractionated radiotherapy; this function has not previously been described, possibly due to the long treatment times associated with early-generation CyberKnife systems. Nevertheless, the Multiplan® (Accuray) treatment planning system is capable of computing very elegant intensity-modulated radiotherapy (IMRT) dose distributions, and improvements in device efficiency have made the delivery of these IMRT plans feasible in clinical practice, thus leading to new CyberKnife treatment applications that would best be described as "Robotic IMRT."

The new CyberKnife VSI™ platform includes a number of enhancements that improve efficiency, including Sequential Optimization treatment planning, the Iris™ Variable Aperture Collimator (which allows for modulation of the beam during treatment [36]), an increased output rate of a 1,000 MU/min linear accelerator, and a 20% increase in robotic traversal speed. In addition, a treatment time reduction tool accessed during plan optimization allows the user to reduce the total number of treatment beams and nodes while still meeting treatment plan objectives. Collectively these enhancements create a device that can reduce treatment times by over half compared with predecessor CyberKnife systems while maintaining the precision and accuracy of the CyberKnife system [37].

A potential further Robotic IMRT enhancement would be a multileaf collimator (MLC)-based CyberKnife robotic IMRT approach, which has been evaluated as a planning exercise in software form only [38]. That evaluation suggested even greater conformality with MLC-based CyberKnife robotic IMRT, versus either conventional coplanar MLC-based IMRT or CyberKnife Iris–based robotic IMRT, which should be deliverable in a more time-efficient manner than the current CyberKnife technology allows. But at the time of this writing, there is not yet a clinical system in use to fully test this hypothesis.

7.8 CyberKnife Robotic IMRT for Prostate Cancer

One potential application of Robotic IMRT is in the treatment of prostate cancer. Although the use of a four- to five-fraction hypofractionated CyberKnife SBRT regimen has been promising for early-stage, localized prostate cancer [32, 33, 35], there are still many clinicians that believe in treating these patients with a more conventional, extended-fractionation approach, perhaps still preferring the long established safety of a conventionally fractionated approach. CyberKnife robotic *IMRT* (as opposed to CyberKnife robotic *SBRT*) will enable clinicians to deliver a conventional fractionation scheme to these patients, yet still retain the benefits of continual intrafraction tracking and beam-aiming correction that enable a reduction in CTV-to-PTV margins, translating to a more precise and accurate IMRT treatment with the potential for less full-dose exposure of collateral tissues compared to other contemporary IGRT/IMRT delivery systems.

A specific robotic IMRT prostate cancer application of interest could be its use in the treatment of patients that present with more advanced yet still clinically localized lesions (e.g., T3N0M0 disease). In such cases, a larger clinical target volume (CTV) that includes full seminal vesicle coverage may be required to account for the greater probability and magnitude of extraprostatic extension. This means a larger volume of adjacent normal tissue is also invariably irradiated, thus providing a rationale for the use of biologically "gentler" conventional-dose fractionation as opposed to the typical CyberKnife robotic extreme hypofractionation (SBRT) approach.

Traditionally, such external radiotherapeutic treatment has been delivered strictly by conventional gantry-based linear accelerators, most recently using image-guided IMRT techniques. With the improved efficiency of the new CyberKnife System, however, an even more exact and customized form of conventionally fractionated image-guided radiation treatment takes form, applying the inherent CyberKnife attributes to maximum advantage. For starters, the Multiplan treatment planning system may design conformal hot spots within the larger PTV, superimposing them where the dominant intraprostatic lesion (DIL) is identified (Figs. 7.1 and 7.2). This concept is known as simultaneous integrated boosting (SIB) and although other IMRT devices are also capable of SIB dose design, the CyberKnife device most accurately delivers this differential dosing pattern to the target volume, because it continuously updates the targeting location by virtue of its automated fiducial-based image-guided detection and correction loop.

In our own practice, the initial model for the Robotic IMRT application is the "Cleveland Clinic Regimen" described by Kupelian et al., delivering a dose of 70 Gy in 28 fractions to the PTV [39]. We have designed treatment plans that satisfy the normal tissue constraints described in this protocol while simultaneously creating intraprostatic SIB dose escalation zones that deliver a mean dose ≥84 Gy in 28 fractions to the DIL, providing a 2-Gy/fraction radiobiologic dose equivalent ≥100 Gy to this area based on an α/β of 3, representing an even more radiobiologically potent dose if the true prostate cancer α/β ratio is lower (Fig. 7.2). Using this "Modified Cleveland Clinic" SIB regimen, we feel we have constructed a regimen that concentrates a more biologically potent dose distribution internally within the prostate CTV and DIL, while simultaneously addressing potential subclinical disease extension beyond the prostate, in a radiobiologically "conventional" manner, which does not currently appear possible to replicate with other IGRT/IMRT treatment systems.

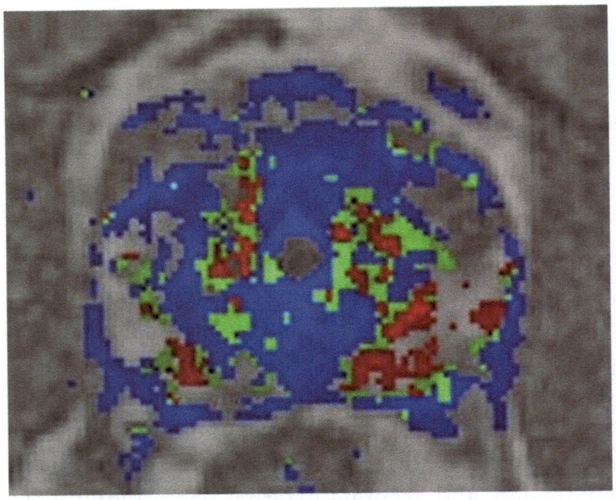

Fig. 7.1 Dynamic perfusion MRI image of prostate. Abnormal gadolinium perfusion, *colorized red*, reveals bilateral dominant intraprostatic lesions (DIL)

Our actual clinical experience with the use of the "Modified Cleveland Clinic" CyberKnife robotic IMRT regimen is currently very preliminary at ten treated patients, with a maximum follow-up of 1 year, limiting possible clinical conclusions, yet some early observations are possible. Thus far in this limited cohort, the acute toxicity appears comparable with other contemporary IMRT methods, with no grade 3 toxicity seen, and a PSA-response that appears favorable, with several of the initial patients reaching PSA nadir levels <0.5 ng/ml in the first 3–6

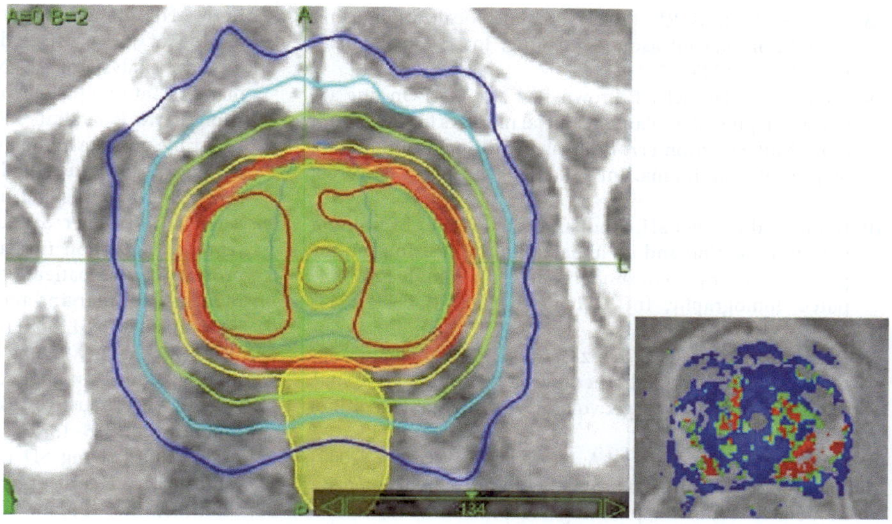

Fig. 7.2 Robotic IMRT prostate isodose plan with simultaneous intraprostatic boosting (Rx = 7,000 cGy/28 fx); DIL regions coincide with intraprostatic dose escalation zones (*red* = 8,400 cGy; *orange* = 7,700 cGy; *yellow* = 7,000 cGy (prescription dose); *green* = 6,000 cGy; *turquoise* = 5,000 cGy; *blue* = 4,000 cGy)

months post-treatment. It is still too soon to assess late toxicity or longer-term effectiveness in this limited patient population, but the preliminary result appears encouraging.

7.9 Conclusion

The next generation of intelligent prostate cancer dose escalation and targeting will be driven by ever accelerating technological progression. The processes of improving image guidance and conformality will allow improvements in the overall concordance of the prescribed dose volume with the planning target volume, not only at the time of set-up (enabled by IGRT), but also throughout the treatment fraction (enabled by tracking). This improved concordance will, in turn, lead to ever increasing differential coverage of the PTV – and even specified segments within the PTV – versus adjacent tissues such as the rectum, further improving the therapeutic ratio.

The final remaining paradox, which may not be so easily solved, is not a physics challenge at all. Rather, it is the fact that we have entered a historical phase in which technology evolves more rapidly than the disease we seek to safely eradicate, which stubbornly sticks to its own plodding yet inexorable timetable to fully play out. To address this final paradox, the medical community will need to come to better agreement as to the appropriate use of carefully considered, more rapidly measurable surrogate endpoints that will serve as the best proxy for the measurement of long-term outcomes.

References

1. Vicini FA, Kestin LL, Martinez AA (1999) The importance of adequate follow-up in defining treatment success after external beam irradiation for prostate cancer. Int J Radiat Oncol Biol Phys 45:553–561
2. Zelefsky MJ, Fuks Z, Hunt M et al (2002) High-dose intensity modulated radiation therapy for prostate cancer: early toxicity and biochemical outcome in 772 patients. Int J Radiat Oncol Biol Phys 53:1111–1116
3. Morgan PB, Hanlon AL, Horwitz EM et al (2007) Radiation dose and late failures in prostate cancer. Int J Radiat Oncol Biol Phys 67:1074–1081
4. Perez CA, Michalski JM, Purdy JA et al (2000) Three-dimensional conformal therapy or standard irradiation in localized carcinoma of prostate: preliminary results of a nonrandomized comparison. Int J Radiat Oncol Biol Phys 47:629–637
5. Kuban DA, Tucker SL, Dong L et al (2008) Long-term results of the M. D. Anderson randomized dose-escalation trial for prostate cancer. Int J Radiat Oncol Biol Phys 70:67–74
6. Cahlon O, Zelefsky MJ, Shippy A et al (2008) Ultra-high dose (86.4 Gy) IMRT for localized prostate cancer: toxicity and biochemical outcomes. Int J Radiat Oncol Biol Phys 71: 330–337
7. Zietman AL, Bae K, Slater JD et al (2010) Randomized trial comparing conventional-dose with high-dose conformal radiation therapy in early-stage adenocarcinoma of the prostate: long-term results from proton radiation oncology group/American college of radiology 95-09. J Clin Oncol 28:1106–1111

8. Trichter F, Ennis RD (2003) Prostate localization using transabdominal ultrasound imaging. Int J Radiat Oncol Biol Phys 56:1225–1233
9. Chung PW, Haycocks T, Brown T et al (2004) On-line aSi portal imaging of implanted fiducial markers for the reduction of interfraction error during conformal radiotherapy of prostate carcinoma. Int J Radiat Oncol Biol Phys 60: 329–334
10. Hammoud R, Patel SH, Pradhan D et al (2008) Examining margin reduction and its impact on dose distribution for prostate cancer patients undergoing daily cone-beam computed tomography. Int J Radiat Oncol Biol Phys 71: 265–273
11. Pilepich MV, Prasad SC, Perez CA (1982) Computed tomography in definitive radiotherapy of prostatic carcinoma, part 2: definition of target volume. Int J Radiat Oncol Biol Phys 8:235–239
12. De Meerleer GO, Vakaet LA, De Gersem WR et al (2000) Radiotherapy of prostate cancer with or without intensity modulated beams: a planning comparison. Int J Radiat Oncol Biol Phys 47:639–648
13. Little DJ, Dong L, Levy LB et al (2003) Use of portal images and BAT ultrasonography to measure setup error and organ motion for prostate IMRT: implications for treatment margins. Int J Radiat Oncol Biol Phys 56:1218–1224
14. Beltran C, Herman MG, Davis BJ (2008) Planning target margin calculations for prostate radiotherapy based on intrafraction and interfraction motion using four localization methods. Int J Radiat Oncol Biol Phys 70:289–295
15. Kuban DA, Levy LB, Cheung MR et al (2011) Long-term failure patterns and survival in a randomized dose-escalation trial for prostate cancer. Who dies of disease? Int J Radiat Oncol Biol Phys 79:1310–1317
16. Nguyen PL, Chen RC, Hoffman KE et al (2010) Rectal dose-volume histogram parameters are associated with long-term patient-reported gastrointestinal quality of life after conventional and high-dose radiation for prostate cancer: a subgroup analysis of a randomized trial. Int J Radiat Oncol Biol Phys 78:1081–1085
17. Enke C, Ayyangar K, Saw CB, Zhen W, Thompson RB, Raman NV (2002) Inter-observer variation in prostate localization utilizing BAT. Int J Radiat Oncol 54:269
18. McNair HA, Mangar SA, Coffey J et al (2006) A comparison of CT- and ultrasound-based imaging to localize the prostate for external beam radiotherapy. Int J Radiat Oncol Biol Phys 65:678–687
19. Langen KM, Willoughby TR, Meeks SL et al (2008) Observations on real-time prostate gland motion using electromagnetic tracking. Int J Radiat Oncol Biol Phys 71:1084–1090
20. King CR, Lehmann J, Adler JR et al (2003) CyberKnife radiotherapy for localized prostate cancer: rationale and technical feasibility. Technol Cancer Res Treat 2:25–30
21. Xie Y, Djajaputra D, King CR et al (2008) Intrafractional motion of the prostate during hypofractionated radiotherapy. Int J Radiat Oncol Biol Phys 72:236–246
22. Ghilezan MJ, Jaffray DA, Siewerdsen JH et al (2005) Prostate gland motion assessed with cine-magnetic resonance imaging (cine-MRI). Int J Radiat Oncol Biol Phys 62:406–417
23. Kotte AN, Hofman P, Lagendijk JJ et al (2007) Intrafraction motion of the prostate during external-beam radiation therapy: analysis of 427 patients with implanted fiducial markers. Int J Radiat Oncol Biol Phys 69:419–425
24. Vapiwala N, Rajendran RR, Plastaras JP, Kassaee A (2008) Real-time prostate motion is highly variable among patients undergoing prostate radiotherapy (RT) with electromagnetic localization and tracking. Int J Radiat Oncol 72:S350–S351
25. Khan DC, Tropper S, Liu P, Mantz CA (2009) Patient-reported reduction in acute GU and GI side effects for prostate cancer patients treated with 81 Gy IMRT using reduced PTV margins and electromagnetic tracking. Int J Radiat Oncol 75:S113–S114
26. Wang X, Zhang X, Dong L et al (2004) Development of methods for beam angle optimization for IMRT using an accelerated exhaustive search strategy. Int J Radiat Oncol Biol Phys 60:1325–1337
27. Adler JR Jr, Chang SD (2009) Cyberknife image-guided radiosurgery. Neurosurgery 64:A1
28. Choi BO, Choi IB, Jang HS et al (2008) Stereotactic body radiation therapy with or without transarterial chemoembolization for patients with primary hepatocellular carcinoma: preliminary analysis. BMC Cancer 8:351
29. Collins BT, Vahdat S, Erickson K et al (2009) Radical cyberknife radiosurgery with tumor tracking: an effective treatment for inoperable small peripheral stage I non-small cell lung cancer. J Hematol Oncol 2:1
30. Gagnon GJ, Nasr NM, Liao JJ et al (2009) Treatment of spinal tumors using cyberknife fractionated stereotactic radiosurgery: pain and quality-of-life assessment after treatment in 200 patients. Neurosurgery 64:297–306; discussion 306–297
31. Hara W, Loo BW Jr, Goffinet DR et al (2008) Excellent local control with stereotactic radiotherapy boost after external beam radiotherapy in patients with nasopharyngeal carcinoma. Int J Radiat Oncol Biol Phys 71:393–400
32. Fuller DB, Naitoh J, Lee C et al (2008) Virtual HDR CyberKnife treatment for localized prostatic carcinoma: dosimetry comparison with HDR brachytherapy and preliminary clinical observations. Int J Radiat Oncol Biol Phys 70:1588–1597
33. King CR, Brooks JD, Gill H et al (2009) Stereotactic body radiotherapy for localized prostate cancer: interim results of a prospective phase II clinical trial. Int J Radiat Oncol Biol Phys 73:1043–1048
34. Koong AC, Le QT, Ho A et al (2004) Phase I study of stereotactic radiosurgery in patients with locally advanced pancreatic cancer. Int J Radiat Oncol Biol Phys 58:1017–1021
35. Katz AJ, Santoro MI (2009) Cyberknife radiosurgery for early carcinoma of the prostate: a three year experience. Int J Radiat Oncol 75:S312–S313
36. Heijmen B, van de Water S, Breedveld S et al (2009) A variable circular collimator: a time-efficient alternative for a multi-leaf collimator in robotic radiosurgery? Int J Radiat Oncol 75(3 Suppl):S674–S675
37. Fuller DB (2009) Comparison of Virtual HDR Prostate Treatment Plans Created with Fixed and Variable Aperture Collimators. Presented to the ASTRO 2009 Annual Meeting, Chicago, IL

38. Fan J, Li J, Price R, Jin L, Wang L, Chen L, Ma C (2010) MLC-based CyberKnife radiotherapy for prostate cancer. American Society of Radiation Oncology, Philadelphia
39. Kupelian PA, Willoughby TR, Reddy CA et al (2007) Hypofractionated intensity-modulated radiotherapy (70 Gy at 2.5 Gy per fraction) for localized prostate cancer: Cleveland Clinic experience. Int J Radiat Oncol Biol Phys 68:1424–1430

Part IV

Hypofractionated Radiation Delivery

Radiobiology of Prostate Cancer

8

Alexandru Daşu

CONTENTS

8.1 Abstract

The 1999 proposal of Brenner and Hall of an α/β value of 1.5 Gy for prostate tumors has rekindled the interest in the traditional radiobiological aspects of time, dose, and fractionation as effective means of modulating the therapeutic window in radiation therapy. It is well established that, depending on the fractionation sensitivity of normal and tumor tissues, one could depart from the usual fractionation pattern and devise schedules that lead to the same tumor results with less complications, or better tumor control with the same level of complications. Nevertheless, radiobiology experience indicates that the success of any fractionation schedule depends on the temporal pattern of dose delivery. From this perspective, the present chapter aims to review the radiobiological aspects that may be relevant for the design of treatment schedules for prostate tumors.

8.2 LQ Modeling in Clinical Radiobiology

The most commonly used model to describe the effects of ionizing radiation on cells and tissues is the linear quadratic (LQ) model. A quadratic relationship between dose and chromosome damage has been recognized as early as 1942 [1]. It was, however, only after the systematic investigation of the fractionation response of irradiated tissues [2, 3] that the LQ model has gained widespread recognition. It is nowadays the most used model to analyze the effect of fractionated schedules and to calculate isoeffect doses for these schemes [4, 5].

According to the LQ model, cell survival (SF) after (n) fractions of dose (d) could be calculated with Eq. 8.1.

$$-\ln(SF) = n(\alpha d + \beta d^2) \tag{8.1}$$

L.E. Ponsky et al. (eds.), *Treating Prostate Cancer and Related Genitourinary Applications*, Robotic Radiosurgery, DOI 10.1007/978-3-642-11495-3_8,

where α and β are parameters of the model. Equation 8.1 could also be used to describe tissue response to radiation as tissue effects are the result of radiation-induced cell killing [6]. To avoid uncertainties in the number of surviving cells in tissues, isoeffect calculations are used in these latter cases that imply the same effect, i.e., the same level of cell survival, for different fractionation regimes employing various numbers and sizes of fractions.

Equation 8.1 could also be adapted to include the effects of proliferation through the addition of a supplementary term as in Eq. 8.2 [5].

$$Effect = n\left(\alpha d + \beta d^2\right) - \frac{T_{elapsed} - T_k}{T_p} \ln 2 \tag{8.2}$$

where T_p is a characteristic proliferation parameter indicating the effective doubling time of the cells, T_{elapsed} is the elapsed time since the beginning of the treatment, and T_k is the time delay for the onset of proliferation [7].

Several theories have been proposed for the mechanistic meaning of the α and β parameters of the LQ model [8–10]. The common interpretation is that the α parameter is related to the unrepairable damage in the cells, while the β parameter is related to the repairable damage in the cells. From this perspective, the ratio of the two parameters gives a measure of the repair potential of the cells for fractionated schedules with long time intervals between fractions. Incomplete repair models like that of Thames [11] have also been proposed to account for the effects of shorter interfraction intervals.

Clinical and experimental observations have yielded an interesting pattern with respect to the repair potential of various normal tissues and tumors quantified as α/β values. Thus, it appears that actively proliferating tissues that express their response to radiation early (the so-called acutely reacting tissues) have generally high α/β values in contrast with tissues with slow proliferation, which express their radiation response rather late (the so-called late-reacting tissues) with low α/β values [3, 12]. Consequently, the generic values $\alpha/\beta=10$ Gy and $\alpha/\beta=3$ Gy are currently used for isoeffect calculations for early- and late-reacting tissues, respectively.

Figure 8.1 shows an illustration of the fractionation effects on various tissues: Early-reacting tissues (left graph) are less sensitive to fractionation than late-reacting tissues (right graph). This observation has provided the basis for the current radiotherapy practice and for the introduction of new fractionation schedules for many tumor sites. As many proliferating

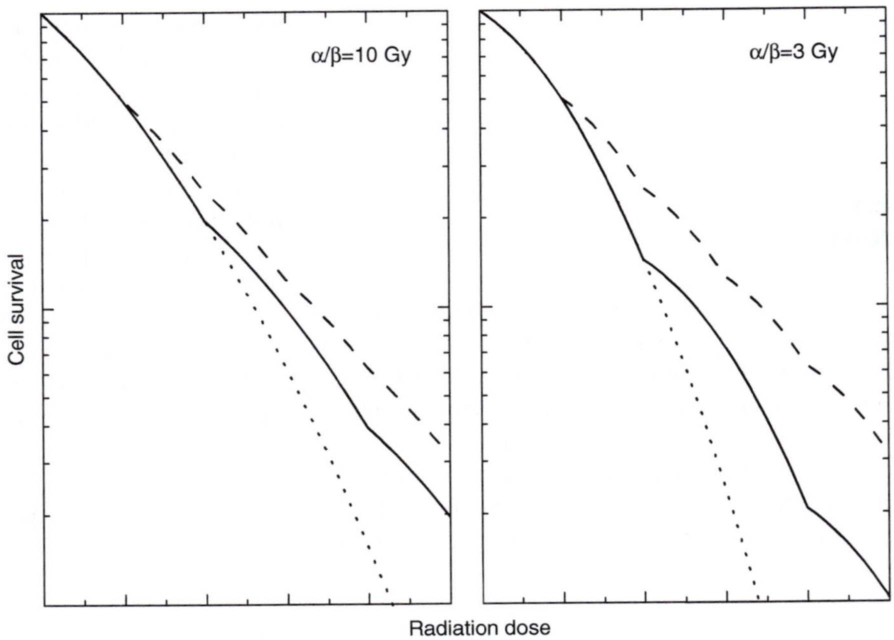

Fig. 8.1 Fractionation effects on early- and late-reacting tissues. Dotted curves, single dose irradiations. Solid curves, fractionated irradiations with dose d per fraction. Dashed curves, fractionated irradiations with dose d/2 per fraction

tumors have high α/β values, similar to early-reacting normal tissues, the conventional practice is to use radiotherapy schedules with many small fractions. As shown by the graphs in Fig. 8.1, such schedules have the potential to reduce significantly the damage to late-reacting normal tissues with low α/β values, while the effects are minimal for tumors with high α/β values. Indeed, hyperfractionation had been successfully used for many sites, such as the highly proliferating head and neck tumors, to increase the cure rate with the same level of complications or to decrease the complication rate with the same level of tumor kill. Consequently, delivering the treatment in many fractions of about 2 Gy has become the clinical norm for the radiation therapy of many tumors with acceptable late effects.

Prostate tumors differ from many other tumors by having a proliferation pattern that resembles that of late-reacting normal tissues [13, 14]. From this perspective, it could be expected that they have a fractionation sensitivity that also resembles that of late-reacting normal tissues. The important question, however, is how low or high their fractionation sensitivity is in comparison to those of the adjacent normal tissues that are usually irradiated during radiation treatment. Thus, if prostate tumors have low α/β values, but still above those of the relevant late-reacting normal tissues, increasing the dose-per-fraction would increase the radiation effect to the prostate, but this would increase the effect to normal tissues even more, leading practically to a narrowing of the existing therapeutic gain by increasing the probability of unacceptably high late complication rates. In contrast, if prostate tumors have α/β values below those of late-reacting normal tissues, the trend would be reversed and hypofractionated regimens could widen the therapeutic window.

8.3 Proliferation of Prostate Tumors

Split-course treatments were common approaches in radiotherapy up to the 1970s and 1980s when the importance of proliferation, and especially that of accelerated repopulation, has been emphasized for rapid-growing tumors like those in the head and neck region or the cervix [7, 15–17]. While clinical studies have shown strong correlations between the duration of the treatment and its outcome for these tumors, similar analyses for prostate tumors did not lead to equally clear conclusions. Analyzing patients treated with split-course treatments, Parsons et al. [18] and Forman et al. [19] did not observe a treatment duration effect for prostate tumors. A later analysis of 780 patients treated with radiotherapy courses extending from less than 7 weeks to more than 9 weeks also failed to show any impact of overall treatment time [20]. In contrast, Amdur et al. [21] have reported a time effect for prostate tumors after reviewing the results from 167 patients. Similarly, Perez et al. [22] have found a correlation between treatment time and the number of pelvic failures in 496 patients with T2 tumors, but not in 587 other patients with T1 or T3 tumors. This data refers to patients treated before the era of prostate-specific antigen (PSA) and they could not easily be extrapolated to patients of the PSA era, as there may be uncertainties in the endpoints used for outcome reporting. Nevertheless, studies also exist about patients treated in the PSA era.

Horwitz et al. [23] have reported no significant effect of treatment time on outcome in 470 patients treated with doses in the range of 58–70.4 Gy. More recent studies, analyzing patients treated with increasingly higher doses suggest that there might be a time factor for prostate tumors. Thus, analyzing 1796 patients treated with doses in the interval of 65–82 Gy, D'Ambrosio et al. [24] found that treatment duration negatively influenced the outcome in low-risk patients, but not in intermediate- or high-risk patients. Similarly, an analysis of biochemical failure in 4,839 patients from nine institutions showed a significant influence of treatment time in low- and intermediate-risk patients treated to doses ≥70 Gy, but not in high-risk patients or in patients treated with doses <70 Gy [25]. This appears to confirm the findings of both Horwitz et al. [23] and D'Ambrosio et al. [24] and suggests that the time delay for the onset of proliferation, T_k, for prostate tumors may be longer than 7 weeks (the time required to deliver 70 Gy with conventional fractionation). Furthermore, Thames et al. [25] have reported a time factor of 0.24 Gy/day representing "one third to one half that estimated for head-and-neck tumors," which supports a pattern of slow proliferation in prostate tumors.

Studies of proliferation kinetics in pretreatment biopsies from prostate tumors have yielded long potential doubling times with a median value of 42 days as the result of low proportions of cycling cells [13, 14]. The potential doubling times determined are in a rather broad interval indicating that some tumors may undergo somewhat more active proliferation than others. An alternative parameter that could quantify the in vivo proliferation potential of clinical prostate tumors is the doubling time of PSA concentration, which correlates with prostate tumor volume. Studies of the temporal kinetics of PSA levels also show long doubling times of the order of 13–16 months, as well as similarly long delays for the rise in PSA levels in patients with biochemical failures, thus confirming the slow proliferation pattern of prostate tumors [26, 27].

The characteristic proliferation time as well as the time to the onset of accelerated repopulation are parameters of interest that could be used to determine an optimal duration for radiotherapy schedules in general, as it has been shown that proliferation may reduce the effectiveness of lengthy schedules [28–30]. While the proliferation of prostate tumors is much slower than that of head and neck tumors, for example, further investigation of its characteristics, and especially variations across different risk groups, is warranted. Indeed, it has been shown that variations in the time to the onset of proliferation could significantly influence the calculation of fractionation sensitivity through comparison of treatment schedules with different durations [31]. In any case, the results available thus far indicate that prostate tumors have a slow proliferation pattern similar to that of late-reacting normal tissues. The important question is whether evidence also exists for a similar sensitivity to fractionation.

8.4 Radiobiologic Derivation of α/β Values for Prostate Cancer

The discussion regarding the clinically relevant α/β value for prostate tumors has been initiated by the publication of Brenner and Hall [32] of a radiobiologic analysis of results from 367 patients from two centers. By comparing results from low dose-rate brachytherapy studies with I-125 seeds to those from external-beam treatments with doses per fraction between 1.8 and 2.0 Gy per fraction, they proposed that the fractionation radiosensitivity of prostate tumors would be described by an α/β value of 1.5 Gy (95% confidence interval 0.8–2.2 Gy). The validity of this proposal was immediately questioned after publication [33, 34] and this marked the beginning of a long debate, where various arguments were brought forth, including patient heterogeneity, relative biological effectiveness of radiation, nonuniform dose distributions, as well as the traditional radiobiological aspects such as proliferation, hypoxia, and repair. An overview of this debate and the variables that could interfere with the derivation of α/β values has been published by Dasu [35] and included a review of clinical data from more than 6,000 patients treated with external-beam radiotherapy, low dose-rate and high dose-rate brachytherapy. The study found a broad range of proposals for the α/β values relevant to prostate tumors, reflecting the generally low number of patients included in the clinical studies and the uncertainties related to radiobiological confounding factors. Nevertheless, the weighted average of the published proposals for α/β values was only 1.85 Gy, suggesting that prostate carcinomas may have a high fractionation sensitivity and could therefore benefit from hypofractionated regimes. The review concluded, however, that the data available then was not robust enough to recommend hypofractionation as the standard treatment for prostate tumors, although the results were promising enough to further investigate in clinical trials the potential of hypofractionation. This chapter aims to provide an update of the clinical radiobiology knowledge on prostate tumors, and the now decade-long debate on their α/β value. It should be stated from the beginning that it will generally be based on published clinical data. As many studies dedicated to hypofractionation of prostate therapy have been initiated only recently and have yet been scarcely presented in the literature or at conferences, this review may not be able to represent all current activity in the field, although further results are eagerly awaited.

The majority of the early radiobiological analyses of the fractionation sensitivity of prostate tumors (Table 8.1) are based on historical clinical datasets [32–46]. As such, there are some limitations as to the number of patients or the fractionation patterns available from some of these datasets, which are reflected in the rather wide confidence intervals of the derived values. Nevertheless, these analyses

Table 8.1 Radiobiological analyses of clinical data

Reference	α/β proposal (Gy)	Confidence interval (Gy)	Number of patients	Treatment	Observations
Brenner and Hall [32]	1.5	0.8–2.2	367	EBRT, LDRBR	
King and Mayo [34]	4.96	4.1–5.6	367	EBRT, LDRBR	Reanalysis of the dataset used by Brenner and Hall [32]
Brenner and Hall [33]	2.1		367	EBRT, LDRBR	Reanalysis of the dataset used by Brenner and Hall [32]
Fowler et al. [39]	1.49	1.25–1.76	1,471	EBRT, LDRBR	
Wang et al. [44]	3.1	1.7–4.5	1,471	EBRT, LDRBR	Analysis of the dataset used by Fowler et al. [39]
Brenner et al. [37]	1.2	0.03–4.1	192	EBRT, HDRBR	
Livsey et al. [41]	(1.5)		705	EBRT	Data compatible with $\alpha/\beta = 1.5$ Gy
Dasu [35]	1.3		705	EBRT	Point estimate from the Livsey et al. [41] dataset
Chappell et al. [38]	1.44	1.22–1.76	2,400	EBRT	Analysis of the Fowler et al. [39] and Lukka et al. [42] datasets
Bentzen and Ritter [36]	1.12	−3.3–5.6	936	EBRT	Analysis of the Lukka et al. [42] dataset
Dasu [35]	2.4		410	EBRT	Point estimate from the Kupelian et al. [40] dataset.
Bentzen and Ritter [36]	8.3	0.7–16	330	EBRT	Analysis of the Valdagni et al. [43] dataset
Yeoh et al. [46]	2.2	−6–10.6	217	EBRT	
Dasu [35]	1.85		4,628	EBRT, HDRBR, LDRBR	Weighted average from the datasets above
Williams et al. [45]	2.6–3.7	0.9–4.8 and 1.1–∞	3,756	EBRT, HDRBR	
Arcangeli et al. [47]	1.4		168	EBRT	
Proust-Lima et al. [48]	1.55	0.46–4.52	5,093	EBRT	
Miralbell et al. [49], (Fowler, personal communication)	1.4	0.9–2.2	5,969	EBRT	
Leborgne et al. [50], Fowler, personal communication)	1.86	0.7–5.1	274	EBRT	
Dasu [51]	1.5–2		4,479	EBRT	Present study

EBRT external beam radiation therapy, *LDRBR* low dose rate brachytherapy, *HDRBR* high dose rate brachytherapy indicate almost unanimously that, in contrast with other tumors, prostate tumors have a high sensitivity to fractionation. The results, however, could not provide a clear answer to the question whether the α/β value for prostate tumors is equal to or lower than the corresponding values of the late-responding normal tissues nearby that are irradiated during treatment. More recent analyses, as for example that of Arcangeli et al. [47] or Proust-Lima et al. [48], appear to support the initial proposal of $\alpha/\beta = 1.5$ Gy for prostate tumors. The analysis by Proust-Lima et al. [48] deserves particular attention as it uses data from a large patient population treated only with external-beam radiotherapy and thus is free of some of the uncertainties that affect intercomparisons of results from different treatment modalities. Still though, the limited range of doses-per-fraction available for analysis (1.7–2.77 Gy) led the authors of the study to conclude that the "data support the use of hypofractionation at fractional doses up to 2.8 Gy, but cannot presently be assumed to accurately represent higher doses per fraction." From this point of view, prospective studies with higher doses per fraction and especially randomized studies designed to compare conventionally fractionated and hypofractionated treatments of the prostate are still of high interest. Two other analyses have just been submitted for publication, one by Miralbell et al. and the other by Leborgne and coworkers (personal correspondence with Prof Jack Fowler). The former of these studies is the largest analysis thus far of a patient population treated with external-beam radiotherapy. It is interesting to note that the α/β value these studies propose and the corresponding confidence interval are strikingly close to the original proposals of Brenner and Hall [32].

8.5 Clinical Trials of Hypofractionation

Hypofractionation has seldom been used for the treatment of malignant tumors in comparison to conventional fractionation schemes due to the high risk of complications in late reacting tissues. This explains, to a certain extent, the scarcity of available historical data for radiobiological analyses of the sensitivity to fractionation of prostate tumors. Nevertheless, as radiobiological evidence in support of a low α/β value for prostate tumors accumulates, the number of studies employing hypofractionated schemes is on the rise. This is illustrated in Fig. 8.2, showing that, not only the number of hypofractionation studies has increased, but so has the size of the doses-per-fraction used in clinical studies of hypofractionation, as summarized in Tables 8.2 and 8.3. Increasing doses-per-fraction and accumulating patient numbers will increase the statistical power of future analyses and will ultimately contribute to better determinations of the relevant α/β value or range of values for prostate tumors.

Figure 8.2 refers to the clinical studies of the PSA era. It should be mentioned, however, that quite high hypofractionation regimens, such as six fractions of

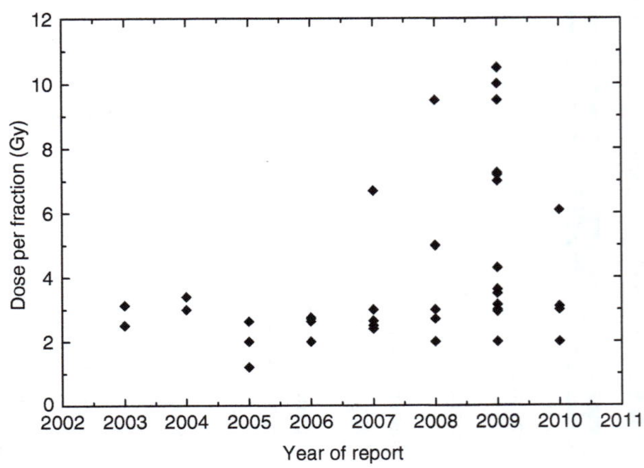

Fig. 8.2 Timeline of the doses per fraction used in clinical fractionation studies for prostate tumors

6 Gy each, have been used for many years in London for the treatment of prostate tumor patients [52, 53]. As a note, the most famous patient receiving this treatment was probably Sir Lawrence Olivier, who was cured of the disease, experiencing no major sequelae and living a further 22 years [54].

When comparing results from clinical studies, one has to take into account the effect of possible confounding factors, some of which will be reviewed later in this study. From this point of view, randomized studies have the advantage of minimizing variations due to these confounding factors between the arms of the study and thus presumably minimizing their impact on the results. Results from only four randomized studies of hypofractionation for prostate treatment are available, totaling 1,421 patients.

Lukka et al. [42] have reported the largest randomized study thus far, although employing rather low total doses by today's standards. In their study, 470 patients were treated with 66 Gy in 33 fractions of 2 Gy each, while 466 patients received 52.5 Gy in 20 fractions of 2.63 Gy each. With a median follow-up of 68.4 months, the 5-year biochemical control defined according to the ASTRO definition was 62.3% in the conventionally fractionated arm and 57.7% in the hypofractionated one. The results from the hypofractionated arm may seem disappointing at first, but a subsequent analysis by Bentzen and Ritter [36] concluded that they were the result of too low a total dose in the hypofractionated arm, and that, in fact, the results supported an α/β value as low as 1.12 Gy (although with confidence intervals extending from −3.3 Gy to 5.6 Gy).

A year later, Yeoh and colleagues presented the results from 217 patients included into two arms with similar fractionation [46]: The 109 patients in the conventionally fractionated arm received 64 Gy in 32 fractions of 2 Gy each, while the 108 patients in the hypofractionated arm received 55 Gy in 20 fractions of 2.75 Gy each. Also using the ASTRO definition of biochemical failure, their 5-year results were similar to those of the Canadian study mentioned above. Thus, 64.2% of the patients in the conventionally fractionated arm and 65.7% in the hypofractionated arm were free from biochemical failures after a median follow-up of 48 months. The equivalence of the results in the two arms led the authors of the study to suggest an α/β value of 2.2 Gy. A subsequent analysis at 7.5 years showed considerably better results in the hypofractionated arm compared to the arm with standard fractionation, suggesting that the α/β value might be as low as 0.7 Gy (Fowler, personal communication).

More recently, Arcangeli and co-workers have reported the results from a randomized study with higher total doses. In their study, they compared the results from 85 patients treated to 80 Gy in 40 fractions of 2 Gy each with those from 83 patients treated with 62 Gy in 20 fractions of 3.1 Gy each [47]. Using the newer Phoenix definition of biochemical failure of nadir + 2 ng/ml, after a median follow-up of 35 months, they reported better control in the hypofractionated arm, 87%, than in the conventionally fractionated arm, 79%. These results led them to conclude that sensitivity to fractionation could be described by an α/β value around 1.4 Gy.

Similar results were also observed by Pollack and colleagues, as reported by Buyyounouski et al. [55], who compared the outcome from 50 patients treated with 76 Gy in 38 fractions of 2 Gy each with 50 patients treated with 70.2 Gy in 26 fractions of 2.7 Gy each. With the same Phoenix definition of biochemical failure and a comparable median follow-up, 39 months, they have seen 79% of patients in the conventionally fractionated arm free from biochemical failure and 83% in the hypofractionated arm. As with the results of the Italian group above, these results are also compatible with a low α/β value.

It has to be mentioned that the randomized studies reported so far have employed moderate hypofractionation, thus contributing to a general uncertainty in deriving a reliable α/β value for prostate tumors. As the total number of patients included in randomized studies increases, the statistical significance of the analyses is expected to increase, especially when results from studies with highly hypofractionated schedules will be included in the analysis.

Despite not having the advantages in design of randomized studies, valuable information can also be obtained from the more numerous non-randomized studies employing hypofractionated schedules.

Livsey et al. [41] reported the results from 705 patients employing one of the highest early hypofractionations, 50 Gy in 16 fractions of 3.13 Gy each ($BED_3 = 102.2\ Gy_3$). With a median follow-up of 48 months, they observed 56% of the patients biochemically free of disease (defined according to the

Table 8.2 Clinical studies reporting tumor response from hypofractionated schedules

Reference	Number of patients	Risk groups	Fractionation pattern (dose/no of fractions)	Dose per fraction (Gy)	Treatment duration (weeks)	Median follow-up (months)	Failure definition	Biochemical control (%)	at years	Hormone therapy
Randomized										
Lukka et al. [42]	470	M	66 Gy/33 fx	2	6.5	68.4	ASTRO	62.3	5	No
	466	M	52.5 Gy/20 fx	2.63	4	68.4	ASTRO	57.7	5	No
Yeoh et al. [46]	109	n/a	64 Gy/32 fx	2	6.5	48	ASTRO	64.2	5	No
	108	n/a	55 Gy/20 fx	2.75	4	48	ASTRO	65.7	5	No
Pollack et al. [99],	50	I+H	76 Gy/38 fx	2	n/a	39	Phoenix	79	5	Yes
Buyyounouski et al. [55]	50	I+H	70.2 Gy/26 fx	2.7	n/a	39	Phoenix	83	5	Yes
Arcangeli et al. [47]	85	H	80 Gy/40 fx	2	8	35	Phoenix	79	3	Yes
	83	H	62 Gy/20 fx	3.1	5	32	Phoenix	87	3	Yes
Non-randomized										
Livsey et al. [41]	705	M	50 Gy/16 fx	3.13	3.1	48	ASTRO	56	5	No
	181	L	50 Gy/16 fx	3.13	3.1	48	ASTRO	82	5	No
	247	I	50 Gy/16 fx	3.13	3.1	48	ASTRO	56	5	No
	277	H	50 Gy/16 fx	3.13	3.1	48	ASTRO	39	5	No
Kitamura et al. [56]	12	M	65 Gy/26 fx	2.5	n/a	37	ASTRO	92	3	No
	19	M	70 Gy/28 fx	2.5	n/a	19	ASTRO	89	1.5	Yes
Akimoto et al. [57]	53	I+H	69 Gy/23 fx	3	7.5	35	ASTRO	78	3	Yes
	53	I+H	69 Gy/23 fx	3	7.5	35	ASTRO	56	5	Yes
Valdagni et al. [43]	179	M	74 Gy/37 fx	2	7.5	25.2	ASTRO	70	5	Yes
	75	L	74 Gy/37 fx	2	7.5	25.2	ASTRO	84.5	5	Yes
	58	I	74 Gy/37 fx	2	7.5	25.2	ASTRO	61.3	5	Yes
	28	H	74 Gy/37 fx	2	7.5	25.2	ASTRO	65.3	5	Yes
	151	M	79.2 Gy/66 fx	1.2	6.5	37.7	ASTRO	82.6	5	Yes
	61	L	79.2 Gy/66 fx	1.2	6.5	37.7	ASTRO	88.3	5	Yes
	62	I	79.2 Gy/66 fx	1.2	6.5	37.7	ASTRO	81.0	5	Yes
	21	H	79.2 Gy/66 fx	1.2	6.5	37.7	ASTRO	67.4	5	Yes
Kupelian et al. [40]	310	M	78 Gy/39 fx	2	7.6	71	ASTRO	78	5	Yes
	68	L	78 Gy/39 fx	2	7.6	71	ASTRO	93	5	Yes
	84	I	78 Gy/39 fx	2	7.6	71	ASTRO	79	5	Yes
	158	H	78 Gy/39 fx	2	7.6	71	ASTRO	72	5	Yes

Kupelian et al. [60]	770	M	70 Gy/28 fx	2.5	5.5	45	ASTRO	82	5	Yes
	262	L	70 Gy/28 fx	2.5	5.5	45	ASTRO	95	5	Yes
	216	I	70 Gy/28 fx	2.5	5.5	45	ASTRO	85	5	Yes
	292	H	70 Gy/28 fx	2.5	5.5	45	ASTRO	68	5	Yes
	770	M	70 Gy/28 fx	2.5	5.5	45	Phoenix	83	5	Yes
	262	L	70 Gy/28 fx	2.5	5.5	45	Phoenix	94	5	Yes
	216	I	70 Gy/28 fx	2.5	5.5	45	Phoenix	83	5	Yes
	292	H	70 Gy/28 fx	2.5	5.5	45	Phoenix	72	5	Yes
Martin et al. [61]	92	M	60 Gy/20 fx	3	4	38	ASTRO	76	3	Yes
	29	L	60 Gy/20 fx	3	4	38	ASTRO	84	3	Yes
	56	I	60 Gy/20 fx	3	4	38	ASTRO	72	3	Yes
	7	H	60 Gy/20 fx	3	4	38	ASTRO	71	3	Yes
	92	M	60 Gy/20 fx	3	4	38	Phoenix	97	1.2	Yes
	29	L	60 Gy/20 fx	3	4	38	Phoenix	100	3	Yes
	56	I	60 Gy/20 fx	3	4	38	Phoenix	85	3	Yes
	7	H	60 Gy/20 fx	3	4	38	Phoenix	71	3	Yes
Madsen et al. [64]	40	n/a	33.5 Gy/5 fx	6.7	1	41	ASTRO	70	4	n/a
	40	n/a	33.5 Gy/5 fx	6.7	1	41	Phoenix	90	4	n/a
Junius et al. [62]	38	M	66 Gy/25 fx	2.64	5	20	ASTRO	92		Yes
	38	M	66 Gy/25 fx	2.64	5	20	Phoenix	100		Yes
Leborgne and Fowler [65]	89	M	60–63 Gy/20 fx	3–3.15	4.7	49	Phoenix	88	5	Yes
	29	L	60–63 Gy/20 fx	3–3.15	4.7	49	Phoenix	96	5	Yes
	45	I	60–63 Gy/20 fx	3–3.15	4.7	49	Phoenix	84	5	Yes
	15	H	60–63 Gy/20 fx	3–3.15	4.7	49	Phoenix	85	5	Yes
	130	M	78 Gy/39 fx	2	7.8	49	Phoenix	90	5	Yes
	56	L	78 Gy/39 fx	2	7.8	49	Phoenix	98	5	Yes
	66	I	78 Gy/39 fx	2	7.8	49	Phoenix	84	5	Yes
	8	H	78 Gy/39 fx	2	7.8	49	Phoenix	87	5	Yes
Higgins et al. [59]	300	M	52.5 Gy/20 fx	2.63	4	58	Phoenix	42.7	5	Yes
	37	L	52.5 Gy/20 fx	2.63	4	58	Phoenix	73.8	5	Yes
	103	I	52.5 Gy/20 fx	2.63	4	58	Phoenix	55.7	5	Yes
	160	H	52.5 Gy/20 fx	2.63	4	58	Phoenix	31.4	5	Yes
King et al. [64]	41	L	36.25 Gy/5 fx	7.25	1/2[a]	33	ASTRO	100	3	No
	41	L	36.25 Gy/5 fx	7.25	1/2[a]	33	Phoenix	100	3	No
Rene et al. [66]	129	L+I	66 Gy/22 fx	3	4.5	51	Phoenix	98	5	No

ASTRO American Society for Therapeutic Radiation Oncology, *L* low risk group, *I* intermediate risk group, *H* high risk group, *M* all three risk groups mixed
[a]The treatment was given either in 1 or in 2 weeks

Table 8.3 Undergoing clinical studies with hypofractionated schedules

Reference	Number of patients	Risk groups	Fractionation pattern (dose/no of fractions)	Dose per fraction (Gy)	Treatment duration (weeks)	Acute toxicity data	Hormone therapy
Non-randomized							
Koukourakis et al. [72]	7	H	51 Gy/15 fx	3.4	3	Yes	Yes
Jereczek-Fossa et al. [70]	10	L+I	72 Gy/30 fx	2.4	6	No	Yes
Lim et al. [73]	66	H	67.5 Gy/25 fx	2.7	5	Yes	Yes
Tang et al. [76]	30	L	35 Gy/7 fx	5	6	Yes	Yes
Fuller et al. [69]	10	L+I	38 Gy/4 fx	9.5	1	Yes	n/a
Arcangeli et al. [67]	102	M	56 Gy/16 fx	3.5	4	Yes	Yes
Friedland et al. [68]	112	L+I	35–36 Gy/5 fx	7–7.2	1	Yes	Yes
Ritter et al. [75]	100	n/a	64.7 Gy/22 fx	2.94	n/a	Yes	n/a
	100	n/a	58.1 Gy/16 fx	3.63	n/a	Yes	n/a
	80	n/a	51.6 Gy/12 fx	4.3	n/a	Yes	n/a
Timmerman et al. (quoted in Ritter et al. [75])	15	n/a	47.5 Gy/5 fx	9.5	n/a	n/a	n/a
	10	n/a	50 Gy/5 fx	10	n/a	n/a	n/a
	–	n/a	52.5 Gy/5 fx	10.5	n/a	n/a	n/a
Randomized							
Khoo and Dearnaley [71]	450[a]	n/a	74 Gy/37 fx	2	7.5	No	n/a
		n/a	57 Gy/19 fx	3	4	No	n/a
		n/a	60 Gy/20 fx	3	4	No	n/a
Norkus et al. [74]	44	L+I	74 Gy/37 fx	2	7.5	Yes	n/a
	47	L+I	57 Gy/17 fx	3–4.5	3.5	Yes	n/a
Per Nilsson, personal communication	296[b]	n/a	78 Gy/39 fx	2	8	n/a	n/a
		n/a	42.7 Gy/7 fx	6.1	2	n/a	n/a

L low risk group, *I* intermediate risk group, *H* high risk group, *M* all three risk groups mixed
[a]This is the total number of patients reported for the three arms of the CHHiP trial
[b]Target number of patients for the ongoing Scandinavian trial

ASTRO criteria), or 82%, 56% and 39% for the low-, intermediate-, and high-risk groups of patients defined according to stage, PSA level, and Gleason score.

With a different fractionation scheme, 65–70 Gy in 26–28 fractions of 2.5 Gy each (BED_3 = 119.2–128.3 Gy_3), Kitamura and colleagues [56] reported 92% biochemical control at 3 years in the 12 patients receiving 65 Gy, and 89% at 1.5 years in the 19 patients receiving 70 Gy (according to the ASTRO criteria). While the reported results are rather preliminary, they also indicate quite a high effectiveness of the fractionation regime used.

A year later, Akimoto et al. [57] reported the results of 53 patients treated with 23 fractions of 3 Gy each to a total of 69 Gy (BED_3 = 138 Gy_3), finding 56% biochemically free patients at 5 years according to the ASTRO definition of biochemical failure.

Another study employing a significant number of patients has been reported by Valdagni et al. [43]. Treating 151 patients with a hyperfractionated scheme of 66 fractions of 1.2 Gy each (110.9 Gy_3) with two fractions per day and comparing them in a non-randomized study with 179 patients treated with 37 fractions of 2 Gy each (123.3 Gy_3), they have found better results in the hyperfractionated arm than the one with conventional fractionation. These results appear to contradict all the other findings regarding the fractionation sensitivity, a statistical analysis indicating an α/β value as high as 8.3 Gy, although with quite large confidence limits, 0.7–16 Gy [36]. It should be mentioned that the authors of the analysis argued that the value they derived could be an overestimate due to incomplete repair in the arm with two daily fractions separated by 6 h or less, and in that case the "observations are just what you would expect if α/β is in the range of 1–2 Gy." The magnitude of the hypothesized effect, however, is difficult to estimate due to uncertainties with respect to the repair time of prostate cells. Fowler et al. [39] proposed a repair half-time of 1.9 h based on clinical data, which would indicate that at 6 h from the morning fraction, 11% of the sublethal damage will still be present (or 16% at 5 h). Failing to account for the remaining damage in this case would significantly influence the derivation of the equivalent normalized total dose for the hyperfractionated schedule and ultimately the fractionation sensitivity of prostate tumors. In contrast to Fowler et al. [39], Wang et al. [44] advanced the hypothesis of a repair half-time of only 16 min, which implies that almost all sublethal damage would be very quickly removed and, therefore, the effect of incomplete repair would be negligible. Studies of prostate cell lines in vitro further complicated the picture, as they yielded significantly slower repair rates with characteristic half-times of 5–6 h [58], which imply that more than 40% of the sublethal damage of the morning fraction may be present when the afternoon fraction is delivered. Even if this would be characteristic to the slow component in a multi-component repair process, the impact on the equivalent normalized total dose and the fractionation sensitivity would still be significant.

Another clinical study with a rather large patient population was reviewed by Higgins et al. [59]. It analyzed 300 patients treated with 52.5 Gy delivered in 20 fractions (98.5 Gy_3). According to the newer Phoenix definition of biochemical failure, the 5-year results reflected the somewhat low total dose. Thus, 42.7% of the patients in the whole population were free of biochemical failures after 5 years, and 73.8%, 55.7%, and 31.4% in the low-, intermediate-, and high-risk groups, respectively.

More recent studies appear to support a high sensitivity to fractionation for prostate tumors. Kupelian et al. [60] found that according to the ASTRO criteria, out of 770 patients treated with 28 fractions of 2.5 Gy each to a total dose of 70 Gy (128.3 Gy_3), 82% were biochemically free of disease at 5 years. When broken down into three risk groups of patients, the hypofractionated schedule led to 95%, 85%, and 68% local control for the low-, intermediate-, and high-risk groups, respectively. These results are quite similar to those reported earlier for 310 patients treated with 39 fractions of 2 Gy each (130 Gy_3) [40]. This study also reported results according to the newer Phoenix definition of biochemical failure, but they were quite similar to those obtained with the ASTRO definition.

Using a somewhat higher dose per fraction, but a lower total dose, 60 Gy in 20 fractions of 3 Gy each (120 Gy_3), Martin et al. [61] reported 76% biochemical control with the ASTRO criteria in 92 patients analyzed at 3 years after treatment. The Phoenix definition of biochemical failure led to better results for the whole population (97%) and for low- and intermediate-risk patients (100% and 85%, respectively).

Somewhat better results with the ASTRO criteria were reported by Junius and colleagues [62] who studied 38 patients treated with 66 Gy in 25 fractions (124.1 Gy_3). After a median follow-up of 20 months, they found 92% of the patients disease-free. According to the Phoenix definition, all patients were free of biochemical failure.

The same year, results of a clinical study with one of the highest fractionation schemes yet were reported. Out of 40 patients treated with 33.5 Gy delivered in five fractions of 6.7 Gy each (108.3 Gy_3), Madsen et al. [63] reported 70% success according to the ASTRO definition and 90% success according to the Phoenix definition.

A similarly short hypofractionation scheme was employed by King and colleagues [64] who treated 41 low-risk patients with five fractions of 7.25 Gy each (123.9 Gy_3) and found all the patients disease-free, using either the ASTRO or the Phoenix definition of biochemical failure.

Leborgne and Fowler [65] recently reported a non-randomized comparison between hypo- and conventional fractionation. They have found similar results with the Phoenix definition in 89 patients treated with 20 fractions of either 3 or 3.15 Gy (average $BED_3 = 123.8\ Gy_3$) and 130 patients treated with 39 fractions of 2 Gy each (130 Gy_3), in both the overall cohort and in the low-, intermediate-, and high-risk subgroups.

The most recent results from a hypofractionation study have been reported by Rene et al. [66]. Using the Phoenix definition of biochemical failure, they found 98% of 129 low- and intermediate-risk patients were disease-free at 5 years after 22 fractions of 3 Gy each ($BED_3 = 132\ Gy_3$).

Several other studies of hypofractionation are ongoing [67–76] as illustrated in Table 8.3. Some of these studies have reported acute toxicity results, while others are still accruing patients. It is important to note that several of these studies employ rather high doses per fraction and thus it is hoped that their results will contribute to a reduction of the confidence intervals of the derived α/β values that are currently rather high.

8.6 Radiobiologic Analysis of the Reported Clinical Results

The results from the 4,479 patients included in the hypofractionation studies summarized in Table 8.2 can be compared with dose–response relationships from conventionally fractionated treatments for prostate tumors to obtain an estimation of the overall fractionation sensitivity of prostate tumors.

Table 8.4 presents a summary of recent biochemical responses reported by prostate treatments with conventional fractionation [40, 42, 43, 46, 47, 65, 77–81]. These could be used to determine interpolated dose–response curves as in Fig. 8.3. The parameters for the interpolated dose–response curves are presented in Table 8.5. It can be seen that the parameters thus derived generally agree with previous determinations of dose response-curves reported by Pollack et al. [79] or Cheung et al. [82].

It should be noted that the dose–response relationships obtained appear to depend on the definition of biochemical failure used, thus stressing the importance of using reliable and consistent criteria for reporting clinical results.

Figures 8.4–8.7 and 8.8–8.11 show the superposition of the derived dose–response curves in Fig. 8.3 and the normalized total doses to 2 Gy per fraction (NTD_2) for the fractionated schedules in Table 8.2 for various assumptions of the fractionation sensitivity of the prostate tumors quantified by the α/β value.

It can be seen that the agreement between dose–response curves for conventional fractionation and individual points corresponding to various fractionation regimens in Table 8.2 deteriorates progressively as the α/β value assumed for calculations increases. This indicates that clinical data supports the hypothesis of a high fractionation sensitivity for prostate tumors and, hence, a correspondingly low α/β value, irrespective of the definition used for biochemical failure. For high-risk patients analyzed according to the ASTRO definition of biochemical failure as well as for low-risk patients analyzed according to the Phoenix definition, the scarcity of data leads to a rather high uncertainty of the derived dose–response relationships. Nevertheless, clinical data from the 4,479 patients reported in Table 8.2 appears to support an α/β value as low as 1.5–2 Gy for prostate tumors, regardless of the risk group to which the patients belong. This is in agreement with the recent findings of Proust-Lima and colleagues [48] and Miralbell and colleagues (Fowler, personal communication) who have also found that the fractionation sensitivity of prostate tumors does not appear to depend on the risk group. A narrower bracketing of the relevant value is not possible with the data available as the points are considerably scattered. Even when future data becomes available, it will most likely indicate levels of success above the linear part of the dose–response curve and, hence, other assumptions would have to be made with respect to the shape of the dose–response curve.

It is interesting to note that clinical results from patients treated with very high doses per fraction, for example the dataset reported by Madsen et al. [63] for mixed risk groups, appear to reveal a clear indication of the fractionation sensitivity of prostate tumors, as their corresponding NTD_2 vary significantly with the α/β value assumed for calculations. This supports an expected improvement in the width of the confidence interval with inclusion in the analysis of the results from highly hypofractionated trials.

8.7 Discussion

As results from clinical studies accumulate, they appear to strengthen the original proposal of Brenner and Hall [32] of a very high fractionation sensitivity of prostate carcinomas. The confidence intervals of the derived values, however, are still rather large and, therefore, one would have to carefully weigh the effects of the possible confounding factors, especially when estimating the expected therapeutic gain from hypofractionation.

One of the most important factors that influence the results from clinical studies appears to be the risk groups of patients analyzed, and especially the pooling of the patients belonging to different risk groups. As illustrated by the results in Table 8.5, different risk groups appear to have different dose–response relationships, and this could hamper comparisons of results from patient populations with different risk compositions. Also related to the influence of the patient subgroups is the administration of hormone therapy to prostate patients undergoing radiotherapy. For example, Valdagni et al. [43] showed different results for the subgroup that did not receive hormone therapy from all patients pooled together. The potential interaction between androgen deprivation and fractionation pattern is therefore an aspect that deserves closer investigation in the future.

Besides patient heterogeneity, dose heterogeneity has also been discussed as a factor with potential implications on the outcome of therapy [83, 84]. This is especially important for modern treatment approaches that could result in increasingly sophisticated and quite often heterogeneous dose distributions. An important question is whether the results of earlier clinical studies obtained from therapy approaches employing almost uniform doses in the target volume are still relevant for the newer treatment approaches. Indeed, it is quite possible that the same prescribed dose would be delivered with dose distributions with different heterogeneities. A most extreme example of dose heterogeneity is for the dose distributions achievable with brachytherapy. While the issue was initially brought under discussion for permanent seed implants [83], high-dose-rate brachytherapy is increasingly used in combination with external-beam radiotherapy and even as monotherapy for the treatment of prostate carcinomas [85–93]. These latter treatment approaches have lately led to very good results due to a combination of favorable dose distribution, increased dose to the target, and, possibly, increased hypofractionation to the target. However, direct comparisons with results from external-beam radiation therapy should be carefully interpreted.

The method for dose prescription is another factor that could lead to target dose heterogeneity. While most studies report the dose to the ICRU reference point, there are also studies that report doses to an isodose surface that envelops the target volume (for example [64]). The potential differences in dose homogeneity between different methods might also influence the analysis of the reported results and the derivation of dose–response relationships.

Many of the problems mentioned above could be avoided with randomized clinical studies, as these minimize the effects of patient heterogeneity and have the potential to reduce the uncertainty of the derived results. However, they are quite difficult to set up as they usually require a lengthy patient accrual time that could delay the analysis of the results. Nevertheless, analyses of non-randomized studies could also be useful if the possible sources of uncertainty are taken into account.

In spite of the mentioned confounding factors, the results of an increasing number of clinical studies appear to support a high fractionation sensitivity of

Table 8.4 Biochemical responses reported from prostate treatments with conventional fractionation

Reference	Number of patients	Risk groups	Total dose (Gy)	Dose per fraction (Gy)	Failure definition	Biochemical control (%)
Pollack et al. [79]	500	M	66	2	ASTRO	54
	495	M	70	2	ASTRO	71
	132	M	78	2	ASTRO	77
Pollack et al. [80]	150	M	70	2	ASTRO	64
	151	M	78	2	ASTRO	70
Lukka et al. [42]	470	M	66	2	ASTRO	62.3
Kupelian et al. [40]	310	M	78	2	ASTRO	78
Valdagni et al. [43]	179	M	74	2	ASTRO	70
Dearnaley et al. [77]	64	M	64	2	ASTRO	59
	62	M	74	2	ASTRO	71
Yeoh et al. [46]	109	M	64	2	ASTRO	64.2
Eade et al. [78]	43	M	69	2	ASTRO	60
	552	M	72.5	2	ASTRO	68
	568	M	77.5	2	ASTRO	76
	367	M	81	2	ASTRO	84
	43	M	69	2	Phoenix	70
	552	M	72.5	2	Phoenix	81
	568	M	77.5	2	Phoenix	83
	367	M	81	2	Phoenix	89
Zelefsky et al. [81]	358	M	70.2	1.8	Phoenix	61
	471	M	75.6	1.8	Phoenix	74
	741	M	81	1.8	Phoenix	85
	477	M	86.4	1.8	Phoenix	82
Leborgne and Fowler [65]	130	M	78	2	Phoenix	90
Kupelian et al. [40]	68	L	78	2	ASTRO	93
Valdagni et al. [43]	75	L	74	2	ASTRO	84.5
Leborgne and Fowler [65]	56	L	78	2	Phoenix	98
Pollack et al. [79]	286	I	64	2	ASTRO	30
		I	66	2	ASTRO	42
		I	68	2	ASTRO	56
		I	70	2	ASTRO	63
		I	78	2	ASTRO	93
Kupelian et al. [40]	84	I	78	2	ASTRO	79

Valdagni et al. [43]	58	I	74	2	ASTRO	61.3
Zelefsky et al. [81]	155	I	70.2	1.8	Phoenix	67
	171	I	75.6	1.8	Phoenix	81
	332	I	81	1.8	Phoenix	88
	191	I	86.4	1.8	Phoenix	85
Leborgne and Fowler [65]	66	I	78	2	Phoenix	84
Kupelian et al. [40]	158	H	78	2	ASTRO	72
Valdagni et al. [43]	28	H	74	2	ASTRO	65.3
Zelefsky et al. [81]	156	H	70.2	1.8	Phoenix	40
	234	H	75.6	1.8	Phoenix	61
	176	H	81	1.8	Phoenix	66
	186	H	86.4	1.8	Phoenix	71
Leborgne and Fowler [65]	28	H	78	2	Phoenix	87
Arcangeli et al. [47]	168	H	80	2	Phoenix	79

ASTRO American Society for Therapeutic Radiation Oncology, *L* low risk group, *I* intermediate risk group, *H* high risk group, *M* all three risk groups mixed

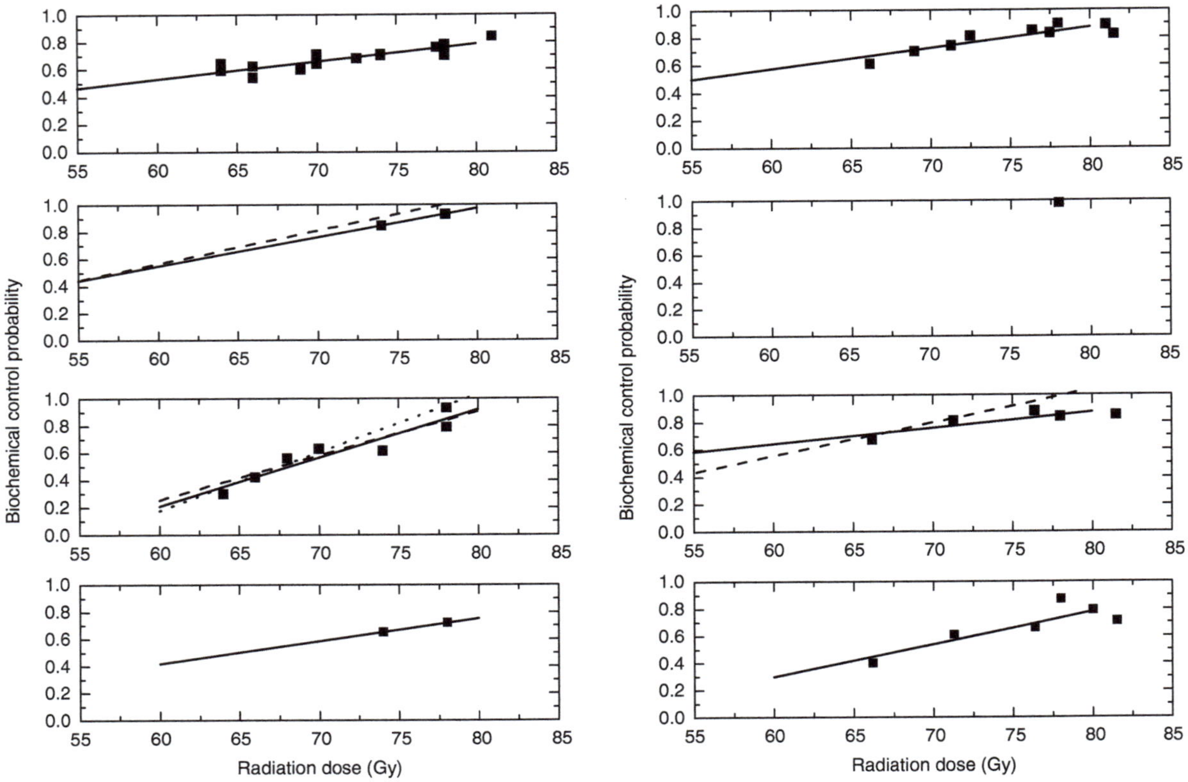

Fig. 8.3 Dose-response relationships from conventional fractionation. Left panels: ASTRO definition of biochemical failure. Right panels: Phoenix definition of biochemical failure. Solid curves, this analysis. Dashed curves, relationships reported by Cheung et al. [82]. Dotted curves, relationships reported by Pollack et al. [79]. Top panels, mixed risk groups. Second from top panels, low-risk patients. Third from top, intermediate-risk patients. Bottom panels, high-risk patients

Table 8.5 Interpolated dose response parameters for prostate treatments with conventional fractionation

Risk group	Failure definition	D_{50} (Gy)	γ	Source
M	ASTRO	57.6	0.74	This study
M	Phoenix	56.0	0.88	This study
L	ASTRO	57.8	1.23	This study
L	ASTRO	57.3	1.4	Cheung et al. [82]
L	Phoenix	n/a	n/a	n/a
I	ASTRO	67.5	2.89	Pollack et al. [79]
I	ASTRO	67.5	2.2	Cheung et al. [82]
I	ASTRO	68.1	2.41	This study
I	Phoenix	57.8	1.4	Cheung et al. [82]
I	Phoenix	47.9	0.56	This study
H	ASTRO	64.9	1.09	This study
H	Phoenix	68.4	1.65	This study

ASTRO American Society for Therapeutic Radiation Oncology, *L* low risk group, *I* intermediate risk group, *H* high risk group, *M* all three risk groups mixed

prostate tumors. This may hold the promise of improved results with shorter, hypofractionated treatments that may be favored both by patients that may face fewer treatment fractions, as well as by radiotherapy departments that may treat a larger number of patients in the same time period. However, a major concern for hypofractionated treatments is the risk of increased toxicity in the late-reacting

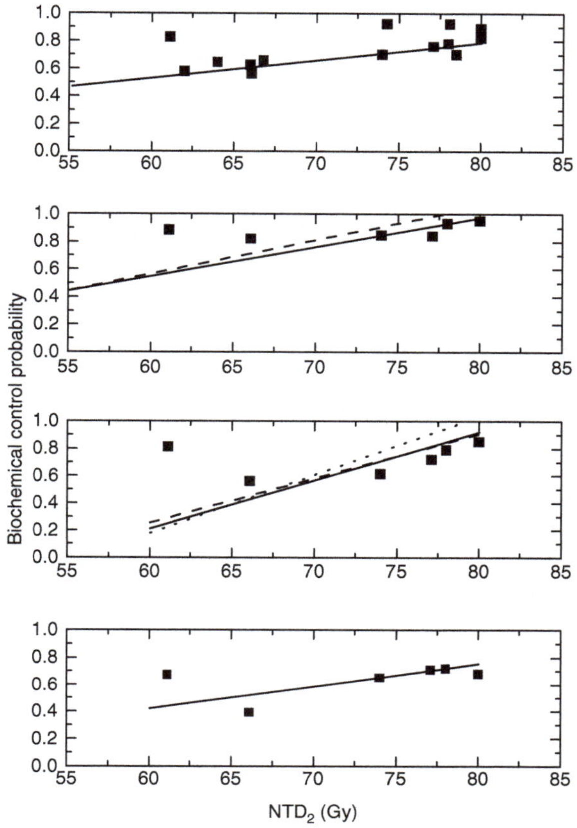

Fig. 8.4 Dose-response relationships for the ASTRO definition of biochemical failure; α/β assumed 1.5 Gy. Top panel, mixed risk groups. Second from top panel, low-risk patients. Third from top, intermediate-risk patients. Bottom panel, high-risk patients

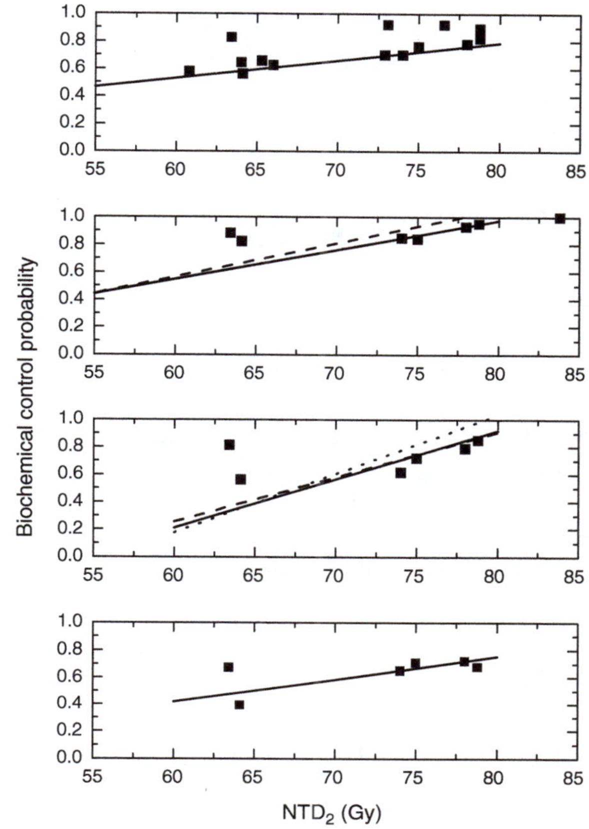

Fig. 8.5 Dose-response relationships for the ASTRO definition of biochemical failure; α/β assumed 2 Gy. Top panel, mixed risk groups. Second from top panel, low-risk patients. Third from top, intermediate-risk patients. Bottom panel, high-risk patients

tissues. For prostate tumors, the tissues of interest for late toxicity are the rectum, the bladder, the urethra, and the neurovascular bundles. The urethra has high radioresistance and it is often included in the high-dose target volume. Furthermore, clinical data indicates that it is also quite insensitive to fractionation [85]. Bladder complications also appear to indicate high α/β values [3]. Most uncertainty exists for the fractionation sensitivity of the rectum. Animal experiments have yielded α/β values for late rectal complications in the range of 4–6 Gy with confidence intervals between 2 and 8 Gy as reviewed by Fowler et al. [94]. A similar value, $\alpha/\beta = 5.4$ Gy, was also found in a later radiobiological analysis of human data on rectal injury [95]. These reports might support a fractionation differential between prostate tumors and late rectal injury and hence a potential therapeutic gain from the use of hypofractionation. However, there are also some studies that appear to indicate quite a high fractionation sensitivity for the rectal tissue. For instance, Yeoh et al. [46] have reported similar complication levels in the two arms of their randomized study calculated to be isoeffective for an α/β value of 3 Gy, thus supporting a comparable fractionation sensitivity. What's more unsettling appears to be the recent analysis of Marzi et al. [96] who found an α/β value for late rectal toxicity as low as 2 Gy, with a confidence interval extending approximately between 1 and 3.5 Gy. Such dangerously low α/β values would overlap onto most of the derivations of α/β values for prostate as well, questioning the direct therapeutic gain from hypofractionation. From this perspective, studies about the fractionation sensitivity of rectal injury appear warranted. Nevertheless, even with a highly fractionation-sensitive rectum, high complication levels could, in principle, be

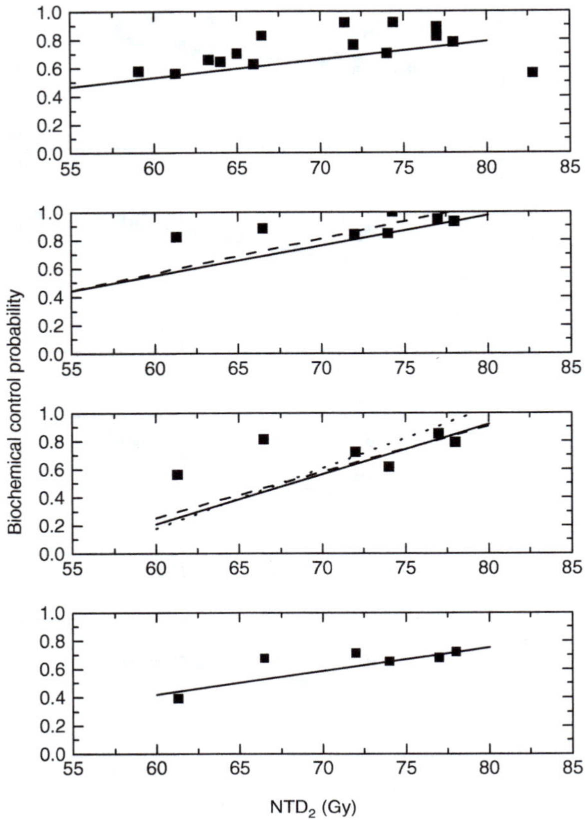

Fig. 8.6 Dose-response relationships for the ASTRO definition of biochemical failure; α/β assumed 3 Gy. Top panel, mixed risk groups. Second from top panel, low-risk patients. Third from top, intermediate-risk patients. Bottom panel, high-risk patients

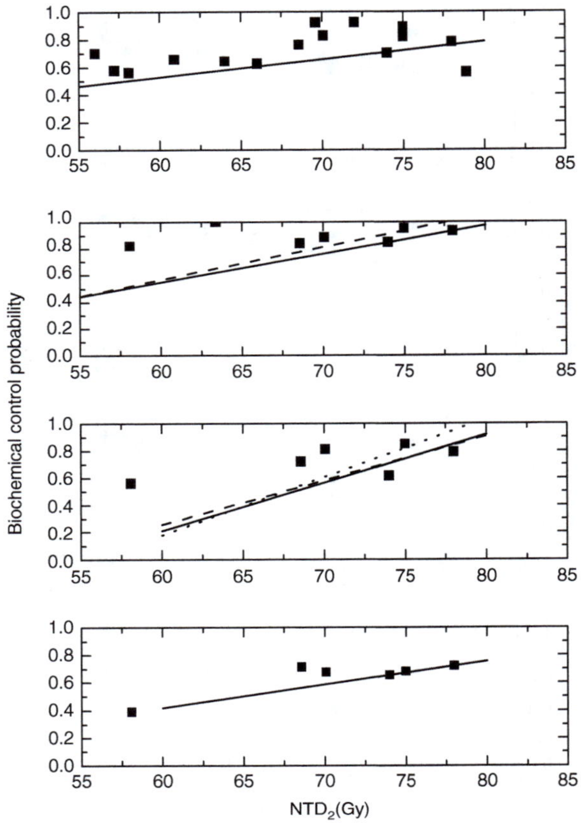

Fig. 8.7 Dose-response relationships for the ASTRO definition of biochemical failure; α/β assumed 5 Gy. Top panel, mixed risk groups. Second from top panel, low-risk patients. Third from top, intermediate-risk patients. Bottom panel, high-risk patients

avoided through limiting the rectum volume or surface receiving high doses, similar to the dose-volume constraints used for dose escalation studies with conventional fractionation. A similar approach would also be valid for the neurovascular bundles for which no data regarding the fractionation sensitivity is available [94]. The problem is that available dose constraints have been derived for conventionally fractionated schedules. Extrapolating these doses to hypofractionated regimens irradiating targets with smaller margins might therefore be pursued with caution. Best results would be obtained if fractionation patterns, normal tissue constraints, and margin definitions would be derived from dedicated clinical studies. The multitude of ongoing hypofractionation studies for prostate carcinomas holds many promises for successful derivation of these parameters.

Care must also be paid to the acute reactions. This might seem surprising at first, as isoeffective hypofractionated treatments calculated for a low tumor α/β would afford most protection to tissues with very high α/β values. However, radiobiological analyses have shown that schedules too short could lead to an increased rate of acute reactions, as they might prevent the protection afforded by compensatory proliferation as shown by Fowler [97, 98].

In spite of the difficulties mentioned above, clinical results available now appear to support further investigations of the opportunity of hypofractionation for radiation treatment of prostate tumors. Only through carefully planned clinical studies, enough evidence will be gathered on the advantages and disadvantages of hypofractionation as a standard form of treatment for prostate tumors.

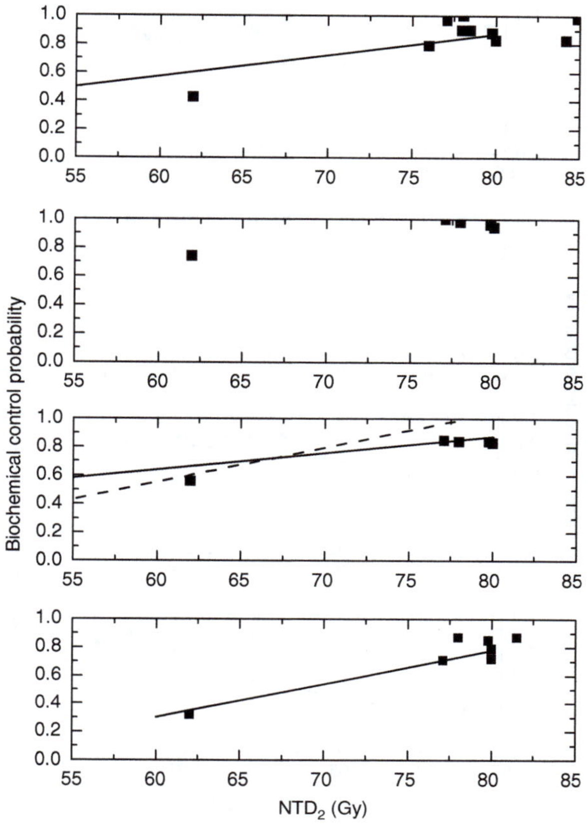

Fig. 8.8 Dose-response relationships for the Phoenix definition of biochemical failure; α/β assumed 1.5 Gy. Top panel, mixed risk groups. Second from top panel, low-risk patients. Third from top, intermediate-risk patients. Bottom panel, high-risk patients

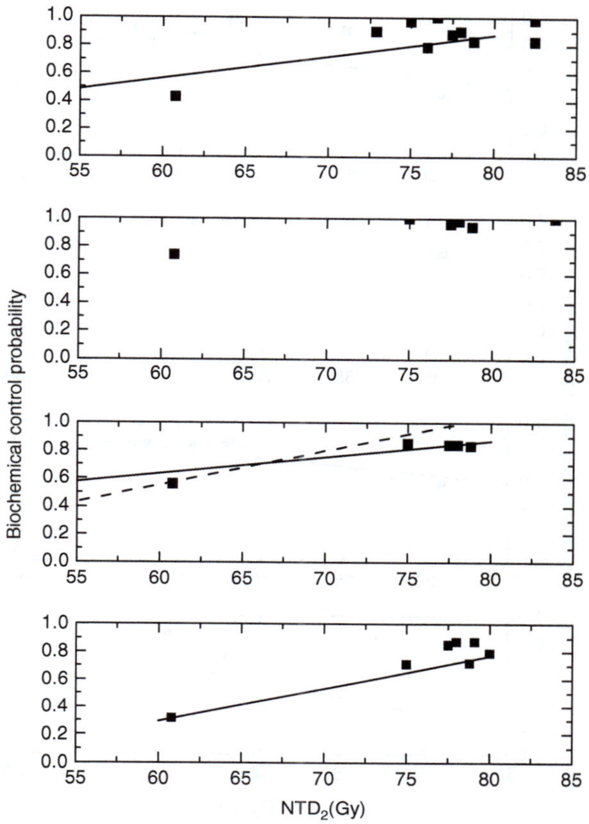

Fig. 8.9 Dose-response relationships for the Phoenix definition of biochemical failure; α/β assumed 2 Gy. Top panel, mixed risk groups. Second from top panel, low-risk patients. Third from top, intermediate-risk patients. Bottom panel, high-risk patients

8.8 Conclusions

This chapter addressed the radiobiological data that may be relevant for the hypofractionation of radiation therapy for prostate tumors. Results from several clinical studies are available and others are expected in the future. Although several confounding factors may interfere with the derivation of the fractionation sensitivity of prostate tumors, the majority of the clinical data appears to support an α/β value for prostate tumors between 1.5 and 2 Gy. This value is below most of the α/β values reported for the relevant late-responding tissues and holds the promise of a significant therapeutic gain that may be achieved from the hypofractionation of prostate treatment. Nevertheless, studies investigating the predicted advantage should be pursued with caution. As more clinical information regarding tumor response and complication rates mature, they will bring evidence on the sensitivity to fractionation of prostate tumors and will, thus, ultimately contribute to the well-being of the patients.

Acknowledgments The author would like to thank Prof. Jack Fowler for many stimulating discussions on the radiobiology of the prostate and for constructively critical comments on the manuscript.

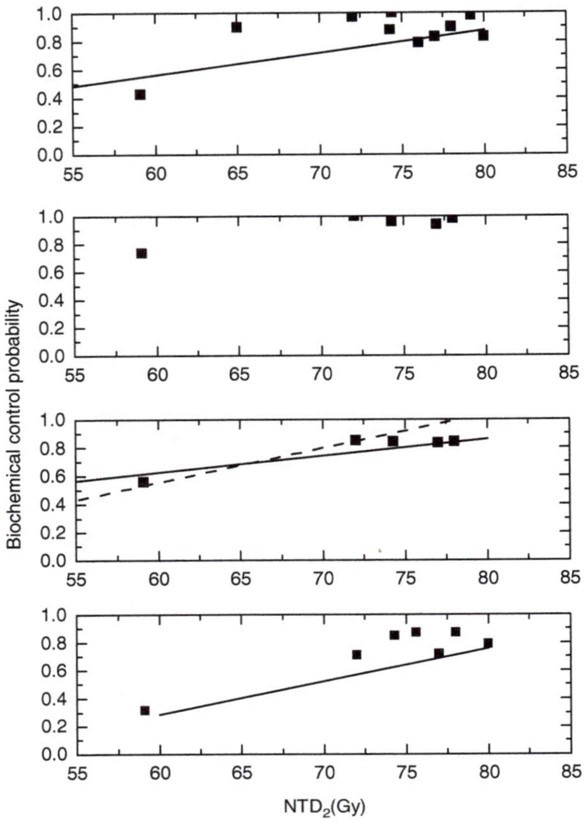

Fig. 8.10 Dose-response relationships for the Phoenix definition of biochemical failure; α/β assumed 3 Gy. Top panel, mixed risk groups. Second from top panel, low-risk patients. Third from top, intermediate-risk patients. Bottom panel, high-risk patients

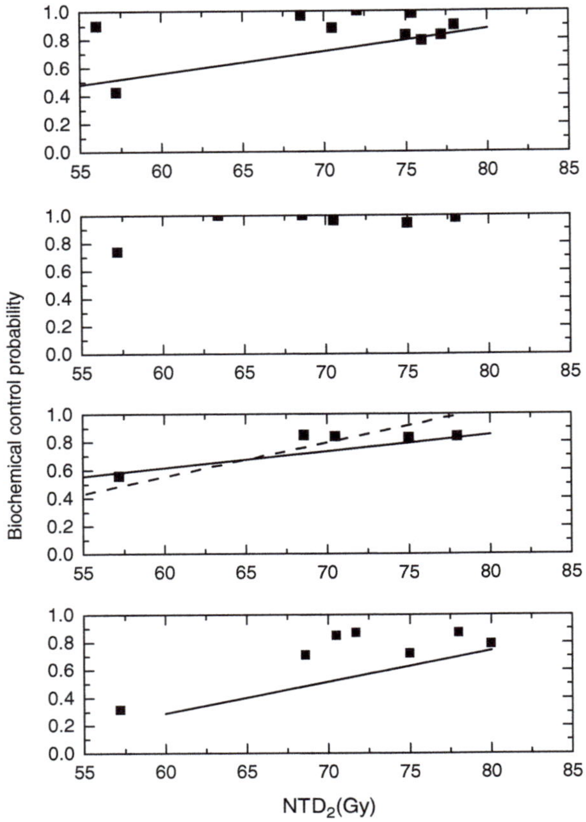

Fig. 8.11 Dose-response relationships for the Phoenix definition of biochemical failure; α/β assumed 5 Gy. Top panel, mixed risk groups. Second from top panel, low-risk patients. Third from top, intermediate-risk patients. Bottom panel, high-risk patients

References

1. Lea DE, Catcheside DG (1942) The mechanism of the induction by radiation of chromosome aberrations in Tradescandia. J Genet 44:216–245
2. Douglas BG, Fowler JF (1975) Letter: fractionation schedules and a quadratic dose-effect relationship. Br J Radiol 48:502–504
3. Thames HD, Hendry JH (1987) Fractionation in radiotherapy. Taylor & Francis, London/New York/Philadelphia
4. Barendsen GW (1982) Dose fractionation, dose rate and iso-effect relationships for normal tissue responses. Int J Radiat Oncol Biol Phys 8:1981–1997
5. Fowler JF (1989) The linear-quadratic formula and progress in fractionated radiotherapy. Br J Radiol 62:679–694
6. Hall EJ, Giaccia AJ (2006) Radiobiology for the radiologist, 6th edn. Lippincott Williams & Wilkins, Philadelphia
7. Withers HR, Taylor JM, Maciejewski B (1988) The hazard of accelerated tumor clonogen repopulation during radiotherapy. Acta Oncol 27:131–146
8. Chadwick KH, Leenhouts HP (1973) A molecular theory of cell survival. Phys Med Biol 18:78–87
9. Curtis SB (1986) Lethal and potentially lethal lesions induced by radiation–a unified repair model. Radiat Res 106:252–270
10. Kellerer AM, Rossi HH (1972) The theory of dual radiation action. Curr Top Radiat Res Q 8:85–158
11. Thames HD (1985) An 'incomplete-repair' model for survival after fractionated and continuous irradiations. Int J Radiat Biol Relat Stud Phys Chem Med 47:319–339
12. Thames HD Jr, Withers HR, Peters LJ et al (1982) Changes in early and late radiation responses with altered dose fractionation: implications for dose-survival relationships. Int J Radiat Oncol Biol Phys 8:219–226
13. Haustermans K, Fowler JF (2000) A comment on proliferation rates in human prostate cancer. Int J Radiat Oncol Biol Phys 48:303
14. Haustermans KM, Hofland I, Van Poppel H et al (1997) Cell kinetic measurements in prostate cancer. Int J Radiat Oncol Biol Phys 37:1067–1070
15. Fyles A, Keane TJ, Barton M et al (1992) The effect of treatment duration in the local control of cervix cancer. Radiother Oncol 25:273–279
16. Lanciano RM, Pajak TF, Martz K et al (1993) The influence of treatment time on outcome for squamous cell cancer of

the uterine cervix treated with radiation: a patterns-of-care study. Int J Radiat Oncol Biol Phys 25:391–397
17. Withers HR, Peters LJ, Taylor JM et al (1995) Local control of carcinoma of the tonsil by radiation therapy: an analysis of patterns of fractionation in nine institutions. Int J Radiat Oncol Biol Phys 33:549–562
18. Parsons JT, Thar TL, Bova FJ et al (1980) An evaluation of split-course irradiation for pelvic malignancies. Int J Radiat Oncol Biol Phys 6:175–181
19. Forman JD, Zinreich E, Lee DJ et al (1985) Improving the therapeutic ratio of external beam irradiation for carcinoma of the prostate. Int J Radiat Oncol Biol Phys 11: 2073–2080
20. Lai PP, Pilepich MV, Krall JM et al (1991) The effect of overall treatment time on the outcome of definitive radiotherapy for localized prostate carcinoma: the Radiation Therapy Oncology Group 75–06 and 77–06 experience. Int J Radiat Oncol Biol Phys 21:925–933
21. Amdur RJ, Parsons JT, Fitzgerald LT et al (1990) The effect of overall treatment time on local control in patients with adenocarcinoma of the prostate treated with radiation therapy. Int J Radiat Oncol Biol Phys 19:1377–1382
22. Perez CA, Michalski J, Mansur D et al (2004) Impact of elapsed treatment time on outcome of external-beam radiation therapy for localized carcinoma of the prostate. Cancer J 10:349–356
23. Horwitz EM, Vicini FA, Ziaja EL et al (1997) An analysis of clinical and treatment related prognostic factors on outcome using biochemical control as an end-point in patients with prostate cancer treated with external beam irradiation. Radiother Oncol 44:223–228
24. D'Ambrosio DJ, Li T, Horwitz EM et al (2008) Does treatment duration affect outcome after radiotherapy for prostate cancer? Int J Radiat Oncol Biol Phys 72:1402–1407
25. Thames HD, Kuban D, Levy LB et al (2010) The role of overall treatment time in the outcome of radiotherapy of prostate cancer: an analysis of biochemical failure in 4839 men treated between 1987 and 1995. Radiother Oncol 96:6–12
26. Buyyounouski MK, Hanlon AL, Horwitz EM et al (2005) Biochemical failure and the temporal kinetics of prostate-specific antigen after radiation therapy with androgen deprivation. Int J Radiat Oncol Biol Phys 61:1291–1298
27. Pollack A, Zagars GK, Kavadi VS (1994) Prostate specific antigen doubling time and disease relapse after radiotherapy for prostate cancer. Cancer 74:670–678
28. Fowler JF (2001) Biological factors influencing optimum fractionation in radiation therapy. Acta Oncol 40:712–717
29. Fowler JF (2008) Optimum overall times II: extended modelling for head and neck radiotherapy. Clin Oncol (R Coll Radiol) 20:113–126
30. Fowler JF, Welsh JS, Howard SP (2004) Loss of biological effect in prolonged fraction delivery. Int J Radiat Oncol Biol Phys 59:242–249
31. Dasu A, Fowler JF (2005) Comments on "Comparison of in vitro and in vivo alpha/beta ratios for prostate cancer". Phys Med Biol 50:L1–4; author reply L5–L8
32. Brenner DJ, Hall EJ (1999) Fractionation and protraction for radiotherapy of prostate carcinoma. Int J Radiat Oncol Biol Phys 43:1095–1101
33. Brenner DJ, Hall EJ (2000) In response to Drs. King and Mayo: low α/β values for prostate cancer appear to be independent of modeling details. Int J Radiat Oncol Biol Phys 47:538–539
34. King CR, Mayo CS (2000) Is the prostrate alpha/beta ratio of 1.5 from Brenner & Hall a modeling artifact. Int J Radiat Oncol Biol Phys 47:536–539
35. Dasu A (2007) Is the alpha/beta value for prostate tumours low enough to be safely used in clinical trials? Clin Oncol (R Coll Radiol) 19:289–301
36. Bentzen SM, Ritter MA (2005) The alpha/beta ratio for prostate cancer: what is it, really? Radiother Oncol 76:1–3
37. Brenner DJ, Martinez AA, Edmundson GK et al (2002) Direct evidence that prostate tumors show high sensitivity to fractionation (low alpha/beta ratio), similar to late-responding normal tissue. Int J Radiat Oncol Biol Phys 52:6–13
38. Chappell R, Fowler J, Ritter M (2004) New data on the value of alpha/beta–evidence mounts that it is low. Int J Radiat Oncol Biol Phys 60:1002–1003
39. Fowler J, Chappell R, Ritter M (2001) Is alpha/beta for prostate tumors really low? Int J Radiat Oncol Biol Phys 50: 1021–1031
40. Kupelian PA, Thakkar VV, Khuntia D et al (2005) Hypofractionated intensity-modulated radiotherapy (70 gy at 2.5 Gy per fraction) for localized prostate cancer: long-term outcomes. Int J Radiat Oncol Biol Phys 63:1463–1468
41. Livsey JE, Cowan RA, Wylie JP et al (2003) Hypofractionated conformal radiotherapy in carcinoma of the prostate: five-year outcome analysis. Int J Radiat Oncol Biol Phys 57:1254–1259
42. Lukka H, Hayter C, Julian JA et al (2005) Randomized trial comparing two fractionation schedules for patients with localized prostate cancer. J Clin Oncol 23:6132–6138
43. Valdagni R, Italia C, Montanaro P et al (2005) Is the alpha-beta ratio of prostate cancer really low? A prospective, non-randomized trial comparing standard and hyperfractionated conformal radiation therapy. Radiother Oncol 75:74–82
44. Wang JZ, Guerrero M, Li XA (2003) How low is the alpha/beta ratio for prostate cancer? Int J Radiat Oncol Biol Phys 55:194–203
45. Williams SG, Taylor JM, Liu N et al (2007) Use of individual fraction size data from 3756 patients to directly determine the alpha/beta ratio of prostate cancer. Int J Radiat Oncol Biol Phys 68:24–33
46. Yeoh EE, Holloway RH, Fraser RJ et al (2006) Hypofractionated versus conventionally fractionated radiation therapy for prostate carcinoma: updated results of a phase III randomized trial. Int J Radiat Oncol Biol Phys 66: 1072–1083
47. Arcangeli G, Saracino B, Gomellini S et al (2010) A prospective phase III randomized trial of hypofractionation versus conventional fractionation in patients with high-risk prostate cancer. Int J Radiat Oncol Biol Phys 78:11–18
48. Proust-Lima C, Taylor JM, Sécher S et al (2011) Confirmation of a low alpha/beta ratio for prostate cancer treated by external beam radiation therapy alone using a post-treatment repeated-measures model for PSA dynamics. Int J Radiat Oncol Biol Phys 79:195–201
49. Miralbell R, Roberts SA, Zubizarreta E, Hendry JH. (2011) Dose-fractionation sensitivity of prostate cancer deduced from radiotherapy outcomes of 5969 patients in seven international institutional datasets: $\alpha/\beta = 1.4$ (0.9-2.2) Gy. Int J Radiat Oncol Biol Phys

50. Leborgne F, Fowler J, Leborgne JH, Mezzera J. (2011) Later outcomes and alpha/beta estimate from hypofractionated conformal three-dimensional radiotherapy versus standard fractionation for localized prostate cancer. Int J Radiat Oncol Biol Phys
51. L.E. Ponsky et al. (eds.), Robotic Radiosurgery Treating Prostate Cancer and Related Genitourinary Applications
52. Collins CD, Lloyd-Davies RW, Swan AV (1991) Radical external beam radiotherapy for localised carcinoma of the prostate using a hypofractionation technique. Clin Oncol (R Coll Radiol) 3:127–132
53. Lloyd-Davies RW, Collins CD, Swan AV (1990) Carcinoma of prostate treated by radical external beam radiotherapy using hypofractionation. Twenty-two years' experience (1962–1984). Urology 36:107–111
54. Brenner DJ (2003) Hypofractionation for prostate cancer radiotherapy–what are the issues? Int J Radiat Oncol Biol Phys 57:912–914
55. Buyyounouski MK, Price RA Jr, Harris EE et al (2010) Stereotactic body radiotherapy for primary management of early-stage, low- to intermediate-risk prostate cancer: report of the American Society for Therapeutic Radiology and Oncology Emerging Technology Committee. Int J Radiat Oncol Biol Phys 76:1297–1304
56. Kitamura K, Shirato H, Shinohara N et al (2003) Reduction in acute morbidity using hypofractionated intensity-modulated radiation therapy assisted with a fluoroscopic real-time tumor-tracking system for prostate cancer: preliminary results of a phase I/II study. Cancer J 9:268–276
57. Akimoto T, Kitamoto Y, Saito J et al (2004) External beam radiotherapy for clinically node-negative, localized hormone-refractory prostate cancer: impact of pretreatment PSA value on radiotherapeutic outcomes. Int J Radiat Oncol Biol Phys 59:372–379
58. Carlson DJ, Stewart RD, Li XA et al (2004) Comparison of in vitro and in vivo alpha/beta ratios for prostate cancer. Phys Med Biol 49:4477–4491
59. Higgins GS, McLaren DB, Kerr GR et al (2006) Outcome analysis of 300 prostate cancer patients treated with neoadjuvant androgen deprivation and hypofractionated radiotherapy. Int J Radiat Oncol Biol Phys 65:982–989
60. Kupelian PA, Willoughby TR, Reddy CA et al (2007) Hypofractionated intensity-modulated radiotherapy (70 Gy at 2.5 Gy per fraction) for localized prostate cancer: Cleveland Clinic experience. Int J Radiat Oncol Biol Phys 68:1424–1430
61. Martin JM, Rosewall T, Bayley A et al (2007) Phase II trial of hypofractionated image-guided intensity-modulated radiotherapy for localized prostate adenocarcinoma. Int J Radiat Oncol Biol Phys 69:1084–1089
62. Junius S, Haustermans K, Bussels B et al (2007) Hypo fractionated intensity modulated irradiation for localized prostate cancer, results from a phase I/II feasibility study. Radiat Oncol 2:29
63. Madsen BL, Hsi RA, Pham HT et al (2007) Stereotactic hypofractionated accurate radiotherapy of the prostate (SHARP), 33.5 Gy in five fractions for localized disease: first clinical trial results. Int J Radiat Oncol Biol Phys 67: 1099–1105
64. King CR, Brooks JD, Gill H et al (2009) Stereotactic body radiotherapy for localized prostate cancer: interim results of a prospective phase II clinical trial. Int J Radiat Oncol Biol Phys 73:1043–1048
65. Leborgne F, Fowler J (2009) Late outcomes following hypofractionated conformal radiotherapy vs. standard fractionation for localized prostate cancer: a nonrandomized contemporary comparison. Int J Radiat Oncol Biol Phys 74:1441–1446
66. Rene N, Faria S, Cury F et al (2010) Hypofractionated radiotherapy for favorable risk prostate cancer. Int J Radiat Oncol Biol Phys 77:805–810
67. Arcangeli S, Strigari L, Soete G et al (2009) Clinical and dosimetric predictors of acute toxicity after a 4-week hypofractionated external beam radiotherapy regimen for prostate cancer: results from a multicentric prospective trial. Int J Radiat Oncol Biol Phys 73:39–45
68. Friedland JL, Freeman DE, Masterson-McGary ME et al (2009) Stereotactic body radiotherapy: an emerging treatment approach for localized prostate cancer. Technol Cancer Res Treat 8:387–392
69. Fuller DB, Naitoh J, Lee C et al (2008) Virtual HDR CyberKnife treatment for localized prostatic carcinoma: dosimetry comparison with HDR brachytherapy and preliminary clinical observations. Int J Radiat Oncol Biol Phys 70:1588–1597
70. Jereczek-Fossa BA, Cattani F, Garibaldi C et al (2007) Transabdominal ultrasonography, computed tomography and electronic portal imaging for 3-dimensional conformal radiotherapy for prostate cancer. Strahlenther Onkol 183:610–616
71. Khoo VS, Dearnaley DP (2008) Question of dose, fractionation and technique: ingredients for testing hypofractionation in prostate cancer–the CHHiP trial. Clin Oncol (R Coll Radiol) 20:12–14
72. Koukourakis MI, Touloupidis S, Manavis J et al (2004) Conformal hypofractionated and accelerated radiotherapy with cytoprotection (HypoARC) for high risk prostatic carcinoma: rationale, technique and early experience. Anticancer Res 24:3239–3243
73. Lim TS, Cheung PC, Loblaw DA et al (2008) Hypofractionated accelerated radiotherapy using concomitant intensity-modulated radiotherapy boost technique for localized high-risk prostate cancer: acute toxicity results. Int J Radiat Oncol Biol Phys 72:85–92
74. Norkus D, Miller A, Kurtinaitis J et al (2009) A randomized trial comparing hypofractionated and conventionally fractionated three-dimensional external-beam radiotherapy for localized prostate adenocarcinoma: a report on acute toxicity. Strahlenther Onkol 185:715–721
75. Ritter M, Forman J, Kupelian P et al (2009) Hypofractionation for prostate cancer. Cancer J 15:1–6
76. Tang CI, Loblaw DA, Cheung P et al (2008) Phase I/II study of a five-fraction hypofractionated accelerated radiotherapy treatment for low-risk localised prostate cancer: early results of pHART3. Clin Oncol (R Coll Radiol) 20:729–737
77. Dearnaley DP, Hall E, Lawrence D et al (2005) Phase III pilot study of dose escalation using conformal radiotherapy in prostate cancer: PSA control and side effects. Br J Cancer 92:488–498
78. Eade TN, Hanlon AL, Horwitz EM et al (2007) What dose of external-beam radiation is high enough for prostate cancer? Int J Radiat Oncol Biol Phys 68:682–689
79. Pollack A, Smith LG, von Eschenbach AC (2000) External beam radiotherapy dose response characteristics of 1127

men with prostate cancer treated in the PSA era. Int J Radiat Oncol Biol Phys 48:507–512
80. Pollack A, Zagars GK, Starkschall G et al (2002) Prostate cancer radiation dose response: results of the M. D. Anderson phase III randomized trial. Int J Radiat Oncol Biol Phys 53:1097–1105
81. Zelefsky MJ, Yamada Y, Fuks Z et al (2008) Long-term results of conformal radiotherapy for prostate cancer: impact of dose escalation on biochemical tumor control and distant metastases-free survival outcomes. Int J Radiat Oncol Biol Phys 71:1028–1033
82. Cheung R, Tucker SL, Lee AK et al (2005) Dose-response characteristics of low- and intermediate-risk prostate cancer treated with external beam radiotherapy. Int J Radiat Oncol Biol Phys 61:993–1002
83. Lindsay PE, Moiseenko VV, Van Dyk J et al (2003) The influence of brachytherapy dose heterogeneity on estimates of alpha/beta for prostate cancer. Phys Med Biol 48:507–522
84. Viani GA, Stefano EJ, Afonso SL (2009) Higher-than-conventional radiation doses in localized prostate cancer treatment: a meta-analysis of randomized, controlled trials. Int J Radiat Oncol Biol Phys 74:1405–1418
85. Akimoto T, Ito K, Saitoh J et al (2005) Acute genitourinary toxicity after high-dose-rate (HDR) brachytherapy combined with hypofractionated external-beam radiation therapy for localized prostate cancer: correlation between the urethral dose in HDR brachytherapy and the severity of acute genitourinary toxicity. Int J Radiat Oncol Biol Phys 63:463–471
86. Demanes DJ, Rodriguez RR, Schour L et al (2005) High-dose-rate intensity-modulated brachytherapy with external beam radiotherapy for prostate cancer: California endocurietherapy's 10-year results. Int J Radiat Oncol Biol Phys 61:1306–1316
87. Galalae RM, Martinez A, Mate T et al (2004) Long-term outcome by risk factors using conformal high-dose-rate brachytherapy (HDR-BT) boost with or without neoadjuvant androgen suppression for localized prostate cancer. Int J Radiat Oncol Biol Phys 58:1048–1055
88. Galalae RM, Martinez A, Nuernberg N et al (2006) Hypofractionated conformal HDR brachytherapy in hormone naive men with localized prostate cancer. Is escalation to very high biologically equivalent dose beneficial in all prognostic risk groups? Strahlenther Onkol 182:135–141
89. Grills IS, Martinez AA, Hollander M et al (2004) High dose rate brachytherapy as prostate cancer monotherapy reduces toxicity compared to low dose rate palladium seeds. J Urol 171:1098–1104
90. Martinez AA, Demanes DJ, Galalae R et al (2005) Lack of benefit from a short course of androgen deprivation for unfavorable prostate cancer patients treated with an accelerated hypofractionated regime. Int J Radiat Oncol Biol Phys 62:1322–1331
91. Martinez AA, Pataki I, Edmundson G et al (2001) Phase II prospective study of the use of conformal high-dose-rate brachytherapy as monotherapy for the treatment of favorable stage prostate cancer: a feasibility report. Int J Radiat Oncol Biol Phys 49:61–69
92. Yoshioka Y, Konishi K, Oh RJ et al (2006) High-dose-rate brachytherapy without external beam irradiation for locally advanced prostate cancer. Radiother Oncol 80:62–68
93. Yoshioka Y, Nose T, Yoshida K et al (2003) High-dose-rate brachytherapy as monotherapy for localized prostate cancer: a retrospective analysis with special focus on tolerance and chronic toxicity. Int J Radiat Oncol Biol Phys 56:213–220
94. Fowler JF, Ritter MA, Chappell RJ et al (2003) What hypofractionated protocols should be tested for prostate cancer? Int J Radiat Oncol Biol Phys 56:1093–1104
95. Brenner DJ (2004) Fractionation and late rectal toxicity. Int J Radiat Oncol Biol Phys 60:1013–1015
96. Marzi S, Saracino B, Petrongari MG et al (2009) Modeling of alpha/beta for late rectal toxicity from a randomized phase II study: conventional versus hypofractionated scheme for localized prostate cancer. J Exp Clin Cancer Res 28:117
97. Fowler JF (2005) The radiobiology of prostate cancer including new aspects of fractionated radiotherapy. Acta Oncol 44:265–276
98. Fowler JF, Harari PM, Leborgne F et al (2003) Acute radiation reactions in oral and pharyngeal mucosa: tolerable levels in altered fractionation schedules. Radiother Oncol 69:161–168
99. Pollack A, Hanlon AL, Horwitz EM et al. (2006) Dosimetry and preliminary acute toxicity in the first 100 men treated for prostate cancer on a randomized hypofractionation dose escalation trial. Int J Radiat Oncol Biol Phys 64:518–526

Hypofractionated Radiation Therapy in Prostate Cancer: Rationale, History, and Outcomes

9

Víctor Macias Hernandez

CONTENTS

9.1 Abstract

About 10 years ago, the first studies supporting the hypothesis that the response of prostate cancer to radiation was similar to that of slow-proliferating normal tissues were published. However, hypofractionation has been a common practice throughout radiotherapy history, mainly in western countries. The results of both experimental and clinical studies suggest that the α/β ratio for prostate cancer cells is lower than the α/β ratio for late-responding cells of the rectum and the bladder. This particularity allows the therapeutic window to be increased through the use of hypofractionated schemes. It has also been possible to establish, based on late toxicity results, that hypofractionated regimens are safe, and even without the use of IMRT or IGRT technology, the slight increases in acute toxicity found in some studies has been well tolerated. Nevertheless, to date, hypofractionation has not proved to be superior to conventionally fractionated therapy in terms of tumor control. Hypofractionation studies have so far been limited by their relatively short follow-up, a modest increase in dose per fraction (usually 2.5–3 Gy), and the difficulty to establish comparisons among different radiation techniques, hypofractionation schemes, and toxicity scales.

L.E. Ponsky et al. (eds.), *Treating Prostate Cancer and Related Genitourinary Applications*, Robotic Radiosurgery,
DOI 10.1007/978-3-642-11495-3_9,

9.2 The Origins of Hypofractionation

By early twentieth century, scientists had become convinced that response of cancer cells and healthy cells to radiation was different. For therapists like Claude Regaud, irradiation in multiple sessions over a few weeks was more appropriate [1]. This method was based on the finding that cancer cells were more radiosensitive in some phases of the cell cycle. Therefore, dose fractionation would make it likelier for radiation exposure to coincide with radiosensitive phases. On the other hand, Hermann Wintz considered that cancer cells had a faster growth rate and a greater ability to recover from radiation-induced damage than did cells of late-response tissues [2]. Therefore, it was more advisable to administer the treatment in one or a few fractions, and this latter school of opinion was prevalent until the Coutard studies [3]. Henri Coutard initially prescribed a high dose per fraction (DPF) over a few weeks, provided that the tumors were relatively small, and used low-dose-rate X-rays. He was largely guided by the severity of the skin and mucosal reactions occurring during radiation therapy, in the belief that the radiosensitivity of tumor cells was the same as that of regenerative cells of tissue where the cancer had originated. Subsequently, to treat larger lesions, he markedly reduced the DPF, and could then use a high dose rate. This regimen was known as simple fractionation (low DPF with high dose rate). Its suitability, given the growing healthcare pressure, and its relatively good outcomes made it an internationally accepted regimen. From this point on, two schools could be considered:

1. The French school, represented by Francois Baclesse [4], which further extended treatments for the purpose of reducing acute epithelitis and mucositis that were often dose-limiting. The treatment was extended substantially to over 2 months, which required increasing the total dose in an attempt to compensate for the overall treatment time (OTT) prolongation and the subsequent accelerated tumor repopulation.
2. The Anglo-Saxon school (UK, Canada, Australia), represented by Ralston Paterson [5] was strongly influenced by certain technological advancements such as a field light to guide irradiation, a mobile treatment table, the multiple-field technique, etc. Radiation therapy was administered over 3–5 weeks with relatively high DPF. To some extent, this hypofractionated regimen has been maintained in these countries to date, as shown in the first modern publications on hypofractionation in prostate cancer [6, 7].

The regimens recommended by the two schools, i.e., conventional fractionation (the French school) and hypofractionation (the Anglo-Saxon school), obtained satisfactory results, both in relation to local control and adverse events, although the former was the prevalent. Hypofractionation re-emerged in the 1950s and 1960s with the advent of two new techniques – radiosurgery, as performed by the pioneering neurosurgeon Lars Leksell in Sweden (1950) [8], and intraoperative radiation therapy at the University of Kyoto (1965). Both were characterized by the administration of high, ablative doses (DPF >8 Gy) to a low volume in a single session. In the 1970–1980s, extreme hypofractionation regimens were used, including those with one to three fractions a week, with negative clinical outcomes [9–13]. These studies were designed assuming that the proliferation potential of normal tissues (based on observation of the epithelium) was higher than tumor proliferation, and that the severity of late effects was closely related to the severity of the acute effects. Late toxicity started after some years instead of a few months, and its severity was not consistent with acute toxicity and was much more severe than expected. In addition, tumor control was also lower than expected, probably due to the rapid interfraction growth of cancer cells, so that the massive cell depletion caused by the high DPF had not entirely counterbalanced the accelerated repopulation. A review of the effect of radiation on healthy tissues, QUANTEC (Quantitative Analysis of Normal Tissue Effects in the Clinic), that quantifies the large dose-volume information from 3D conformal radiation therapy, has recently been published [14]. It is a valuable resource that allows the definition of tolerance doses of organs at risk and represents a significant input so as not to repeat previous errors in the design of current hypofractionation regimens.

9.3 The Four Rs of Radiation Therapy and Hypofractionation

The so-called four Rs of radiation therapy are: Repair (of radiation-induced damage, chiefly in the DNA chain), redistribution (grouping of irradiated cells in certain phases of the cell cycle), repopulation (based on the accelerated proliferation of surviving cells), and cell reoxygenation (by improving supply after inactivation of part of the tumor mass). The four Rs are similar for cancer and healthy tissues. The more similar they are, the lower the therapeutic window.

9.3.1 Repair

Acute-response tissues (ARTs; typically cancers), and late-response tissues (LRTs) have different dose–response curve shapes, which express their different levels of sensitivity to fractionation changes. LRTs have low α/β, that is, their cell death rate largely follows the quadratic component of the linear quadratic model. ARTs/cancers have a comparatively high α/β; therefore, their cell death rate largely follows the linear component. Hence, LRTs are more sensitive to fractionation than most ARTs/cancers [15].

As the DPF of a radiation therapy regimen increases, the effective dose for LRT increases, so that the total absolute dose that can be prescribed (provided the same late toxicity rate as in the equivalent conventionally fractionated regimen is maintained) is lower. The lower the dose administered to the treatment volume, the lower is the local control. Based on these considerations, it may be concluded that a hypofractionated regimen is only advisable when the α/β ratio is equal to or below the α/β ratio for LRTs that are near the treatment target.

9.3.2 Repopulation

The impact of the time factor is low or absent for LRT. Compensating proliferation starts many months after the start of radiation therapy. The OTT increase does not prevent late toxicity and OTT reduction does not increase it. For some cancers/ARTs, the time factor is important if the variation is of the order of at least several days. The compensating proliferation starts a few weeks after the start of radiation. Acute toxicity is reduced by increasing OTT over 2 weeks, and it is increased when OTT is decreased by 1.5–2 weeks.

As discussed above, several hypofractionated regimens of one to three sessions a week, with some OTT protraction, led to a local control decrease, possibly because tumor repopulation was more rapid than expected. Withers et al. have calculated that, over 4 weeks of OTT, it is necessary to increase the total dose to compensate for tumor repopulation [16]. Attention should be paid to not reducing OTT too much to avoid, for example, an increase in the severity of acute toxicity to the extent of necessitating breaks in the course of the radiation therapy. Therefore, Fowler recommends not reducing OTT to much less than 5 weeks [17].

9.3.3 Redistribution

Cells surviving a radiation dose are grouped mainly in the most radioresistant cell cycle phases. The higher the DPF, the more marked is the effect. This reduces the cytotoxic efficacy of the next dose if the cells have fast cell cycles, as in clonogenic cells of many tumors. However, redistribution has little influence if target cells show a slow cell cycle, as in LRTs and some cancers.

9.3.4 Reoxygenation

The appropriate oxygen and nutrient supply to cancer cells increases their radiosensitivity. Following the inactivation of some tumor cells after a treatment session, the surviving fraction is more highly oxygenated, and thus more susceptible to the next fraction. This is an argument against hypofractionation. On the other hand, reoxygenation also enhances repopulation of the surviving fraction of the tumor cells [18]. One of the theories that aims to explain the difference between the observed and the theoretically expected response after radiosurgery treatment of brain lesions is reoxygenation-induced cell death. According to this theory, massive tumor cell destruction after administration of a very high single dose, and the subsequent reoxygenation, results in the production of excessive amount of oxygen radicals resulting in cell death [19].

9.4 Radiobiology of Prostate Cancer and Adjacent Organs

Technological innovations in the last several decades have led to the re-emergence of hypofractionated radiation therapy from its familiar, "classic" applications (e.g., palliative radiation therapy, high-dose-rate (HDR) brachytherapy, radiosurgery, and intraoperative radiation therapy) to be applied in the curative treatment of prostate cancer and bronchopulmonary cancer, for example. It may be argued that this rebirth is based on the principles of the School of Manchester: Administration of high DPF to a small treatment volume, enabled by the technological improvements that allow accurate radiation delivery and relatively better sparing of organs at risk. The growing acceptance of hypofractionated regimens for the treatment of prostate cancer is based on both these technological possibilities and on the unusual radiobiology of prostate cancer that theoretically makes it highly sensitive to high DPF. Conventionally fractionated regimens are based on the assumption that cancers are less sensitive to an increase in DPF than LRTs (i.e., cancers have a high α/β ratio, usually ≥ 8 Gy, and LRTs have a low α/β ratio, on the order of 2–4 Gy). A low α/β ratio is related to a higher ability to repair between fractions. Therefore, under these conditions, in order to enlarge the therapeutic window, it is more favorable to use multiple, relatively small fractions.

However, recent analyses point out that the α/β ratio for prostate cancer is similar or lower than the α/β ratio for rectal LRTs (dose-limiting organ of risk); therefore, it should be more beneficial to use a hypofractionated regimen.

9.4.1 The α/β Ratio for Prostate Carcinoma

There is clear evidence of the low proliferation rate of low- and intermediate-grade cells in prostate cancer based on direct measurements of the time of cell duplication and analysis of PSA increase kinetics [20, 21]. The main arguments about a lower α/β ratio for prostate cancer have been based largely on clinical studies comparing tumor control obtained after different radiation therapy treatments. As most of these are not randomized studies designed specifically to test the effects of dose and fractionation, the ability of the data from these studies to allow a reasonable mathematical calculation of α/β ratio has been vigorously questioned. Dasu [22] published a review of the intense debate concerning the radiobiology of prostate cancer that focused on the basis for arguments concerning its actual α/β ratio.

9.4.1.1 Radiobiological Analysis of Studies that Mix Different Modalities

In 1999, Brenner and Hall [23] calculated the α/β ratio for prostate cancer cells comparing 3-year disease-free survival in two groups of patients treated at two different sites (367 patients). Some patients were treated with I-125 low-dose-rate (LDR) brachytherapy at a dose of 145 Gy, while others with external radiation at a DPF of 1.82 Gy up to 70–74 Gy. The patients in both groups had similar initial PSA and Gleason scores. Using the linear-quadratic model, an α/β of 1.5 Gy was reached with a 95% confidence interval of 0.8–2.2 Gy. Similarly, Fowler et al. compared the results of 1,471 patients from ten sites after HDR and LDR brachytherapy, estimating the α/β ratio as 1.49 Gy, with a 95% confidence interval of 1.25–1.76 Gy [24]. Both articles were discussed, leading to many arguments in favor and against the methods used, which are summarized as follows:

1. *The data was not sufficiently mature*:

   In the initial study by Brenner and Hall [23], the number of patients analyzed was relatively small (367 patients), and follow up was only 3 years.

2. *Heterogeneity*:

   Most of the arguments against the proposals of Brenner and Hall dealt with the need to correct for heterogeneity. King and Mayo [25], considering partially the heterogeneity (assuming that the α parameter of the linear quadratic equation is heterogeneously distributed), obtained, after reanalysis of Brenner and Hall's data, an α/β ratio of 4.96 Gy (95% CI 4.1–5.6). Brenner and Hall reanalyzed their series, this time assuming complete heterogeneity, and found an α/β ratio of 2.1 Gy. In subsequent studies on the effect of heterogeneity, it was concluded that the difference between the use of a homogeneous or heterogeneous model was too small to be detected in the clinical practice [26, 27].

3. *Distribution of non-homogeneous dose in brachytherapy*:

Other critics claimed that calculations of the α/β ratio assumed a homogeneous dose distribution in brachytherapy. An analysis of the matter concluded that, even considering the heterogeneity in the distribution of brachytherapy dose, the α/β ratios are low, though slightly higher than the previous ones [28].

4. *Tumor cell repopulation*:

Wang et al. [29] analyzed again the initial series of Fowler et al. correcting the values of some parameters and obtaining an α/β ratio of 3.1 Gy (95% CI 1.7–4.5 Gy). It is higher than those obtained by Brenner and Hall, and by Fowler et al., but not as disagreeing, considering the confidence intervals of the ratio in the three studies. The differences are largely due to the fact that Brenner and Hall, and Fowler et al. did not take into account tumor cell repopulation, as they considered it to be irrelevant in prostate cancer, while Wang et al. used the parameters of repopulation in head and neck cancer. A low repopulation rate for prostate cancer is suggested by PSA increase kinetics seen in relapses after radiation therapy, where PSA duplication times are long [21], and by post-treatment potential doubling time (TPOT) values, obtained from human prostate cancer biopsies, that are much higher than those of head and neck cancer [30]. However, it is still unknown whether high-risk prostate cancer has a faster proliferation rate and will behave as ART and, consequently, have a higher α/β ratio than low-intermediate risk prostate cancer.

5. *Relative biologic efficacy of different treatments:*

It has been claimed that LDR brachytherapy has a greater biologic efficacy against ART, and that this may have affected the calculation of the α/β ratio. To prevent this error, Brenner et al. [31] performed an analysis in patients treated with a combination of standard external radiation therapy and a dose-escalated boost through different HDR brachytherapy regimens (with three and two fractions of 5.5- to 10.5-Gy DPF). The resulting α/β ratio was 1.2 Gy (95% CI, 0.03–4.1 Gy). It was obtained through comparing the biochemical control rates of the groups at 3 years, after adjusting for age, T stage, Gleason index, PSA, and follow-up time.

It has been suggested that grouping the patients in accordance with the above variables may have not necessarily removed all possible confounding factors. Another limitation was the uncertainty resulting from the dose heterogeneity intrinsic to HDR brachytherapy.

Similarly, Williams et al. [32] designed a study in order to measure the α/β ratio directly based on the influence of DPF and the total dose on the probability for biochemical recurrence. They treated 3,571 patients with external-beam radiotherapy with the DPF 1.8–2.86 Gy. One hundred and eighty-five of the patients were also given an HDR brachytherapy boost with the DPF 5.5–12 Gy. The estimated α/β ratio was 3.7 Gy (95% CI, 1.1–∞ Gy) based on the recurrence rate after external radiation therapy. The α/β ratio was 2.6 Gy (95% CI 0.9–4.8 Gy) however, when the brachytherapy patients were included. The conclusion supported the concept of a low α/β ratio, but, as in the study of Brenner et al., it could not be estimated precisely because of the dependence of the calculation on the homogeneity correction factor of brachytherapy. Studies on only external radiation therapy with high DPF were necessary.

6. *Hypoxia*:

From the irradiation of cell cultures of prostate cancer, and taking into account the effects of hypoxia on local control, Nahum et al. [33] estimated an α/β ratio of 8.3 Gy (95% CI 1.2–15.5). It has been subsequently shown that the α/β ratio of in vitro cells is not related to the α/β ratio of in vivo cells, which are subject to hormonal and other regulations [34]. Furthermore, the hypoxia associated with poor nutrient supply would slow down cell proliferation even further and thus the α/β ratio increase secondary to hypoxia would be compensated. Carlson et al. estimated an α/β ratio between 1.1 and 6.3 Gy.

In short, a radiobiological analysis of retrospective studies comparing clinical results after external normofractionated radiation therapy and/with LDR or HDR brachytherapy, and experimental studies, appear to point to a low α/β ratio for prostate carcinoma, but with relatively large confidence intervals which do not allow for establishing exactly how low the ratio is in relation to the surrounding LRT. Prospective in vivo studies are required for comparing hypofractionation and normofractionation regimens.

9.4.1.2 Analysis of Studies with Hypofractionated External Radiation Therapy

Although virtually only in English-speaking countries, hypofractionated radiation therapy has always been used for treating prostate cancer with a very low late complication rate, as shown in the publication of a London hospital on their experience since 1962 [35]. In general, analysis of biochemical relapse-free survival and late toxicity in a number of studies comparing various hypofractionation and normofractionation regimens shows a low α/β ratio for prostate cancer [7, 36–39]. The α/β ratios calculated based on these comparative studies, reviewed briefly below, range from 1.12 to 2.4 Gy (mean 1.80 Gy), with confidence intervals that are very wide (e.g., from 6 to 10.6 Gy in the study by Yeoh et al. [37]). These studies are also limited by the use of moderately hypofractionated treatment regimens, with DPFs ranging from 2.5 to 3.1 Gy and do not have the statistical power to estimate α/β ratios clearly. Nevertheless, they clearly are consistent with the hypothesis of an α/β ratio for prostate cancer that is lower than for adjacent LRTs.

9.4.1.3 Analysis of Studies with Hyperfractionated External Radiation Therapy Regimens

An α/β ratio for prostate carcinoma that is not consistent with the values obtained in the studies mentioned above resulted from a non-randomized study of 370 patients receiving either conventional fractionation or a hyperfractionated regimen [40]. The hyperfractionation group was treated with two daily fractions of 1.2 Gy at 6-h intervals. The dose administered to both groups was isoeffective assuming a tumor α/β ratio of 10 Gy. Grade ≥2 genitourinary (GU) toxicity was higher in the normofractionated group (48.6% vs. 37.3%, $p=0.03$), but gastrointestinal (GI) toxicity did not differ between the two treatments. Biochemical control at 5 years was 70% and 82.6% in the normofractionated and hyperfractionated arms, respectively. Based on these findings, an α/β ratio of 8.3 Gy (95% CI, 0.7–16 Gy) emerged. This value was similar to that described for most malignant tumors, though its large confidence interval does not preclude very low α/β values. Bentzen et al. have pointed out that this very high α/β ratio could be an overestimation resulting from incomplete repair of the sublethal damage in the hyperfractionated group [41]. In conclusion, both retrospective analyses of studies comparing external normofractionated radiation therapy to brachytherapy, and those including external hypofractionated radiation therapy and HDR brachytherapy, do not lead to a final conclusion regarding the value of the α/β ratio for prostate cancer. Although most of the analyses suggest a lower value than usual for carcinomas at other sites, the crux of the matter is to define how low it is as compared to the α/β ratio for LRT around the prostate. Five and 10-year results of ongoing prospective randomized clinical trials on external hypofractionated radiation therapy would help clarify this question.

9.4.2 The α/β Ratio for Late-Response Tissues of the Rectum and Bladder

Most radiobiological calculations assume, without distinguishing between organs (except for the central nervous system), that the LRT α/β is 3 Gy.

9.4.2.1 The α/β Ratio for Late-Response Tissues of the Rectum

Experimental studies in rodents [42–44] have suggested an α/β ratio for rectum in the range of 2.67–6.65 Gy. Fowler et al. [17], after reviewing the data from experimental studies, reported an α/β ratio between 4 and 6 Gy (95% CI, 2–8 Gy). Brenner et al. [45] analyzed late toxicity in the Akimoto et al. series of 100 patients treated with a combination of external-beam radiotherapy and different HDR brachytherapy fractionations [38], and reported an α/β ratio for rectal LRT in humans of 5.4 Gy. It has been suggested that late rectal damage would largely result from severe acute toxicity [46–48], which is consistent with an α/β ratio for rectum between the classical values for ART and LRT. On the other hand, Fiorino et al. [49] claimed that α/β ratio cannot be measured accurately based on the varying dose distributions in the rectum among patients and the different treatment patterns among sites. Studies comparing moderate hypofractionation vs. normofractionation in prostate cancer, where both arms have similar rectal late toxicity (though with a moderate hypofractionation regimen), suggest α/β ratios for prostate cancer and for rectal LRT not very different.

Deore et al. [50] analyzed data from 203 patients with stage IIIB cervical cancer treated with external-beam radiotherapy and various hypofractionated HDR brachytherapy regimens (DPF between 2 and 5.4 Gy). Nineteen percent of the patients suffered from late rectosigmoid toxicity significantly more frequently in patients that received a high DPF. An α/β ratio for the rectum of 3.87 ± 0.74 Gy was estimated. Marzi et al. also calculated an α/β ratio close to 3 Gy after comparing rectal toxicity in 162 patients treated after randomization between 80 Gy/40 fractions/8 weeks or 62 Gy/20 fractions/5 weeks, with a median follow-up of 2.5 years [51]. In conclusion, the evidence available shows that the α/β ratio for rectal LRT is probably higher than the α/β ratio for prostate cancer.

9.4.2.2
The α/β Ratio of Late-Response Tissues of the Genitourinary Tract

The values proposed for the bladder range from 2 to 4 Gy, based on clinical studies on brachytherapy for uterine cervical cancer [51, 52]. This is consistent with the study of Akimoto et al. [53], who correlated the urethral late complication rate to the dose distribution delivered by prostate HDR brachytherapy and found the urethra was insensitive to fractionation changes. The data from experimental studies with rodents also estimated the bladder α/β ratio range between 3 and 7 Gy.

9.5
Theoretical Advantages of Hypofractionation in Prostate Cancer

The use of normofractionated regimens (low DPF to reach relatively high total doses) is based on the assumption that some cancers, with typically high α/β ratios (>8 Gy), are less sensitive to fractionation than LRTs, where a low α/β ratio is assumed (≈3 Gy). The situation may be contrary to that of prostate cancer, where the evidence suggests a low α/β ratio (about 1.5–2.0 Gy) as compared to rectal and lower urinary tract tissues (3 Gy or higher). Under these conditions, prostate cancer would be more sensitive to DPF increases than the close-by LRTs, allowing the possibility of increasing the therapeutic window. A model to calculate isoeffective doses between treatments with different fractionations is required [54]. The current model is the Linear-Quadratic Model (L-QM), a mechanistic binary model that assumes that cell death is the dominant process that explains both early and late, and even vascular effects of radiation. The L-QM is considered more reliable within the DPF range of 2–10 Gy. It may also be acceptable, though possibly less precise, to be used in the design of clinical trials with DPF up to 15–18 Gy.

The lower the α/β ratio for prostate cancer relative to the α/β ratio for rectal tissue, the wider is the therapeutic window of a hypofractionated regimen. The higher the DPF, the greater the benefit that can be obtained from the regimen.

Conventional regimens used to date offer an acceptable late toxicity rate, such as RTOG grade ≥2 toxicities in ≤5% of patients, but a higher rate of biochemical control is desirable. If we assume an α/β ratio for prostate cancer of 1.5 Gy and an α/β ratio for rectal LRT of 3 Gy, and equivalent dose distributions between regimens, we can devise a hypofractionated regimen that increases local control while maintaining the same rate of late toxicity. As the DPF increases, the L-QM predicts an increase in BED1.5 for cancer. To keep the same toxicity, we may adjust the total dose to keep the same BED3 in the rectum. For example, a regimen of 2.5 Gy/fraction to a total of 70 Gy is equivalent for the prostate to about 80 Gy delivered in 2 Gy per fraction, while a regimen of 58.1 Gy in fractions of 3.63 Gy is equivalent to about 86 Gy in fractions of 2 Gy; both regimens maintain a dose equivalent to 76 Gy/2 Gy per fraction to the rectum.

Similarly, if we assume the same α/β ratio and dose distribution as above, as DPF increases, the L-QM predicts a reduction in the BED3 for the rectum provided that we ensure the same BED1.5 is delivered to the prostate cancer to maintain local control. For instance, a regimen of 2.3 Gy/fraction to a total of 69 Gy is equivalent for the rectum to about 74 Gy in 2-Gy fractions, while a regimen of 4.46 Gy/fraction to 44.6 Gy is equivalent to about 66 Gy in 2-Gy fractions; both regimens maintain a 2-Gy dose equivalent in the prostate of 76 Gy.

In clinical practice, most hypofractionated regimens result in a lower total dose when a treatment regimen of five fractions in 5 days a week is used. Fowler et al. advise not to reduce the total treatment time below 5 weeks so as not to cause an unacceptable acute toxicity [17]. Yeoh et al. report that part of the late toxicity seen in their study on external hypofractionated radiation therapy may have been caused by severe acute toxicity [6].

9.6 Clinical Experience in External Hypofractionated Radiation Therapy in Prostate Cancer

Following the influential 1999 paper of Brenner and Hall, suggesting an unusually low α/β ratio for prostate cancer [23], the first study was published in 2000 reporting the preliminary results of the Cleveland Clinic Foundation [55]. In 2003, the first large modern series with 705 patients treated between 1995 and 1998 at the Christie Hospital, Manchester, UK [7], was published. That same year, the results of the first randomized study comparing hypofractionated to normofractionated regimens were published; no differences were found in late toxicity after a 3.5-year follow up in 120 patients [6]. In 2005, the second phase III study was published [39], with a series of 936 patients treated in Canada with similar late toxicity after a 5.7-year follow-up. In 2006, the preliminary results on acute toxicity of the Fox Chase Cancer Center study were published [56]. In 2010, a new randomized study performed in Italy was published [57]; the authors reported for the first time a possible advantage in terms of biochemical failure-free survival favorable to hypofractionation, though the results were preliminary (median follow-up of 3 years). Thus in the last 10 years, several studies have been published using hypofractionation regimens, alone or compared with normofractionation, with radical or adjuvant intention. Many of these used the IMRT technique, but 3D-CRT was also used in some, often with image guidance support. Generally, the studies tested moderately hypofractionated regimens, but a few of them did involve accelerated hypofractionation.

9.6.1 Randomized Clinical Trials Comparing External-Beam Hypofractionation to Conventional Fractionation

In the past 7 years, four studies have been published (summarized in Table 9.1). Close to ten phase III studies are currently in different stages of completion. When their mature results are published, the question of the theoretical advantage of hypofractionation will be clarified; they will enable a more precise determination of the α/β ratio for prostate carcinoma, advance our understanding of fractionation, total dose, and the most appropriate OTT in irradiation of this tumor.

9.6.1.1 Tumor Control

Australian and Canadian studies prohibited androgen deprivation therapy, while in the US and Italian studies, where only patients at intermediate/high risk were recruited, androgen blockade was prescribed. In the US study, hormone therapy was permitted only in high-risk patients until 4 months before randomization and could continue for 24 additional months after that. In the Italian study, all patients were treated with anti-androgen bicalutamide along with a quarterly LHRH analogue for 9 months, starting 2 months before the start of the radiation therapy. The DPF was moderately hypofractionated in the four studies, with 2.75 Gy in the Australian, 2.625 Gy in the Canadian, 2.7 Gy in the US, and 3.1 Gy in the Italian one. For all dose equivalence calculations, the α/β ratio for prostate cancer was considered 1.5 Gy, which was used by Pollack et al. and Arcangeli et al. in the design of their studies.

A phase III study conducted in Australia by Yeoh et al. [6, 37] included 217 T1–T2 patients, 156 of whom were treated with 2D technique, and 61 with 3D-CRT. Fifty-five Gray/20 fractions/4 weeks (BED1.5 = 156 Gy) was compared to 64 Gy/32 fractions/6.5 weeks (BED1.5 = 149 Gy). The primary objective was to establish late toxicity. The study had some limitations, including a low rate of long-term follow-up (5-year biochemical follow-up was available for only 96 of the 182 surviving patients), a higher 2-Gy-per-fraction normalized total dose (NTD2) was used in the hypofractionation arm (66.8 Gy vs. 64 Gy), and the hypofractionation arm included a higher number of high-risk patients. Still, at a median follow-up of 4 years, the 5-year actuarial survival rate was 86.4% for the hypofractionation and 84.1% for the normofractionation groups, a non-significant difference, and the 5-year actuarial biochemical/clinical relapse-free survival was 57.4% versus 55.5% for the two groups, respectively, also not significant. After excluding high-risk patients, the results

Table 9.1 Characteristics of randomized studies comparing hypofractionated radiation therapy to normofractionated radiation therapy

		Canada [39]	Australia [37]	U.S [56]	Italy [57]
N	–	936	217	100	168
Technique	–	2D	2D/3D$_{(22\%)}$	IMRT + IGRT	3D
Toxicity scale	–	NCIC	$_m$LENT-SOMA	$_m$RTOG/LENT	LENT-SOMA
DPF (Gy)	HYPO	2.625	2.75	2.7	3.1
OTT (weeks)	NF	6.5	6.5	7.6	8
	HYPO	4	4	5.2	5
$BED_{1.5}$ ($Gy_{1.5}$)	NF	154	149	213[a]	187
	HYPO	144	156	197	190
BED_3 (Gy_3)	NF	110	107	127[a]	133
	HYPO	98	105	133	126
BED_{10} (Gy_{10})	NF	79	77	91[a]	96
	HYPO	66	70	89	81
Acute GI Tox	NF	≥3: 2.6%	–	≥2: 8%	–
	HYPO	≥3: 4.1%	[b]	≥2: 18%	[c]
Acute GU Tox	NF	≥3: 4.9%	–	≥2: 54%	–
	HYPO	≥3: 8.6%	[b]	≥2: 40%	[c]
Median follow-up (years)		5.7	4	–	2.8
Late GI Tox	NF	≥3: 1.3%	–	–	≥2: 14%
	HYPO	≥3: 1.3%	[c]	–	≥2: 17%
Late GU Tox	NF	≥3: 1.9%	–	–	≥2: 11%
	HYPO	≥3: 1.9%	[c]	–	≥2: 16%
Relapse 5 years	NF	52.95%	35.77%[d]	–	21%[e]
	HYPO	59.95%	34.25%[d]	–	13%[e]

BEDα/β biological equivalent dose calculated through L-QM. *α/β* ratios = 1.5, 3 and 10 Gy, for prostate cancer, LRTs and ARAs, respectively, *NF* normofractionated radiation therapy arm, *HYPO* hypofractionated radiation therapy arm, *NCIC* National Cancer Institute of Canada, *m* modified, *Acute GI Tox* acute gastrointestinal toxicity, *Acute GU Tox* acute genitourinary toxicity, *Late GI Tox* late gastrointestinal toxicity, *Late GU Tox* late genitourinary toxicity
[a]Minimum dose at PTV
[b]Toxicity was significantly higher in this arm
[c]No significant differences between arms
[d]Biochemical or clinical failure
[e]Biochemical failure at 3 years

remained similar. PSA nadirs and curves of the two arms were superimposable.

In the Canadian multicenter study of Lukka et al. [39], a total of 936 T1–T2 patients were treated with a 2D technique. Minimum follow-up was 4.5 years and the median was 5.7 years. The arms were well balanced. A hypofractionated regimen of 52.5 Gy/20 fractions/4 weeks (BED1.5 = 144 Gy) was compared to 66 Gy/33 fractions/6.5 weeks (BED1.5 = 154 Gy). However, the total equivalent dose prescribed to the PTV was lower in the hypofractionated arm (61.9 Gy vs. 66 Gy). The primary objective was to compare recurrence between the two study arms, using a non-inferiority design with pre-established tolerance levels of −7%. Recurrence was defined as biochemical failure, clinical relapse, institution of hormonal therapy, and death related to cancer. The estimated 5-year biochemical or clinical failure rate was not significantly higher in the hypofractionated arm (59.95% vs. 52.95%). There were no substantial differences in overall survival (87.6% in the hypofractionated group vs. 85.2%) or in the percentage of positive biopsies at 2 years after radiation therapy (50.9% vs. 53.2% normofractionation).

In the US study, Pollack et al. [56] treated 100 T1-T3 patients with IMRT and US-guided IGRT.

The hypofractionated regimen was 70.2 Gy/26 fractions/5.2 week (BED1.5 = 197 Gy) compared to 76 Gy/38 fractions/7.6 weeks (BED1.5 = 177 Gy). The study was designed to test whether dose escalation via hypofractionation results in an increase in biochemical failure-free survival without increasing acute toxicity. Given the short follow-up, no data were available on late toxicity and tumor control.

In the Italian study of Arcangeli et al. [57], 168 high-risk patients were treated with 3D-CRT. The hypofractionated regimen was 62 Gy/20 fractions/5 weeks (BED1.5 = 190 Gy) was compared to 80 Gy/40 fractions/8 weeks (BED1.5 = 187 Gy). The primary objective was to establish late toxicity. Unlike the first two studies, which were designed before the specific response to prostate cancer fractionation was known, this study aimed to determine whether a hypofractionated regimen, designed to be equivalent in local control to a normofractionated regimen, can reduce late toxicity without reducing biochemical relapse-free survival. Median follow-up was 2.8 years. Three-year actuarial metastasis-free survival was similar in both arms (82% in the hypofractionated arm vs. 88%, non-significant) and the actuarial biochemical relapse-free survival rate was significantly different in favor of the hypofractionated arm at 3 years (87% vs. 79%, $p = 0.035$) and 4 years (82% vs. 60%, $p = 0.004$).

In conclusion, there is not enough evidence for assuring the appropriateness of one or the other treatment regimen for tumor control, due to the short follow-up (median follow-up of the studies within 3–5 years). The 5-year actuarial biochemical/clinical relapse-free survival rates of the Australian and Canadian studies are low in both arms for the current standard (close to 50%), but consistent with the low total equivalent dose administered (<70 Gy).

9.6.1.2 Late Toxicity

Most patients developing late toxicity have done so within the first 2 years [58, 59]. In three out of the four randomized studies [37, 39, 57], median follow-up exceeded 30 months and late toxicity data were provided. The Australian and Italian groups used the SOMA-LENT scale [60], while the Canadian study used the National Cancer Institute of Canada (NCIC) scale [61]. The CTV was contoured in the US study after fusing the simulation CT with a pelvic MR. This is the only study using IMRT and IGRT by US for daily localization of the prostate. The Italian study and some patients of the Australian one were planned with 3D technique. The rest were planned using a 2D technique.

The Fox Chase Centre study [21] was the only one where prophylactic irradiation of pelvic node chains was performed (in 35% of the patients), to a dose of ≥50–52 Gy in the hypofractionated arm and ≥56 Gy in the normofractionated arm. The normalized total doses in fractions of 2 Gy (NTD2) for rectal and bladder LRTs were 63.25 Gy, 59.1 Gy, and 75.6 Gy in the Australian, Canadian, and Italian studies, respectively. For the calculation, we used the simple formulation of L-QM, assuming that the α/β ratio for LRTs is 3 Gy. The expected therapeutic gain in the hypofractionated arm of the Australian and Canadian studies was very low, due to the moderate hypofractionation (DPF ≤2.7 Gy) and the low total dose prescribed (<67 Gy). Comparing NTD2 for prostate cancer and for LRTs, using α/β ratios of 1.5 Gy and 3 Gy respectively, there is about a 3-Gy difference. The BED3 for rectal and bladder LRTs is similar in hypofractionated vs. normofractionated regimens in the Australian (105 Gy3 vs. 107 Gy3, respectively) and Italian studies (133 Gy3 vs. 126 Gy3, respectively); the BED3 was lower in the hypofractionated regimen of the Canadian study (98 Gy3 vs. 110 Gy3). No significant differences were seen in any of the three studies in terms of late gastrointestinal (GI) or genitourinary toxicity (GU) between the two arms. The Australian study reported that, after a 2-year follow-up, there were not only significant differences between the two regimens in the scores of GI symptoms, both considered individually and overall, but also the effects of sequels in daily activities were similar. A "consequential effect" was seen between the severity of acute and chronic toxicity. The increased acute GU and GI toxicity at 1 month of completing radiation therapy were independent prognostic factors for late GU or GI toxicity increase at 2 years and after 4 years of follow-up [37]. The only dosimetric prognostic factor for late toxicity was a significant relationship found between treatment volume and urinary urgency at 4 years [37].

In conclusion, the studies cannot currently identify a late toxicity reduction, as predicted theoretically by the use of a hypofractionated regimen. The therapeutic gain (calculated with α/β ratios of 1.5 and 3 Gy) in the Australian and Canadian studies may be too low to be detected clinically, or the number of patients may not provide enough statistical power (168 patients included in the Italian study). In any case, the hypofractionated regimens have been shown to be safe in terms of late toxicity, with no increase in the side effects as compared to conventional fractionation.

9.6.1.3 Acute Toxicity

Four randomized studies have provided acute toxicity data. The Australian and Canadian studies evidenced a significantly greater increase in acute GI and GU toxicity in the hypofractionated group vs. the normofractionated group, relative to baseline. The overall treatment time of 6.5 weeks in the normofractionated branch decreased to 6 weeks in the hypofractionated branch. The BEDs for ARTs were higher in the normofractionated arms in the Australian study (BED10 = 70 Gy vs. BED10 = 77 Gy) and the Canadian study (BED10 = 66 Gy vs. BED10 = 79 Gy).

In the US study, a significant increase was seen in Grade 2 or higher GI toxicity in the hypofractionated arm (18% versus 8%). Paradoxically, a significant reduction Grade 2 or higher GU toxicity was also observed in the same arm (48% vs. 56%). The overall treatment time decreased from 7.6 weeks to 5.2 weeks. The BEDs for ARTs were similar between the two regimens. The highest acute RTOG grade was reached earlier in the hypofractionated arm, mainly for bowel symptoms, decreasing promptly after the end of radiation therapy.

In the Italian study, Grade 2 toxicity was slightly higher in the hypofractionated arm. Only one patient developed Grade 3 toxicity and there was no Grade 4 toxicity. The overall treatment time decreased from 8 weeks to 5 weeks. But BEDs for ARTs were higher in the normofractionated regimen (BED10 = 81 Gy10 vs. BED10 = 96 Gy10). In the US study, multivariate analysis of the possible predictive factors of acute toxicity showed that the probability of Grade 2 or higher GI toxicity was increased in both arms as a function of rectal V65Gy/V50Gy ratio; small bladder volume in the planning CT was associated with an increase in acute GU toxicity. The possibility that late GI toxicity could be a "consequential effect" of acute GI toxicity was supported by the result of the multivariate analysis in the Australian study (described in the above Sect. 9.6.1.2). In short, although the results of studies on acute toxicity are not conclusive, hypofractionated radiation therapy may cause a slight but potentially significant increase in acute toxicity, which appears earlier in the treatment course. The only study that did not show this effect on acute toxicity was the US study. This may be related to prescription of similar BEDs for ARTs in both arms, with protraction over 5 weeks or with the use of IMRT with IGRT. In the other three, acute toxicity was higher in the hypofractionated arm, though not significantly so in the Italian study. In any case, hypofractionated treatment was well tolerated in all studies, with acute toxicity rates similar to conventional regimens.

9.6.2 Non-randomized Clinical Trials on External Hypofractionated Radiation Therapy (Moderate Fractionation)

The results related to late and acute toxicity of non-randomized prospective studies on hypofractionated photon radiation therapy with curative intention are shown in Table 9.2. In most studies, one DPF from 2.5 to 3.5 Gy was administered, reaching an NTD ranging from 56.5 to 90.6 Gy. The percentage of both late and acute Grade ≥3 toxicity was generally below 10%. The data is not mature enough to provide information on tumor control. Many studies included a small sample or had a limited follow-up. Two of the 15 studies included in Table 9.2 summarize findings from a sample of near 700 patients with an approximate follow-up of 48 months [7, 36]. Livsey et al. [7] treated 705 patients with 3D-CRT in 3.13-Gy fractions over prostate and seminal vesicles to a nominal dose of 50 Gy in 3.1 weeks (equivalent to 66.1 Gy). No hormonal treatment was included. The mean follow-up was 4 years. The actuarial biochemical disease-free survival rates, according to the ASTRO definition, were 82%, 56%, and 39% for low-, intermediate-, and high-risk patients, respectively. The authors concluded that their results were comparable to those published with normofractionated radiation therapy for the same dose level. To compensate for the fact that it was a retrospective study, where mild late toxicity is usually not established precisely, a total of 101 patients were randomly selected and interviewed in depth. No Grade 3 RTOG toxicity was seen. Grade 2 or higher GI and GU toxicity was 5% and 9%, respectively.

Table 9.2 Characteristics of hypofractionated studies on external hypofractionated radiation therapy

Author ref.	N	FU	Technique (d)	D/OTT	$BED_{1.5}$	BED_3	BED_{10}	Failure	Late Tox	Acute Tox
Akimoto et al. [38]	53	35	3D (3)	69/7.6	207	138	90	3BF = 34	GI3 = 2[a,b] GI2 = 15[a,b] GI1 = 2[a,b]	GU3 = 13 GU2 = 17
Arcangeli et al. [64]	102	–	3D/IM (3.5)	56/4	187	121	77	–	–	GI2 = 38 GI1 = 36 GU2 = 39 GU1 = 42
Arcangeli et al. [57]	168	34	3D (3.1)	/5	190	126	81	3BF = 13[b]	GI3 = 0.6[b] GI ≥ 2 = 17[b] GU3 = 0[b] GU ≥ 2 = 16[b]	–
Coote et al. [65]	60	24	IM (3)	57—60/3.8—4	180	120	78	–	GI2 = 0—10 GI1 = 10—27 GU3 = 0—4 GU2 = 0—4 GU1 = 26—32	GI2 = 9—20 GI1 = 7—13
Di Muzio et al. [66]	60	–	TO (2.55—2.65)	71.4—74.2/5.6	199	136	92	–	–	GI1 = 30 GU3 = 3 GU2 = 20 GU1 = 35
Faria et al. [67]	72	30	3D (3)	66/4.2	198	132	86	14%	GI3 = 13% GI2 = 5% GI1 = 21% GU2 = 18% GU1 = 36%	–
Higgins et al. [68]	300	58	3D (2.625)	52.5/4	144	98	66	5BF = 57[b] (26—68)	–	–
Kupelian et al. [36]	770	45	3D-IG (2.5)	70/5	187	128	87	5BF = 17 (6—28)[b]	GI4 = 0.1 GI3 = 1.3 GI2 = 3.1 GI1 = 5.9 GU3 = 0.1 GU2 = 5.1 GU1 = 4.3	GI2 = 9 GI1 = 40 GU3 = 1 GU2 = 18 GU1 = 48

Leborgne et al. [62]	89	49	3D-IG (3—3.15)	60—63/4.7	186	123	79	5BF = 4—15	5GI3 = 1.1[b] 5GI2 = 4.5[b] 5GI1 = 25[b] 5GU3 = 2.2[b] 5GU2 = 2.2[b] 5GU1 = 1.1[b]	G≥2 = 6—17
Lim et al. [63]	66	–	3D/IM (2.7)	67.5/5	189	128	86	–	–	GI2 = 37 GU3 = 7.6 GU≥2 = 36
Livsey et al. [7]	705	48	3D (3.125)	50/4.4	154	102	66	5BF = 18—61[b]	GI2 = 5 GU2 = 9	–
Martin et al. [69]	92	38	IM-IG (3)	60/4	180	120	78	3BF = 3[b]	GI3 = 1.2 GI2 = 5.1 GI1 = 11.8 GU2 = 10 GU1 = 17.6	GI3 = 1 GI2 = 11 GI1 = 22 GU2 = 25 GU1 = 43
Pervez et al. [70]	66	–	TO (2.72)	68/5	191	130	86	–	–	GI2 = 35 GI1 = 52 GU3 = 7 GU2 = 33 GU1 = 47
Pollack et al. [56]	100	–	IM-IG (2.7)	/5.2	197	133	89	–	–	GI≥2 = 18 GU≥2 = 40
Zilli et al. [71]	88/48	–	IM (4)	56—60/7—7.5	213	135	81	–	–	GI2 = 12 GI1 = 35 GU3 = 1 GU2 = 24 GU1 = 64

N number of patients treated with hypofractionated radiation therapy, *FU* median follow-up (months), *d* dose per fraction (Gy), *3D* 3D conformal radiation therapy, *IM* intensity-modulated radiotherapy *TO* tomotherapy, *D* total dose (Gy), *n* number of fractions, *s* total treatment time (weeks), *BED* α/β biological equivalent dose calculated with the simple formulation of the Linear-Quadratic Model for a given α/β ratio (Gy), *5BF* biochemical failure at 5 years (%), *Late Tox.* late toxicity, *Acute T. Tox* acute toxicity, *GI* gastrointestinal toxicity, *GU* genitourinary toxicity (%), example: *2GU3* grade 3 genitourinary toxicity at 2 years

[a] Rectal bleeding

[b] Actuarial calculation (Kaplan-Meier)

On the other hand, Kupelian et al. [36] treated 770 consecutive patients with US-guided IMRT. The DPF was 2.5 Gy to reach the nominal dose of 70 Gy in 5 weeks (equivalent to 80 Gy). The mean follow-up in this prospective study was 3.75 years. The actuarial biochemical disease-free survival rates, according to the ASTRO definition, were 95%, 85%, and 68% for low-, intermediate-, and high-risk patients. The rates of late RTOG Grade 2, 3, and 4 GI toxicities were 3.1%, 1.3%, and 0.1%; and GU toxicities were 5.1%, 0.1%, and 0%, respectively. With regard to acute side effects, the percentages were 9% Grade 2 and 0% Grade 3 or higher GI toxicity, and 18% Grade 2 and 1% Grade 3 or higher for GU toxicity.

The preliminary results of a non-randomized study comparing three contemporaneous cohorts using fractionations of 2 Gy, 3 Gy, and 3.15 Gy to deliver a nominal dose of 76–80 Gy, 60 Gy, and 63 Gy, respectively, have been published [62]. Fast hypofractionated radiation therapy for 4 days/week over 5 weeks, in 3-Gy fractions, was a safe alternative, particularly with regard to acute rectal toxicity similar to that seen with a normofractionated regimen. However, with the regimen of 3.5 Gy/fraction, the rate of Grade 2 toxicity was higher than that with 3-Gy fractionation (though not significantly so) and that with conventional fractionation ($p<0.001$).

Lim et al. [63] used mixed fractionation in the treatment of 66 high-risk patients. Pelvic node areas received 25 fractions of 1.8 Gy over 5 weeks using a conventional box technique, with a concomitant boost of 0.9 Gy to the prostate using an IMRT technique. The treatment was well tolerated; the rate of GI toxicity (using Common Terminology Criteria for Adverse Events v.3.0) of Grade 2 was 39% and Grade 3 was 0%, and GU toxicity occurred at rates of 36% for grade ≥2 and 7.6% for grade ≥3. Still, this data shows that hypofractionated regimens appear to be relatively safe, as they do not increase late adverse effects or worsen acute toxicity substantially, even without using IMRT or IGRT. To date, it has not been demonstrated whether hypofractionation improves tumor control. It should be noted that these studies include relatively short follow-up (not longer than 5 years), small increases in DPF (usually up to 2.5–3 Gy), and make comparisons among protocols difficult due to the use of different techniques, regimens, and toxicity scales.

9.7 Conclusions

The results to date support the conclusion that hypofractionated radiation therapy is relatively safe for the treatment of localized prostate cancer. No significant increase has been seen in the late adverse events or the acute toxicity. The data from hypofractionation studies appear to indicate that the α/β ratio for prostate cancer is not very different from the α/β ratio for late-response tissues of the bladder and rectum. Ongoing randomized studies designed specifically to demonstrate the possible superiority of hypofractionation over conventional fractionation will better define the role of hypofractionated radiation therapy in the cure of carcinoma of the prostate.

References

1. Regaud C (1977) The influence of the duration of irradiation on the changes produced in the testicle by radium. Int J Radiat Oncol Biol Phys 2:565–567
2. Wintz H (1931) Results obtained with carcinoma uteri treated by Rontgen-rays from 1915–1925. Ann Surg 93: 428–435
3. Coutard H (1937) The results and methods of treatment of cancer by radiation. Ann Surg 106:584–598
4. Baclesse F (1953) Fractionated roentgenotherapy of epitheliomas of the pharynx, larynx, uterus, vagina and breast; study of 1449 cases. Acta Unio Int Contra Cancrum 9: 29–33
5. Paterson R (1954) Radiotherapy in cancer of the cervix; rising cure rates follow improvement in technique. Acta Radiol Suppl 116:395–404
6. Yeoh EE, Fraser RJ, McGowan RE et al (2003) Evidence for efficacy without increased toxicity of hypofractionated radiotherapy for prostate carcinoma: early results of a phase III randomized trial. Int J Radiat Oncol Biol Phys 55: 943–955
7. Livsey JE, Cowan RA, Wylie JP et al (2003) Hypofractionated conformal radiotherapy in carcinoma of the prostate: five-year outcome analysis. Int J Radiat Oncol Biol Phys 57: 1254–1259
8. Leksell L (1951) The stereotaxic method and radiosurgery of the brain. Acta Chir Scand 102:316–319
9. Macbeth FR, Wheldon TE, Girling DJ et al (1996) Radiation myelopathy: estimates of risk in 1048 patients in three randomized trials of palliative radiotherapy for non-small cell lung cancer. The Medical Research Council Lung Cancer Working Party. Clin Oncol (R Coll Radiol) 8:176–181
10. Harrison D, Crennan E, Cruickshank D et al (1988) Hypofractionation reduces the therapeutic ratio in early glottic carcinoma. Int J Radiat Oncol Biol Phys 15:365–372

11. Ashby MA, Ago CT, Harmer CL (1986) Hypofractionated radiotherapy for sarcomas. Int J Radiat Oncol Biol Phys 12: 13–17
12. Overgaard M, Bentzen SM, Christensen JJ et al (1987) The value of the NSD formula in equation of acute and late radiation complications in normal tissue following 2 and 5 fractions per week in breast cancer patients treated with postmastectomy irradiation. Radiother Oncol 9:1–11
13. Singh K (1978) Two regimes with the same TDF but differing morbidity used in the treatment of stage III carcinoma of the cervix. Br J Radiol 51:357–362
14. Bentzen SM, Constine LS, Deasy JO et al (2010) Quantitative Analyses of Normal Tissue Effects in the Clinic (QUANTEC): an introduction to the scientific issues. Int J Radiat Oncol Biol Phys 76:S3–S9
15. Thames HD Jr, Withers HR, Peters LJ et al (1982) Changes in early and late radiation responses with altered dose fractionation: implications for dose-survival relationships. Int J Radiat Oncol Biol Phys 8:219–226
16. Withers HR, Taylor JM, Maciejewski B (1988) The hazard of accelerated tumor clonogen repopulation during radiotherapy. Acta Oncol 27:131–146
17. Fowler JF, Ritter MA, Chappell RJ et al (2003) What hypofractionated protocols should be tested for prostate cancer? Int J Radiat Oncol Biol Phys 56:1093–1104
18. Petersen C, Zips D, Krause M et al (2001) Repopulation of FaDu human squamous cell carcinoma during fractionated radiotherapy correlates with reoxygenation. Int J Radiat Oncol Biol Phys 51:483–493
19. Nakamura K, Brahme A (1999) Evaluation of fractionation regimens in stereotactic radiotherapy using a mathematical model of repopulation and reoxygenation. Radiat Med 17:219–225
20. Haustermans KM, Hofland I, Van Poppel H et al (1997) Cell kinetic measurements in prostate cancer. Int J Radiat Oncol Biol Phys 37:1067–1070
21. Pollack A, Zagars GK, Kavadi VS (1994) Prostate specific antigen doubling time and disease relapse after radiotherapy for prostate cancer. Cancer 74:670–678
22. Dasu A (2007) Is the alpha/beta value for prostate tumours low enough to be safely used in clinical trials? Clin Oncol (R Coll Radiol) 19:289–301
23. Brenner DJ, Hall EJ (1999) Fractionation and protraction for radiotherapy of prostate carcinoma. Int J Radiat Oncol Biol Phys 43:1095–1101
24. Fowler J, Chappell R, Ritter M (2001) Is alpha/beta for prostate tumors really low? Int J Radiat Oncol Biol Phys 50: 1021–1031
25. King CR, Mayo CS (2000) Is the prostrate alpha/beta ratio of 1.5 from Brenner & Hall a modeling artifact. Int J Radiat Oncol Biol Phys 47:536–539
26. Carlone M, Wilkins D, Nyiri B et al (2003) Comparison of alpha/beta estimates from homogeneous (individual) and heterogeneous (population) tumor control models for early stage prostate cancer. Med Phys 30:2832–2848
27. Moiseenko V (2004) Effect of heterogeneity in radiosensitivity on LQ based isoeffect formalism for low alpha/beta cancers. Acta Oncol 43:499–502
28. Lindsay PE, Moiseenko VV, Van Dyk J et al (2003) The influence of brachytherapy dose heterogeneity on estimates of alpha/beta for prostate cancer. Phys Med Biol 48:507–522
29. Wang JZ, Guerrero M, Li XA (2003) How low is the alpha/beta ratio for prostate cancer? Int J Radiat Oncol Biol Phys 55:194–203
30. Dasu A, Fowler JF (2005) Comments on "Comparison of in vitro and in vivo alpha/beta ratios for prostate cancer". Phys Med Biol 50:L1–L4; author reply L5–L8
31. Brenner DJ, Martinez AA, Edmundson GK et al (2002) Direct evidence that prostate tumors show high sensitivity to fractionation (low alpha/beta ratio), similar to late-responding normal tissue. Int J Radiat Oncol Biol Phys 52:6–13
32. Williams SG, Taylor JM, Liu N et al (2007) Use of individual fraction size data from 3756 patients to directly determine the alpha/beta ratio of prostate cancer. Int J Radiat Oncol Biol Phys 68:24–33
33. Nahum AE, Movsas B, Horwitz EM et al (2003) Incorporating clinical measurements of hypoxia into tumor local control modeling of prostate cancer: implications for the alpha/beta ratio. Int J Radiat Oncol Biol Phys 57:391–401
34. Carlson DJ, Stewart RD, Li XA et al (2004) Comparison of in vitro and in vivo alpha/beta ratios for prostate cancer. Phys Med Biol 49:4477–4491
35. Lloyd-Davies RW, Collins CD, Swan AV (1990) Carcinoma of prostate treated by radical external beam radiotherapy using hypofractionation. Twenty-two years' experience (1962–1984). Urology 36:107–111
36. Kupelian PA, Willoughby TR, Reddy CA et al (2007) Hypofractionated intensity-modulated radiotherapy (70 Gy at 2.5 Gy per fraction) for localized prostate cancer: Cleveland Clinic experience. Int J Radiat Oncol Biol Phys 68:1424–1430
37. Yeoh EE, Holloway RH, Fraser RJ et al (2006) Hypofractionated versus conventionally fractionated radiation therapy for prostate carcinoma: updated results of a phase III randomized trial. Int J Radiat Oncol Biol Phys 66:1072–1083
38. Akimoto T, Muramatsu H, Takahashi M et al (2004) Rectal bleeding after hypofractionated radiotherapy for prostate cancer: correlation between clinical and dosimetric parameters and the incidence of grade 2 or worse rectal bleeding. Int J Radiat Oncol Biol Phys 60:1033–1039
39. Lukka H, Hayter C, Julian JA et al (2005) Randomized trial comparing two fractionation schedules for patients with localized prostate cancer. J Clin Oncol 23:6132–6138
40. Valdagni R, Italia C, Montanaro P et al (2005) Is the alpha-beta ratio of prostate cancer really low? A prospective, non-randomized trial comparing standard and hyperfractionated conformal radiation therapy. Radiother Oncol 75:74–82
41. Bentzen SM, Ritter MA (2005) The alpha/beta ratio for prostate cancer: what is it, really? Radiother Oncol 76:1–3
42. Dubray BM, Thames HD (1994) Chronic radiation damage in the rat rectum: an analysis of the influences of fractionation, time and volume. Radiother Oncol 33:41–47
43. Gasinska A, Dubray B, Hill SA et al (1993) Early and late injuries in mouse rectum after fractionated X-ray and neutron irradiation. Radiother Oncol 26:244–253
44. van der Kogel AJ, Jarrett KA, Paciotti MA et al (1988) Radiation tolerance of the rat rectum to fractionated X-rays and pi-mesons. Radiother Oncol 12:225–232
45. Brenner DJ (2004) Fractionation and late rectal toxicity. Int J Radiat Oncol Biol Phys 60:1013–1015

46. Jereczek-Fossa BA, Vavassori A, Fodor C et al (2008) Dose escalation for prostate cancer using the three-dimensional conformal dynamic arc technique: analysis of 542 consecutive patients. Int J Radiat Oncol Biol Phys 71:784–794
47. Dorr W, Hendry JH (2001) Consequential late effects in normal tissues. Radiother Oncol 61:223–231
48. Wang CJ, Leung SW, Chen HC et al (1998) The correlation of acute toxicity and late rectal injury in radiotherapy for cervical carcinoma: evidence suggestive of consequential late effect (CQLE). Int J Radiat Oncol Biol Phys 40:85–91
49. Fiorino C, Sanguineti G, Valdagni R (2005) Fractionation and late rectal toxicity: no reliable estimates of alpha/beta value for rectum can be derived from studies where different volumes of rectum are irradiated at different dose levels: in regard to Brenner (Int J Radiat Oncol Biol Phys 2004;60:1013–1015.). Int J Radiat Oncol Biol Phys 62:289–290; author reply 290–281
50. Deore SM, Shrivastava SK, Supe SJ et al (1993) Alpha/beta value and importance of dose per fraction for the late rectal and recto-sigmoid complications. Strahlenther Onkol 169:521–526
51. Marzi S, Saracino B, Petrongari MG et al (2009) Modeling of alpha/beta for late rectal toxicity from a randomized phase II study: conventional versus hypofractionated scheme for localized prostate cancer. J Exp Clin Cancer Res 28:117
52. Guerrero M, Li XA (2006) Halftime for repair of sublethal damage in normal bladder and rectum: an analysis of clinical data from cervix brachytherapy. Phys Med Biol 51:4063–4071
53. Akimoto T, Ito K, Saitoh J et al (2005) Acute genitourinary toxicity after high-dose-rate (HDR) brachytherapy combined with hypofractionated external-beam radiation therapy for localized prostate cancer: correlation between the urethral dose in HDR brachytherapy and the severity of acute genitourinary toxicity. Int J Radiat Oncol Biol Phys 63:463–471
54. Dale RG (1985) The application of the linear-quadratic dose-effect equation to fractionated and protracted radiotherapy. Br J Radiol 58:515–528
55. Mohan DS, Kupelian PA, Willoughby TR (2000) Short-course intensity-modulated radiotherapy for localized prostate cancer with daily transabdominal ultrasound localization of the prostate gland. Int J Radiat Oncol Biol Phys 46:575–580
56. Pollack A, Hanlon AL, Horwitz EM et al (2006) Dosimetry and preliminary acute toxicity in the first 100 men treated for prostate cancer on a randomized hypofractionation dose escalation trial. Int J Radiat Oncol Biol Phys 64: 518–526
57. Arcangeli G, Saracino B, Gomellini S et al (2010) A prospective phase III randomized trial of hypofractionation versus conventional fractionation in patients with high-risk prostate cancer. Int J Radiat Oncol Biol Phys 78:11–18
58. Smit WG, Helle PA, van Putten WL et al (1990) Late radiation damage in prostate cancer patients treated by high dose external radiotherapy in relation to rectal dose. Int J Radiat Oncol Biol Phys 18:23–29
59. Schultheiss TE, Hanks GE, Hunt MA et al (1995) Incidence of and factors related to late complications in conformal and conventional radiation treatment of cancer of the prostate. Int J Radiat Oncol Biol Phys 32:643–649
60. Pavy JJ, Denekamp J, Letschert J et al (1995) EORTC Late Effects Working Group. Late effects toxicity scoring: the SOMA scale. Radiother Oncol 35:11–15
61. Brundage MD, Pater JL, Zee B (1993) Assessing the reliability of two toxicity scales: implications for interpreting toxicity data. J Natl Cancer Inst 85:1138–1148
62. Leborgne F, Fowler J (2009) Late outcomes following hypofractionated conformal radiotherapy vs. standard fractionation for localized prostate cancer: a nonrandomized contemporary comparison. Int J Radiat Oncol Biol Phys 74:1441–1446
63. Lim TS, Cheung PC, Loblaw DA et al (2008) Hypofractionated accelerated radiotherapy using concomitant intensity-modulated radiotherapy boost technique for localized high-risk prostate cancer: acute toxicity results. Int J Radiat Oncol Biol Phys 72:85–92
64. Arcangeli S, Strigari L, Soete G et al (2009) Clinical and dosimetric predictors of acute toxicity after a 4-week hypofractionated external beam radiotherapy regimen for prostate cancer: results from a multicentric prospective trial. Int J Radiat Oncol Biol Phys 73:39–45
65. Coote JH, Wylie JP, Cowan RA et al (2009) Hypofractionated intensity-modulated radiotherapy for carcinoma of the prostate: analysis of toxicity. Int J Radiat Oncol Biol Phys 74:1121–1127
66. Di Muzio N, Fiorino C, Cozzarini C et al (2009) Phase I-II study of hypofractionated simultaneous integrated boost with tomotherapy for prostate cancer. Int J Radiat Oncol Biol Phys 74:392–398
67. Faria SL, Souhami L, Joshua B et al (2008) Reporting late rectal toxicity in prostate cancer patients treated with curative radiation treatment. Int J Radiat Oncol Biol Phys 72:777–781
68. Higgins GS, McLaren DB, Kerr GR et al (2006) Outcome analysis of 300 prostate cancer patients treated with neoadjuvant androgen deprivation and hypofractionated radiotherapy. Int J Radiat Oncol Biol Phys 65:982–989
69. Martin JM, Rosewall T, Bayley A et al (2007) Phase II trial of hypofractionated image-guided intensity-modulated radiotherapy for localized prostate adenocarcinoma. Int J Radiat Oncol Biol Phys 69:1084–1089
70. Pervez N, Small C, MacKenzie M et al (2010) Acute toxicity in high-risk prostate cancer patients treated with androgen suppression and hypofractionated intensity-modulated radiotherapy. Int J Radiat Oncol Biol Phys 76:57–64
71. Zilli T, Rouzaud M, Jorcano S et al (2010) Dose escalation study with two different hypofractionated intensity modulated radiotherapy techniques for localized prostate cancer: acute toxicity. Technol Cancer Res Treat 9:263–270

High-Dose-Rate Brachytherapy for the Treatment of Low-, Intermediate-, and High-Risk Prostate Cancer

10

Mackenzie McGee, Mihai Ghilezan, and Alvaro Martinez

CONTENTS

10.1 Abstract

Brachytherapy is a type of radiation therapy that allows for the delivery of highly conformal radiation for prostate cancer in the setting of monotherapy for low-risk disease and as a boost for intermediate- to high-risk patients. There are two types of brachytherapy, high-dose-rate (HDR) and low-dose-rate (LDR) brachytherapy, both of which may be used as monotherapy or boost. HDR brachytherapy may offer advantages over LDR including improved accuracy of treatment, toxicities, and radiation safety issues. Brachytherapy has been shown to have similar biochemical control (BC) compared to radical prostatectomy (RP) or external-beam radiotherapy (EBRT) and therefore is a good therapeutic option for appropriately selected patients. We have reviewed the results of 474 patients treated with HDR monotherapy at William Beaumont Hospital, and the results show that BC rates are similar to that of RP or EBRT with low rates of high-grade chronic genitourinary or gastrointestinal toxicities.

Intermediate-risk prostate cancer may be treated with multiple treatment modalities including surgery, EBRT, or EBRT in combination with HDR brachytherapy boost as a means of dose escalation. We present multi-institutional data from Kiel University, California Endocurietherapy Cancer Center and William Beaumont Hospital. For all patients, 5- and 10-year overall survival (OS) was 92.3% and 79.4%, respectively, with BC rates of 89.5% and 81.9%. Cause specific survival at 5 and 10 years was 99.0% and 97.5%, respectively.High-risk prostate cancer patients from the above institutions in addition to Universidad de Navarra who were treated with HDR brachytherapy boost are also presented. OS rates at 5- and 10- years were 87.9% and 67.1%, respectively. BC rates at 5- and 10-years were 79.2% and 61.1%, respectively, with cause-specific survival rates of 94.9% and 87.4%, respectively.

Overall, HDR brachytherapy is an excellent means of delivering highly conformal radiotherapy to the prostate as monotherapy or in combination with EBRT as boost in appropriately selected patients.

10.2 Introduction

Traditionally, radiation therapy and surgery have been the standard-of-care treatment modalities most

L.E. Ponsky et al. (eds.), *Treating Prostate Cancer and Related Genitourinary Applications*, Robotic Radiosurgery,
DOI 10.1007/978-3-642-11495-3_10,

frequently used in the treatment of prostate cancer patients. However, within the field of radiation oncology, it is important to recognize the potential advantages brachytherapy treatment may provide. Patterns of care utilization from The American Urologic Society [1] and the American College of Radiology [2] have reported a significant increase with respect to brachytherapy. This chapter will focus specifically on a type of brachytherapy called high-dose-rate (HDR) brachytherapy as monotherapy or as boost therapy in combination with pelvic external beam radiation, as appropriate.

There are two prostate brachytherapy techniques used to deliver treatment, low-dose-rate (LDR) or HDR brachytherapy. LDR brachytherapy involves the placement of multiple, permanent radioactive seeds into the prostate, typically utilizing Iodine-125, Palladium-103, or Cesium-131 sources. An important difference between these methods is that with permanent seeds, the prescribed dose is delivered over weeks to months. During this period, the patient remains radioactive and must comply with state rules and regulations for patients harboring radioactive material. In contrast, HDR brachytherapy utilizes a single high-intensity radioactive source stored in a remote afterloader, a robot-like machine. Iridium-192 is typically used as the radioactive source and controlled by the afterloader to enter into and retract from interstitial catheters in the patient. The total radiation prescription dose is delivered in a period of typically 10–20 min. Once the afterloader retracts the source from the patient following treatment, he is no longer radioactive.

10.2.1 Advantages of HDR Brachytherapy

Comparatively, HDR has a number of patient- and target-specific advantages over LDR therapy. They are summarized below:

1. The overall treatment time reduction with HDR eliminates the uncertainties related to prostate volume changes that occur during the weeks following a procedure (typical with LDR) due to trauma and swelling, or subsequent shrinkage due to post-radiation fibrosis.
2. HDR allows for improved accuracy of needle placement and radiation dose distribution through the use of intraoperative optimization software that modulates the dose, improves control over spatial source position, and dwell times during the shorter treatments, and potentially limits treatment-related toxicities.
3. A single radioactive source may deliver treatment to large numbers of patients with HDR, whereas LDR requires radioactive sources to be purchased on a per case basis, leading to increased cost of treatment as compared to HDR.
4. From a radiation safety perspective, HDR is ideal, because patients are not radioactive when they return home. As such, patients do not need to follow special precautions such as limiting distance or duration of contact with another individual, children, or pregnant women as is necessary with LDR patients.
5. From a radiobiology perspective, HDR may be favored as treatment delivery over a period of minutes, instead of weeks to months; it does not allow malignant cells to repopulate, advance through the cell cycle, or recover from sublethal damage.

10.3 Early-Stage, Low-Risk Prostate Cancer

According to the National Comprehensive Cancer Network (NCCN) guidelines, low-risk prostate cancer is defined as those patients with stage T1-T2a, Gleason score (GS) ≤6, and PSA < 10 ng/mL [3]. In the modern era, these patients are afforded the opportunity to choose from a variety of appropriately selected treatment options, including active surveillance, radical prostatectomy (RP), EBRT, or brachytherapy as monotherapy with either HDR or LDR treatment. Perhaps, one of the greatest sources of controversy in these patients is determining which patients for whom prostate cancer will never be clinically relevant. The Radiation Therapy Oncology Group (RTOG) is currently partnering with the National Cancer Institute Clinical Trials Group (NCIC) to conduct a phase III randomized trial, randomizing patients to active surveillance versus radical treatment (surgery or radiation therapy) (NCIC 2007). With the current information available to clinicians, one can only hope to make the best recommendations to patients with regard to anticipated side effects and outcomes with each treatment modality and allowing individualized therapy decisions based on this information. In this section, we will focus on the outcomes and possible side effects of HDR brachytherapy as monotherapy.

10.3.1 Brachytherapy as Monotherapy

Brachytherapy as monotherapy is a viable option for appropriately selected low-risk early-stage prostate cancer patients. As previously discussed, this modality may be delivered as HDR or LDR treatments. William Beaumont Hospital (WBH), Michigan [4] and the Cleveland Clinic Foundation [5] have reported single institution experiences with similar outcomes for favorable-risk patients undergoing either EBRT or RP. Several other institutions have reported that patients undergoing interstitial brachytherapy have similar biochemical control rates when compared to reports of patients who have been treated with EBRT or RP [6–11]. Currently, the majority of institutions continue to practice LDR technique utilizing ^{103}Pd or ^{125}I while HDR technique, with ^{192}Ir as its radioactive source, has been gaining popularity [12–14].

Based on the radiobiologic advantages of HDR described above, our institution has traditionally used a twice-daily accelerated hypofractionated regimen with intraoperative conformal intensity-modulated dosimetry with transrectal ultrasound (TRUS) guidance. Traditionally, patients have been selected for monotherapy according to protocol guidelines approved by the WBH Human Investigational Committee (HIC). Patient selection for monotherapy includes clinical stage II (T1c-T2b) disease, Gleason score ≤ 7 (3 + 4 or 2 + 5), pretreatment PSA ≤ 15 ng/mL, and prostate size <65 cm^3. Exclusion criteria for monotherapy includes significant transurethral resection of prostate (TURP) defect, significant urinary obstructive symptoms, blood dyscrasias, or collagen vascular disorders. Prior to scheduling of a procedure, each patient is assessed for anatomic criteria by TRUS done in the treatment lithotomy position.

10.3.1.1 Brachytherapy Procedure and Methods

Prior to the procedure, each patient undergoes spinal anesthesia with placement of a Foley catheter under sterile conditions. The patient is then placed into the lithotomy position and the biplanar ultrasound probe is placed in the rectum. The location of the urethra, bladder, and rectum are assessed with TRUS guidance and a contour of the prostate gland is obtained. Needle placement is then done with ultrasound guidance utilizing a predetermined pattern originated by real-time treatment planning computer software "Swift." Figure 10.1a depicts a real-time implant via the Nucletron Swift guidance system. Figure 10.1b depicts the spatial dwell positions that cover the prostate, seminal vesicles, and periprostatic tissues. Once all needles are placed, a cytoscopy is performed by the patient's urologist to ensure no needles entered the bladder. Two-three visicoils are placed in the prostate at the time of the first treatment to verify needle position during subsequent fractions. Figure 10.2a depicts a final dosimetry for HDR monotherapy with excellent conformality coverage of the prostate with sparing of the urethra and rectum. Historically, patients have been given the option of HDR or LDR brachytherapy; however, our recent experience focuses almost exclusively on HDR brachytherapy.

10.3.1.2 The William Beaumont Hospital Experience

We have previously reported the results of LDR and HDR monotherapy patients. Our experience reported by Grills et al. [15] compared not only biochemical control rates of the two techniques, but also that of toxicity. Similar 3-year biochemical control rates were reported between the two techniques (98% HDR, 97% LDR). Significantly lower rates of acute grade 1–3 urinary and gastrointestinal toxicities were reported for HDR versus LDR including dysuria (36% versus 76%), urinary frequency or urgency (54% versus 92%), and

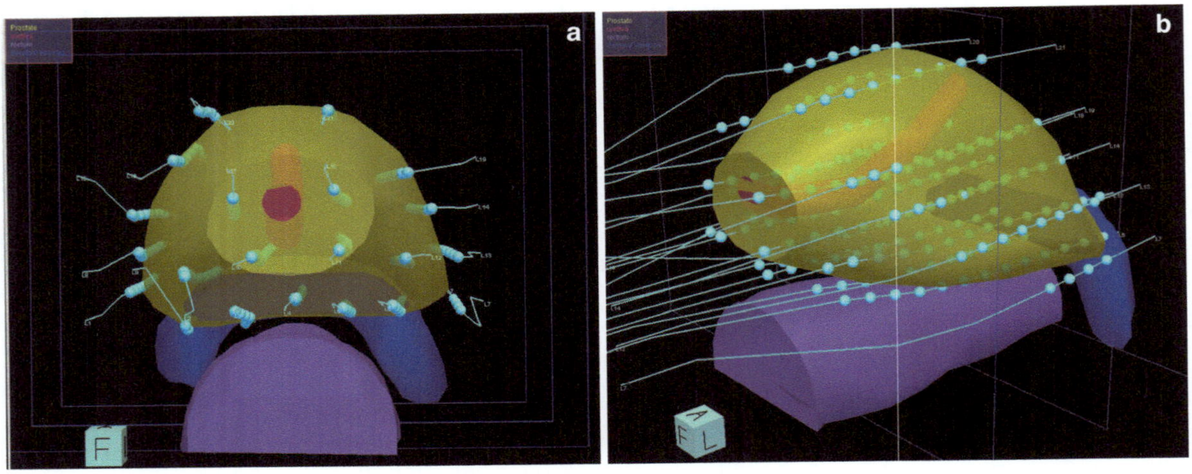

Fig. 10.1 (**a**) Intraoperative 3D rendering of the prostate (*yellow*), urethra (*red*), seminal vesicles (*blue*), and rectum (*purple*) showing ideal needle positions and the spatial dwell positions. (**b**) Real-time 3D TRUS image depicting the HDR spatial dwell positions covering the prostate, seminal vesicles and periprostatic tissues

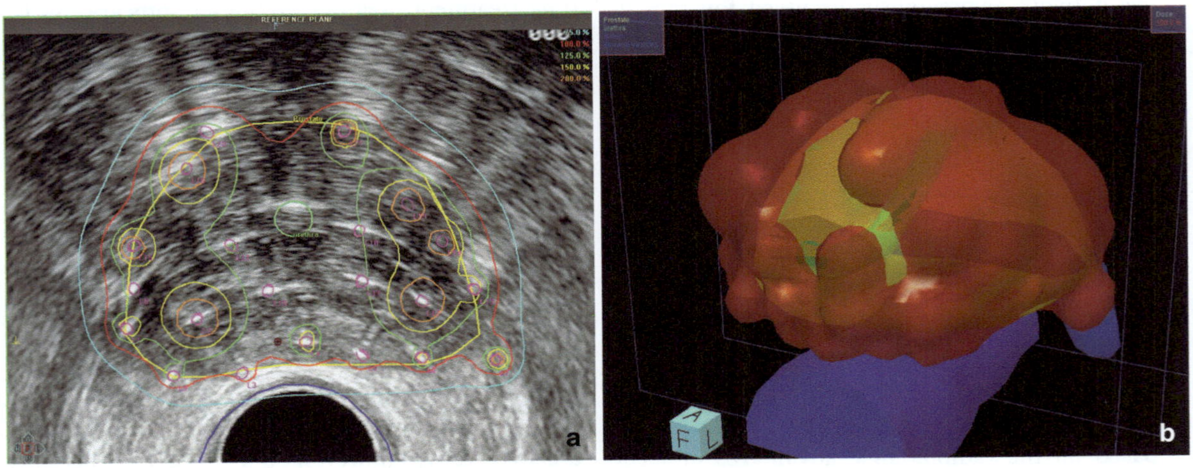

Fig. 10.2 (**a**) Intraoperative final dosimetry with excellent conformality coverage of the prostatic volume (*yellow*) by the 100% isodose line in *red* and 125% isodose line in *green*. (**b**) 3D dose cloud rendering of the 100% isodose line in *red*, sparing the urethra and rectum

rectal pain (6% versus 20%). There was a significantly lower rate of chronic urinary frequency or urgency for the HDR group (32% versus 56%). An important finding for many men considering brachytherapy was that of a nearly three-fold decrease in the 3-year actuarial impotence rate among the HDR alone group (16% versus 45%).

Similarly, we recently reported results regarding success of HDR as monotherapy for favorable prostate cancer [16]. We reviewed 248 patients treated with HDR to a dose of 38 Gy in four fractions twice daily at William Beaumont Hospital (WBH), and 42 Gy in six fractions in two separate implants 1 week apart at California Endocurietherapy Cancer Center (CET) versus 206 patients treated with LDR brachytherapy at WBH. Review of these patients showed that although the 5-year biochemical control rates (Phoenix definition) were not significantly different (89% WBH-LDR, 91% WBH-HDR, 88% CET-HDR), HDR was associated with less acute and chronic genitourinary (GU) and gastrointestinal (GI) toxicities.

Here, we review the results of 474 patients treated during 1999–2010 with HDR brachytherapy as monotherapy at WBH. Acute GU and GI toxicities were analyzed for 264 patients and chronic toxicity for 233 patients who had longer than 6 months and more than two PSA follow-ups. WBH patients were treated with three different fractionation schemes according to a dose escalation trial. One hundred and eighty-nine patients were treated with a prescription dose of 38 Gy in four fractions done as a single implant with treatments twice daily, with a minimum inter-fraction time of 6 h. The prescribed dose was based on an assumed α/β ratio of 3 corresponding to an EBRT minimum tumor dose of 74 Gy with 2.0 Gy/fraction. Progressively, we have investigated decreasing the overall number of fractions with a corresponding increase in dose per fraction. As such, 63 patients were treated with two 12-Gy fractions with the treatment delivered as above. An additional 70 patients were treated with two 13.5-Gy fractions with a single implant. At the time of publication, our protocol was set to investigate HDR single-fraction therapy at a dose of 19 Gy. TRUS-guided planning was used with the dose being delivered to the prostate alone without additional margins.

Overall, the low-risk group of patients had a mean follow-up of 3.3 years (range, 0.01–10.8 years) with a median stage of T1c, Gleason 6 (range, 3–6), and mean pre-treatment PSA of 4.8 ng/ml (range, 0.7–9.9 ng/ml). Toxicity was scored according to CTC version 3.0. Review of acute toxicities showed a single event of grade 4 urinary retention in the 9.5 Gy × 4 group. The most frequent acute toxicity was that of increased urinary frequency and urgency across all treatment groups. There was no significant difference in acute GI or GU toxicity among treatment groups except for an increased rate of grade 2 hematuria for the 13.5 Gy × 2 group ($p = 0.002$). Table 10.1a, b summarize acute grade 1–2 and acute grade 3–4 GU toxicities, respectively. Table 10.2 summarizes acute GI toxicities.

With regard to chronic toxicity rates were excellent with no chronic grade 4 urinary toxicities reported and low rates of grade 1–3 GI and GU toxicities. Table 10.3a summarizes chronic grade 1–2 GU toxicity for all patients, and Table 10.3b summarizes grade 3–4 GU toxicity. The most common toxicities were low-grade urinary frequency and/or urgency, and impotence. There was an increased rate of grade 1 dysuria among the 12 Gy × 2 group versus other treatment regimens. Additionally, there seemed to be an increased rate of grade 2 impotence in the 13.5 Gy × 2 group as compared to other fractionation schemes. Table 10.4a, b show the rates of grade 1–2 and grade 3–4 chronic GI toxicity among each treatment group. The rate of chronic high-grade GI toxicity among all groups was ≤1%. Overall, this study shows that even with increased hypofractionation regimens for HDR monotherapy, there is an acceptable rate of acute toxicity with minimal high-grade toxicity seen. Figure 10.3 shows Kaplan–Meier curve of OS, cause-specific survival, and BC rates for all patients. This study further supports the use of HDR brachytherapy as monotherapy with excellent rates of disease control and with well tolerated side effects.

Table 10.1 Acute grades 1 & 2 (a) and grades 3 & 4 (b) GU toxicity for low-risk patients treated with HDR monotherapy at WBH

(a)						
	9.5 Gy × 4 (%)		12 Gy × 2 (%)		13.5 Gy × 2 (%)	
Toxicity/grade	1	2	1	2	1	2
Dysuria	30	8	18	5	19	5
Frequency/urgency	38	15	29	18	31	20
Urinary retention	16	12	24	5	14	0
Incontinence	5	2	0	0	0	0
Hematuria	6	0	3	0	0	9
(b)						
	9.5 Gy × 4 (%)		12 Gy × 2 (%)		13.5 Gy × 2 (%)	
Toxicity/grade	3	4	3	4	3	4
Dysuria	0	0	3	0	0	0
Frequency/urgency	5	0	0	0	3	0
Urinary retention	1.5	0.5	0	0	0	0
Incontinence	0.5	0	0	0	0	0
Hematuria	0	0	0	0	0	0

Table 10.2 Acute GI toxicity for low-risk patients treated with HDR monotherapy at WBH

	9.5 Gy × 4 (%)		12 Gy × 2 (%)		13.5 Gy × 2 (%)	
Toxicity/grade	1	2	1	2	1	2
Diarrhea	10	2	8	0	5	0
Rectal bleeding	2	0	0	0	0	0
Proctitis	0.8	0.8	0	0	0	3
Rectal pain/tenesmus	6.5	0.5	5	0	0	3
Rectal fistula	0	0	0	0	0	0
Anal fissure	0	0	0	0	0	0

Table 10.3 Grades 1 & 2 (a) and grades 3 & 4 (b) chronic GU toxicity for low-risk patients treated with HDR monotherapy at WBH

(a)	9.5 Gy × 4 (%)		12 Gy × 2 (%)		13.5 Gy × 2 (%)	
Toxicity/grade	1	2	1	2	1	2
Dysuria	1	2	13	0	4	3
Frequency/urgency	20	4	16	2	29	8
Urinary retention	7	0	5	0	13	0
Incontinence	2	0	0	0	3	0
Hematuria	2	0	2	0	0	3
Urethral stricture	0	0	0	0	1	1
Impotence ($n = 206$)	25	15	25	3	8	23

(b)	9.5 Gy × 4 (%)		12 Gy × 2 (%)		13.5 Gy × 2 (%)	
Toxicity/grade	3	4	3	4	3	4
Dysuria	0	0	2	0	0	0
Frequency/urgency	0	0	0	0	0	0
Urinary retention	0	0	0	0	0	0
Incontinence	0	0	0	0	0	0
Hematuria	0	0	0	0	0	0
Urethral stricture	0	0	0	0	0	0

Table 10.4 Grades 1 & 2 (a) and grades 3 & 4 (b) chronic GI toxicity for low-risk patients treated with HDR monotherapy at WBH

(a)	9.5 Gy × 4 (%)		12 Gy × 2 (%)		13.5 Gy × 2 (%)	
Toxicity/grade	1	2	1	2	1	2
Diarrhea	1	0	2	2	3	0
Rectal Bleeding	0	0	0	0	0	0
Proctitis	1	0	2	0	0	0
Rectal pain/tenesmus	2	0	0	0	1	0
Rectal fistula	0	0	0	0	0	0
Anal fissure	0	0	0	0	0	0

(b)	9.5 Gy × 4 (%)		12 Gy × 2 (%)		13.5 Gy × 2 (%)	
Toxicity/grade	3	4	3	4	3	4
Diarrhea	0	0	0	0	0	0
Rectal bleeding	0	0	0	0	0	0
Proctitis	0	0	0	0	0	0
Rectal pain/tenesmus	0	0	0	0	0	0
Rectal fistula	0	0	0	0	0	0
Anal fissure	0	0	0	0	0	0

10.4 Intermediate- to High-Risk Prostate Cancer

As compared with low-risk prostate cancer, the management of intermediate- to high-risk disease is far less standardized with a wide variety of treatments including multi-modality approaches in order to improve patient outcomes. Literature regarding treatment of T3 disease with RP [17–19] and/or the use of low-dose EBRT show suboptimal outcomes thus encouraging ongoing research into the treatment of these patients. Ongoing discussions include appropriate selection of patients for surgery versus radiotherapy, and the use of androgen deprivation therapy (ADT) and its appropriate patient population, as well as the duration and timing of these modalities.

Regarding androgen deprivation therapy, the concern regarding previous clinical trials showing a benefit of combined ADT plus radiotherapy is whether the benefit of ADT is secondary to suboptimal radiotherapy. A phase III EORTC trial of patients with T1–2 prostate adenocarcinoma, grade 3 or T3-T4 tumors of any grade were randomized to EBRT alone versus EBRT with long-term androgen deprivation therapy (ADT) with 10-year follow-up [20]. ADT was LHRH agonist, goserelin, which was started on the first day of RT and continued for three years. Cyproterone actetate was started one week before goserelin injection and continued for one month to prevent flare phenomenon. The updated data reports significant improvement in 10-year diseasefree survival (47.7% versus 22.7%) and overall survival (58.1% versus 39.8%) favoring the combined therapy group. These updated results support the current treatment paradigm of combined long term ADT with RT for high risk patients, however the benefit of ADT remains uncertain in intermediate-risk patients. The ongoing RTOG 0815 phase III randomized trial aims to answer this question by randomizing patients undergoing dose-escalated RT with 6 months of short-term ADT versus RT alone.

In EBRT, three approaches have been tested to improve patient outcomes: Neoadjuvant ADT with EBRT [19, 20], addition of particle-beam therapy as a boost to EBRT [21, 22], and dose escalation by 3-dimensional conformal radiotherapy (3D-CRT) [23, 24]. In this section, we will focus on the use of brachytherapy

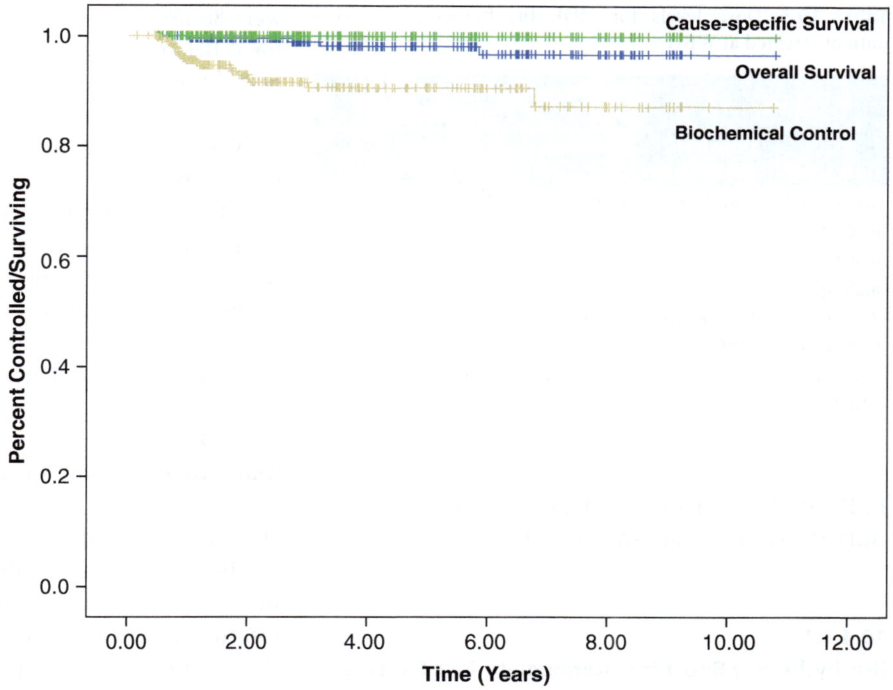

Fig. 10.3 Kaplan–Meier curve of overall survival, cause-specific survival, and biochemical control outcomes for low-risk prostate cancer patients treated with HDR brachytherapy as monotherapy at WBH

boost in addition to 3D-CRT to the pelvis in this patient population as a means of dose escalation [25, 26].

10.4.1 HDR Brachytherapy as a Boost

In 1991, the WBH HIC approved a prospective clinical trial, which was designed to test the hypothesis that for patients with intermediate and/or poor prognostic factors, local failure is related to the large volume of cell mass and radioresistant cell clones, both of which require biologically higher radiation doses than those conventionally used. Thus, we selected a hypofractionated 3D conformal HDR brachytherapy boost as the method of dose escalation in combination with radiotherapy to the pelvis. We have published our results previously [27, 28]. We reported an update combining the data from Kiel University (KU) and WBH, which used similar treatment programs [29]. In this chapter, we report collaborative data from CET, KU, and WBH.

The treatment technique has been previously described by each institution [12, 25–28]. All patients underwent pretreatment pelvic computed tomography (CT) with contrast to assist in defining the prostate and normal tissue volumes. Pelvic EBRT was interdigitated with TRUS-guided transperineal conformal interstitial ^{192}Ir implants. The overall treatment time was compressed to only 5 weeks.

Patients with a prostate gland volume >65 cm^3 or gland length >5.5 cm were initially ineligible for the protocol. These patients underwent downsizing with a short course of hormonal therapy (for less than 6 months) and were analyzed separately [25, 29]. Dosimetry and optimal needle positions within the reference plane were determined intraoperatively using our real-time interactive optimization program [27, 28]. After placement of all needles, cystoscopy was performed to reconfirm the prostate treatment length with adequate depth by virtue of bladder mucosa tenting. To reconfirm the gland apex during cystoscopy, the TRUS probe was placed in the sagittal plane. The veru-montanum (1 cm behind) was used to correlate with the TRUS probe position in the longitudinal plane. On each transverse TRUS image, the 100% isodose line encompassed the contoured prostate volume (Fig. 10.2). The urethra was limited to <125% of the prostate dose and a DVH was used to assess dosimetry quality as seen in Fig. 10.2. The rectal wall dose was limited to 75% of the prostate.

For the WBH patients, dose escalation was used and patients were stratified according to biologic equivalent dose (BED) level. The low dose level was

Table 10.5 Dose levels for HDR brachytherapy boost in patients treated at WBH

		Intermediate risk	High risk patients	BED (Gy)
Dose level	Dose level stratification	# patients (%)	# patients (%)	α/β=1.2
5.50 Gy × 3	Low dose	66 (22%)	48 (27%)	80.2
6.00 Gy × 3				86.1
6.50 Gy × 3				92.5
8.25 Gy × 2				94.2
8.75 Gy × 2	Intermediate dose	97 (32%)	55 (31%)	99.9
9.50 Gy × 2				108.9
10.50 Gy × 2	High dose	138 (46%)	73 (42%)	122.0
11.50 Gy × 2				136.3

BED < 95 Gy and intermediate-high dose level was BED ≥ 95 Gy. BEDs are shown in Table 10.5.

10.4.1.1
Brachytherapy Boost for Intermediate-Risk Patients

The collaborative long-term group included 1,016 patients from CET, KU, and WBH. Patients included in the study had one or more intermediate risk factors as classified by NCCN guidelines (T2b-T2c, or Gleason score 7, or PSA 10–20 ng/ml) and had at least one PSA measurement after treatment completion. Patient characteristics are shown in Table 10.6. For all patients, median age at diagnosis was 67, median pre-treatment PSA 7.6 ng/ml, and median follow-up 4.5 years (range, 0.5–17.0 years). Four hundred and seventy-four patients had 5-year, 216 patients 8-year, and 111 patients had ≥10-year follow-up data. Fifty-six percent of patients had Gleason score <7 versus 44% of patients were with Gleason score of 7 or greater. Significantly more patients in this group had T2b-T2c stage (64%) versus stage T1a-T2b (36%, $p < 0.001$).

Outcomes data at 5 and 10 years is presented for all patients, and by institution, Table 10.7. For all institutions, the 5-year overall survival (OS) was 92.3% and 10 year OS was 79.4%. Cause-specific survival (CSS) at 5 years was 99.0% and 97.5% at 10 years. Local recurrence (LR) rate, calculated by the Kaplan-Meier method, was 1.0% and 2.6% at 5 years and 10 years, respectively. Rate of distant metastases at 5 and 10 years were 2.3% and 4.1%, respectively. Clinical disease-free survival (DFS) was computed utilizing LR, distant metastases (DM), and patient deaths for which 5- and 10-year rates were 88.1% and 71.7%. Biochemical control (BC) data for WBH and CET had combined 5- and 10-year rates of 89.5% versus 81.9%. Figure 10.4 shows Kaplan-Meier curve of OS, CSS, and BC to 10 years for all patients.

Among patients treated at WBH, Table 10.8 shows follow-up and BC rates stratified by dose, low (5.5 Gy × 3–8.25 Gy × 2), intermediate (8.75 Gy × 2–9.50 Gy × 2), and high (10.50 Gy × 2–15 Gy × 2). Five-year BC for the low dose group was 79.4% and 65.0% at 10 years. Intermediate- and high-dose groups had 92.2% and 88.0% BC rates at 5 years and 10-year BC rates were 88.9% and 78.8%, respectively.

10.4.1.2
Brachytherapy Boost for High-Risk Patients

High-risk prostate cancer patients make up the smallest number of treated patients versus low- and intermediate-risk disease. Unfortunately, optimal treatment continues to be a clinical challenge for these patients. Here we present collaborative data for high-risk patients and review pertinent literature regarding HDR boost in combination with EBRT.

Using the NCCN guidelines definition of high-risk disease (≥T3a, Gleason score 8–10, or PSA > 20 ng/ml), we evaluated outcomes of patients treated according to four prospective studies of HDR boost conducted at WBH, CET, KU, and Universidad de Navarra in Spain (UN). The 606 patients had one or more high-risk features with a minimum follow up of 6 months and at least one PSA measurement post treatment. Table 10.9 shows patients characteristics stratified by institution. Median age at diagnosis was 69 years (range, 42–85 years). Median follow-up was 4.4 years (range, 0.7–17.0 years). Sixty-nine patients had 5-year, 147 patients had 8-year and 269 patients had ≥10-year follow-up. Median pre-treatment PSA was 17.8 ng/ml (range, 5.6–418 ng/ml). Gleason score was <8 in 41% of patients versus 59% of patients with Gleason score ≥8. Significantly more patients had a T stage <T2c (60%) versus patients with T stage ≥T2c (40%). Sixty-one percent of the patients had begun hormonal therapy prior to radiation therapy.

Outcomes data for all institutions are presented in Table 10.10, which shows overall survival at 5- and 10-years of 87.9% and 67.1%, respectively. Cause-specific survival for all groups was quite good with rates at 5 years of 94.9% versus 87.4% at 10 years. LR at 5-years was 5.0% versus 9.9% at 10 years. The rate of distant

Table 10.6 Intermediate-risk patient characteristics treated with HDR Boost at CET, KU, and WBH

	All (n = 1,016)	CET (n = 623)	KU (n = 92)	WBH (n = 301)
Age at diagnosis				
Median	67	67	69	67
Mean	66	66	68	67
Range	39–87	39–87	45–83	42–83
≤60	250 (25%)	169 (27%)	18 (20%)	63 (21%)
>60	551 (75%)	454 (73%)	74 (80%)	23 (79%)
Pre-tx PSA (n = 1,015)				
Median	7.6	7.5	7.0	7.9
Mean	8.3	8.2	7.9	8.7
Range	0.37–19.9	0.9–19.7	0.37–19.9	0.4–19.9
<10 ng/ml	719 (71%)	460 (74%)	58 (63%)	201 (67%)
>10–20 ng/ml	296 (29%)	163 (26%)	34 (36%)	99 (33%)
Gleason				
<7	565 (56%)	398 (64%)	41 (45%)	126 (42%)
7	451 (44%)	225 (36%)	51 (55%)	175 (58%)
T-Stage				
T1a-T2b	369 (36%)	447 (72%)	42 (46%)	158 (54%)
T2b-T2c	647 (64%)	176 (28%)	50 (54%)	143 (48%)
Follow-up (years)				
Median	4.5	3.7	4.7	8.0
Mean	5.2	4.0	5.5	7.7
Range	0.5–17.0	0.5–11.0	1.1–15.7	0.5–17.0

Table 10.7 Outcome data at 5 and 10 years for intermediate-risk patients treated with HDR boost

	All		CET (n = 623)		KU (n = 92)		WBH (n = 301)	
	5 years	10 years	5 years	10 years	5 years	10 years	5 years	10 years
Overall survival (%)	92.3	79.4	93.9	82.3	88.9	75.8	91.5	78.6
Cause-specific survival (%)	99.0	97.5	99.6	98.5	98.4	93.7	98.7	97.5
Local recurrence (%)	1.0	2.6	0.2	1.4	2.0	2.6	2.1	4.0
Distant metastases (%)	2.3	4.1	1.2	2.0	7.8	7.8	2.8	5.1
Disease free survival[a] (%)	88.1	71.7	90.0	70.1	82.6	74.2	86.5	71.9
Biochemical control[b] (%)	89.5	81.9	90.7	76.0	–	–	87.9	79.6

[a]Computed as local recurrence, distant metastases, and all patient deaths. Does not include biochemical failures
[b]No PSA sequence for KU

metastases at 5-years was 9.2% and 15.6% at 10 years. Five and 10-year rates of DFS were 76.7% and 51.0%, respectively. Biochemical control rates at 5- and 10-years were 79.2% and 61.1%, respectively (excluding KU due to insufficient available data). Figure 10.5 shows the Kaplan–Meier curve for OS, CSS, and BC for all patients.

At WBH, 48 patients were treated with low dose (5.5 Gy x 3 - 8.25 Gy x 2), and 55 and 73 patients were treated in the intermediate- (8.75 Gy x 2 - 9.5 Gy x 2) and high-dose (10.5 Gy x 2- 11.5 Gy x 2) groups, respectively Table 10.5. Mean follow-up for low-dose patients was 9.8 years, and 8.5 and 6.1 years for the intermediate and high-dose groups, respectively. Five- and 10-year BC rates for low-dose patients were 63.1% and 40.1%, respectively. Intermediate-dose patients had 5- and 10-year BC rates of 76.0% and 65.4% versus the high-dose rates of 86.4% and 63.5%, respectively (Table 10.11).

Recently, we evaluated the 10-year outcome data of patients with localized prostate cancer with high-risk features of Gleason Score 8–10 with promising results for EBRT plus HDR brachytherapy boost (unpublished data by Martinez et al.). This study evaluated four prospective studies of HDR boost conducted at WBH, CET, KU, and

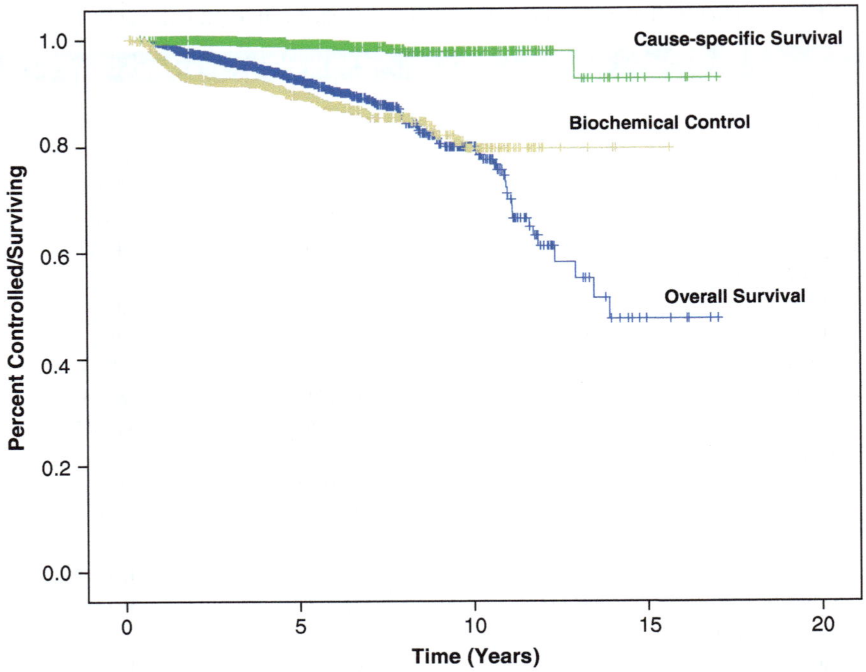

Fig. 10.4 Kaplan–Meier curve of overall survival, cause-specific survival, and biochemical control outcomes for intermediate-risk prostate cancer patients treated with HDR brachytherapy boost in combination with external-beam radiotherapy at CET, KU, and WBH

Table 10.8 Biochemical control rates and follow-up for intermediate-risk patients treated with HDR boost at WBH

	Low-dose group	Intermediate-dose group	High-dose group
Dose group	5.5 Gy × 3–8.25 Gy × 2	8.75 Gy × 2–9.50 Gy × 2	10.50 Gy × 2–15 Gy × 2
Follow-up			
Mean	9.2	8.5	6.4
Median	10.2	9.9	6.8
Range	1.1–17.0	1.6–12.3	0.5–11.0
Biochemical control			
5 years	79.4%	92.2%	88.0%
10 years	65.0%	88.9%	78.8%

UN. Overall, there were a total of 1,910 patients, 488 of whom had a Gleason score of 8–10. Patients were treated with pelvic EBRT to a dose of 46–50.4 Gy with an HDR brachytherapy boost for an overall combined BED of 234–511.7 Gy (presumed α/β ratio of 1.2). Patients had a mean initial PSA of 19.3 ng/ml with a mean follow-up of 5.5 years (134 patients with 8 years or greater follow up). With regard to Gleason score, 70.3% of the patients had Gleason 8, 27.9% had Gleason 9, and 1.8% had Gleason 10 disease. ADT was given in 74.1% of patients.

Overall, this study found a 10-year OS rate of 65.1%, BC rate of 57.4% (Phoenix definition), distant metastasis rate of 22.1%, and clinical failure rate of 28%. Outcomes were further stratified according to initial PSA ≤ 40 versus >40 ng/ml. After stratification, there was a statistically significant difference between groups with respect to OS (67.5% vs. 48.0%), BC (61.8% vs. 0%), freedom from distant metastasis (81.5% vs. 49.5%), cause-specific survival (86.4% vs. 61.9%), and freedom from clinical failure (75.6% vs. 45.9%). Overall, 13% of the patients required adjuvant/salvage ADT. On further analysis, it was found that hormonal therapy didn't improve BC, DM, CSS, or OS; only improvements in freedom from local recurrence and clinical failure at 5 and 10 years were seen. Overall, this study shows good rates of 10-year OS and disease control even in the setting of high initial PSA. This is a prospective study with a large number of patients that may further encourage the study of this subset of patients in a randomized setting.

Table 10.9 High-risk patient characteristics treated with HDR Boost at CET, KU, UN, and WBH

	All ($n=606$)	CET ($n=247$)	KU ($n=111$)	UN ($n=72$)	WBH ($n=176$)
Age at diagnosis					
Median	69	68	69	69	70
Mean	68	68	69	69	69
Range	42–85	42–81	56–84	53–80	44–85
≤60	81 (13%)	32 (13%)	13 (12%)	11 (15%)	25 (14%)
>60	525 (87%)	215 (87%)	98 (88%)	61 (85%)	151 (86%)
Pre-tx PSA (ng/ml)					
Median	17.8	12.2	21.8	22.3	16.8
Mean	23.7	21.9	23.0	23.1	28.2
Range	5.6–418	5.6–345	5.8–120	16.6–34	5.7–418
<20	347 (57%)	170 (69%)	49 (44%)	21 (29%)	107 (61%)
≥20	259 (43%)	77 (31%)	62 (56%)	51 (71%)	69 (39%)
Gleason					
<8	249 (41%)	81 (33%)	61 (55%)	47 (65%)	60 (34%)
≥8	357 (59%)	166 (67%)	50 (45%)	25 (35%)	116 (66%)
T-Stage					
<T2c	362 (60%)	173 (70%)	52 (47%)	25 (35%)	112 (64%)
≥T2c	244 (40%)	74 (30%)	59 (53%)	47 (65%)	64 (36%)
Follow-up (years)					
Median	4.4	4.6	4.3	3.5	4.8
Mean	5.4	5.5	5.0	4.8	5.8
Range	0.7–17.0	0.6–17.0	0.6–15.9	0.8–16.1	0.9–16.3
Pre-RT hormones ($n=453$)					
No	177 (39%)	82 (41%)	22 (30%)	16 (36%)	57 (42%)
Yes	246 (61%)	117 (59%)	51 (70%)	26 (64%)	79 (58%)

Table 10.10 Outcome data at 5 and 10 years for high-risk patients treated with HDR boost

	All ($n=606$) (%)	CET ($n=247$) (%)	KU ($n=111$) (%)	UN ($n=72$) (%)	WBH ($n=176$) (%)
Overall survival					
5 years	87.9	88.8	84.7	88.9	87.4
10 years	67.1	73.5	66.5	–	66.9
Cause specific survival					
5 years	94.9	95.2	91.0	–	95.0
10 years	87.4	88.4	77.1	–	89.9
Local recurrence					
5 years	5.0	0.6	7.8	3.6	8.7
10 years	9.9	0.6	9.9	3.6	15.4
Distant metastases					
5 years	9.2	5.2	24.2	5.5	10
10 years	15.6	19.1	24.2	5.55	14
Disease free survival					
5 years	76.7	81.2	72.5	70.1	74.1
10 years	51.0	35.2	61.1	0	52.4
Biochemical control					
5 years	79.2	82	–	79.1	76.1
10 years	61.1	67.9	–	63.3	57.9

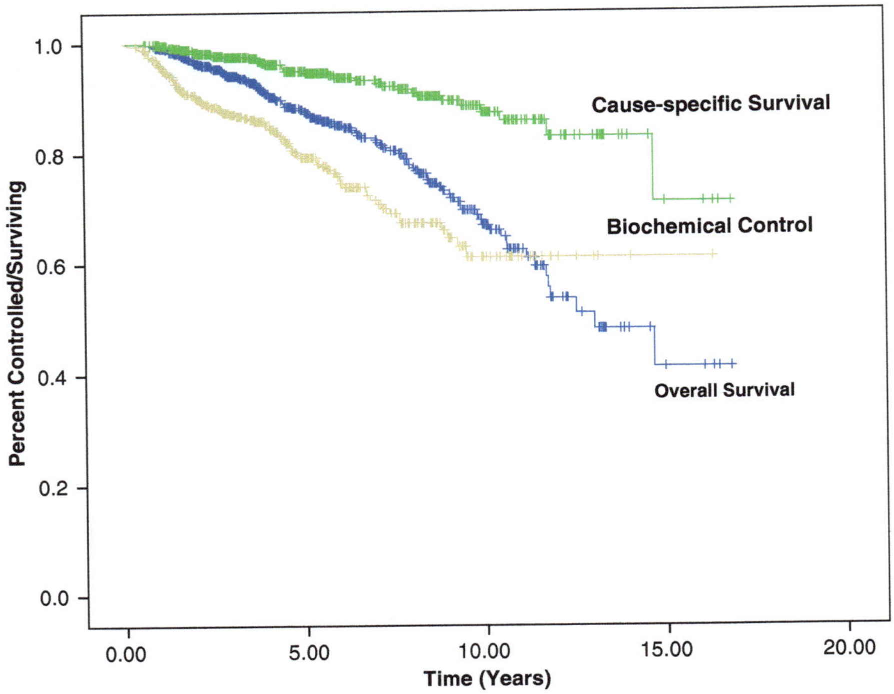

Fig. 10.5 Kaplan–Meier curve of overall survival, cause-specific survival, and biochemical control outcomes for high-risk prostate cancer patients treated with HDR brachytherapy boost in combination with external-beam radiotherapy at CET, KU, UN, and WBH

Table 10.11 Biochemical control rates and follow-up for high-risk patients treated with HDR boost at WBH

	Low-dose group ($n=48$)	Intermediate-dose group ($n=55$)	High-dose group ($n=73$)
Dose group	5.5 Gy × 3–8.25 Gy × 2	8.75 Gy × 2–9.5 Gy × 2	10.50 Gy × 2–15.0 Gy × 2
Follow-up			
Mean	9.8	8.5	6.1
Median	10.6	9.4	6.5
Range	1.9–16.8	1.2–12.7	1.5–10.8
Biochemical control			
5 years	63.1%	76.0%	86.4%
10 years	40.1%	65.4%	63.5%

Further support for brachytherapy boost in the setting of high-risk disease has also been provided by the LDR boost experience at Mt. Sinai [30]. They described a series of 181 patients with Gleason 8–10 prostate cancer treated from 1994 to 2006 with ^{103}Pd to 100 Gy in addition to 45-Gy EBRT and 9 months of ADT. The 8-year outcome data showed an OS of 79%, freedom from DM rate of 80%, freedom from biochemical failure rate of 73% (Phoenix definition), and cause-specific survival of 87%. Similarly, they report that the initial PSA has a significant effect on BC when stratified according to PSA ≤10, >10–20, or >20 ng/ml, with rates of 72%, 82%, and 58%, respectively. This stratification did not correlate to rate of distant metastases. Rather, on multivariate analysis, Gleason score was the only factor to affect the rate of DM, and was a more significant predictor of BC. The BC and freedom from distant metastasis rates for Gleason score 8 were 84% and 86%, Gleason score 9, 55% and 76%, and for Gleason 10, 30% and 30%, respectively. This study provides further long-term data on a large number of patients supporting the use of brachytherapy boost in this patient population.

A retrospective review of surgical patients from Johns Hopkins and the SEARCH database has evaluated whether a subset of high-risk patients would be appropriate candidates for RP as monotherapy [31]. In this study, 220 patients from Johns Hopkins and 149 patients from the SEARCH database were retrospectively reviewed. Favorable surgical pathology outcome was organ-confined disease with final negative margins. Favorable pathology was present in 21% of the Johns Hopkins patients and 41% of the SEARCH patients. On multivariate analysis, elevated initial PSA was the only significant predictor of final pathology in both subsets of patients. Estimated biochemical failure-free survival at 5 and 10 years were 40% and 27% among Johns Hopkins patients, and 32% and 28% among SEARCH patients, respectively. Overall, this study concludes that patients with Gleason score 8–10 are good candidates for multimodality therapy given the high rates of biochemical progression post RP. Analysis of patients with favorable final pathology or Gleason <8 showed biochemical failure rates of ≥50%.

Overall, the literature supports the use of brachytherapy as a boost for intermediate- and high-risk patients. Given the need for multimodality therapy in many of these patients, HDR as boost may provide a viable alternative to surgery in those patients who would be a high-risk for recurrence in the absence of post-operative RT. Further evaluation of these patients is warranted in order to establish best care practices to minimize morbidity while improving patient outcomes.

References

1. Mettlin CJ, Murphy GP, McDonald CJ et al (1999) The National Cancer Data base Report on increased use of brachytherapy for the treatment of patients with prostate carcinoma in the U.S. Cancer 86:1877–1882
2. Lee WR, Moughan J, Owen JB et al (2003) The 1999 patterns of care study of radiotherapy in localized prostate carcinoma: a comprehensive survey of prostate brachytherapy in the United States. Cancer 98:1987–1994
3. Mohler J, Bahnson RR, Boston B et al (2010) NCCN clinical practice guidelines in oncology: prostate cancer. J Natl Compr Canc Netw 8:162–200
4. Martinez AA, Gonzalez JA, Chung AK et al (2000) A comparison of external beam radiation therapy versus radical prostatectomy for patients with low risk prostate carcinoma diagnosed, staged, and treated at a single institution. Cancer 88:425–432
5. Kupelian P, Katcher J, Levin H et al (1997) External beam radiotherapy versus radical prostatectomy for clinical stage T1–2 prostate cancer: therapeutic implications of stratification by pretreatment PSA levels and biopsy Gleason scores. Cancer J Sci Am 3:78–87
6. Blasko JC, Grimm PD, Sylvester JE et al (2000) Palladium-103 brachytherapy for prostate carcinoma. Int J Radiat Oncol Biol Phys 46:839–850
7. D'Amico AV, Whittington R, Malkowicz SB et al (1998) Biochemical outcome after radical prostatectomy, external beam radiation therapy, or interstitial radiation therapy for clinically localized prostate cancer. JAMA 280:969–974
8. Eade TN, Horwitz EM, Ruth K et al (2008) A comparison of acute and chronic toxicity for men with low-risk prostate cancer treated with intensity-modulated radiation therapy or (125) I permanent implant. Int J Radiat Oncol Biol Phys 71:338–345
9. Kupelian PA, Potters L, Khuntia D et al (2004) Radical prostatectomy, external beam radiotherapy <72 Gy, external beam radiotherapy > or =72 Gy, permanent seed implantation, or combined seeds/external beam radiotherapy for stage T1-T2 prostate cancer. Int J Radiat Oncol Biol Phys 58:25–33
10. Stock RG, Stone NN, Tabert A et al (1998) A dose-response study for I-125 prostate implants. Int J Radiat Oncol Biol Phys 41:101–108
11. Wallner K, Merrick G, True L et al (2002) I-125 versus Pd-103 for low-risk prostate cancer: morbidity outcomes from a prospective randomized multicenter trial. Cancer J 8:67–73
12. Demanes DJ, Rodriguez RR, Altieri GA (2000) High dose rate prostate brachytherapy: the California Endocurietherapy (CET) method. Radiother Oncol 57:289–296
13. Martinez AA, Pataki I, Edmundson G et al (2001) Phase II prospective study of the use of conformal high-dose-rate brachytherapy as monotherapy for the treatment of favorable stage prostate cancer: a feasibility report. Int J Radiat Oncol Biol Phys 49:61–69
14. Yoshioka Y, Nose T, Yoshida K et al (2000) High-dose-rate interstitial brachytherapy as a monotherapy for localized prostate cancer: treatment description and preliminary results of a phase I/II clinical trial. Int J Radiat Oncol Biol Phys 48:675–681
15. Grills IS, Martinez AA, Hollander M et al (2004) High dose rate brachytherapy as prostate cancer monotherapy reduces toxicity compared to low dose rate palladium seeds. J Urol 171:1098–1104
16. Martinez AA, Demanes J, Vargas C et al (2010) High-dose-rate prostate brachytherapy: an excellent accelerated-hypofractionated treatment for favorable prostate cancer. Am J Clin Oncol 33:481–488
17. Oefelein MG, Smith ND, Grayhack JT et al (1997) Long-term results of radical retropubic prostatectomy in men with high grade carcinoma of the prostate. J Urol 158:1460–1465
18. Hanks GE, Diamond JJ, Krall JM et al (1987) A ten year follow-up of 682 patients treated for prostate cancer with

radiation therapy in the United States. Int J Radiat Oncol Biol Phys 13:499–505
19. Pilepich MV, Caplan R, Byhardt RW et al (1997) Phase III trial of androgen suppression using goserelin in unfavorable-prognosis carcinoma of the prostate treated with definitive radiotherapy: report of Radiation Therapy Oncology Group Protocol 85–31. J Clin Oncol 15:1013–1021
20. Bolla M, Van Tienhoven G, Warde P et al (2010) External irradiation with or without long-term androgen suppression for prostate cancer with high metastatic risk: 10-year results of an EORTC randomised study. Lancet Oncol 11:1066–1073
21. Forman JD, Duclos M, Sharma R et al (1996) Conformal mixed neutron and photon irradiation in localized and locally advanced prostate cancer: preliminary estimates of the therapeutic ratio. Int J Radiat Oncol Biol Phys 35:259–266
22. Shipley WU, Verhey LJ, Munzenrider JE et al (1995) Advanced prostate cancer: the results of a randomized comparative trial of high dose irradiation boosting with conformal protons compared with conventional dose irradiation using photons alone. Int J Radiat Oncol Biol Phys 32:3–12
23. Zelefsky MJ, Leibel SA, Gaudin PB et al (1998) Dose escalation with three-dimensional conformal radiation therapy affects the outcome in prostate cancer. Int J Radiat Oncol Biol Phys 41:491–500
24. Hanks GE, Lee WR, Hanlon AL et al (1996) Conformal technique dose escalation for prostate cancer: biochemical evidence of improved cancer control with higher doses in patients with pretreatment prostate-specific antigen > or = 10 NG/ML. Int J Radiat Oncol Biol Phys 35:861–868
25. Martinez A, Gonzalez J, Spencer W et al (2003) Conformal high dose rate brachytherapy improves biochemical control and cause specific survival in patients with prostate cancer and poor prognostic factors. J Urol 169:974–979
26. Galalae RM, Martinez A, Mate T et al (2004) Long-term outcome by risk factors using conformal high-dose-rate brachytherapy (HDR-BT) boost with or without neoadjuvant androgen suppression for localized prostate cancer. Int J Radiat Oncol Biol Phys 58:1048–1055
27. Edmundson GK, Rizzo NR, Teahan M et al (1993) Concurrent treatment planning for outpatient high dose rate prostate template implants. Int J Radiat Oncol Biol Phys 27:1215–1223
28. Edmundson GK, Yan D, Martinez AA (1995) Intraoperative optimization of needle placement and dwell times for conformal prostate brachytherapy. Int J Radiat Oncol Biol Phys 33:1257–1263
29. Martinez AA, Demanes DJ, Galalae R et al (2005) Lack of benefit from a short course of androgen deprivation for unfavorable prostate cancer patients treated with an accelerated hypofractionated regime. Int J Radiat Oncol Biol Phys 62:1322–1331
30. Stock RG, Cesaretti JA, Hall SJ et al (2009) Outcomes for patients with high-grade prostate cancer treated with a combination of brachytherapy, external beam radiotherapy and hormonal therapy. BJU Int 104:1631–1636
31. Bastian PJ, Gonzalgo ML, Aronson WJ et al (2006) Clinical and pathologic outcome after radical prostatectomy for prostate cancer patients with a preoperative Gleason sum of 8 to 10. Cancer 107:1265–1272

Stereotactic Treatment for Prostate Cancer: An Overview

11

Mohammad Attar and Eric Lartigau

CONTENTS

11.1 Abstract

In recent years, strong progress in the field of radiotherapy has been made, especially in treatment delivery. Close attention has been paid to prostate cancer in particular because of its high incidence and potential curability. During the last decades, strategies of radiotherapy of prostate cancer have improved with regard to dose escalation, the introduction of modern techniques such as intensity-modulated radiotherapy (IMRT) and hypofractionation by stereotactic techniques, or high-dose-rate (HDR) brachytherapy.

11.2 Rationale for Stereotactic Radiotherapy in Prostate Cancer

Better tumor control has been demonstrated with dose escalation [1–9], but at the expense of some toxicity to the surrounding normal tissues, e.g., bladder and rectum [7–9], which led physicians to seek more sophisticated techniques such as IMRT that may allow increasing the dose to the prostate with some protection of the surrounding sensitive structures, thereby keeping the toxicity to a minimum. Even with these gains, dose escalation efforts were stunted by the need to use relatively large margins around the prostate to account for prostatic motion.

Another interesting issue has been the sensitivity of prostate cancer to the effect of the dose delivered per faction, i.e., the α/β ratio. Several studies suggest that the α/β ratio of prostate cancer is as low as late-responding tissue, unlike the usually high α/β ratio of other tumor cells [10–14]. In some studies, the α/β ratio of prostate cancer was estimated as low as 1.5 Gy [10, 12], which is even lower than the α/β ratio of the surrounding late-responding normal tissues. This means prostate cancer cells are more sensitive to dose per fraction (high EQD_2) than the surrounding normal tissues. Therefore, hypofractionated treatment

L.E. Ponsky et al. (eds.), *Treating Prostate Cancer and Related Genitourinary Applications*, Robotic Radiosurgery,
DOI 10.1007/978-3-642-11495-3_11, © Springer-Verlag Berlin Heidelberg 2012

may increase tumor-cell-killing effect for a lower or similar risk of late toxicity. Hypofractionation has been tried in several randomized studies [15–17] and some have even tried accelerated hypofractionation schedules (five to six fractions).

Substantial late toxicity to bladder and rectum was not observed in the long-term with these accelerated hypofractionation treatments; yet, the importance of accurate treatment delivery with minimal margins has become paramount.

Stereotactic radiotherapy of prostate cancer is used to insure the accuracy of this type of treatment to a localized volume, with limited necessary margins, by using highly precise stereotactic localization systems.

11.3 Techniques of SBRT for Prostate Cancer

Accurate treatment delivery to the prostate with maximal sparing of the normal tissues is not easy, first due to the location of the prostate in the pelvis in contact with the bladder and rectum, and second because of the uncertainty of the prostate's exact position at a given moment. Uncertainty can be due to inter- and intrafraction organ motion and rotation, or due to patient set-up error.

In daily practice, an added margin surrounding the PTV is used to account for this uncertainty. The size of this margin is dictated by the particular technique's precision with which it can localize the prostate, and/or the ability to track its motion. Transabdominal ultrasound and in-room kV-CT have been used for prostate localization. Prostate motion can be tracked radiographically by the insertion of three or four fiducials (markers) in the gland. To this end, portal images are performed before each fraction and compared with the initial planning CT; prostate displacement is calculated by matching the internal fiducials, and the correction is done. Insertion of a balloon filled with a fixed volume of gas into an empty rectum before each fraction can reduce any geometric uncertainties related to the effect of rectal condition. Other immobilization systems or devices, such as a customized vacuum mattress, can also help decrease set-up error.

Stereotactic body radiotherapy (SBRT) with prostate markers can be performed with non-dedicated linear accelerators, or with the linear accelerator-based robotic radiosurgery system, CyberKnife® Accuray Incorporated, Sunnyvale, CA). CyberKnife is the only integrated system capable of target position verification, real-time tracking, and automatic correction during delivery of treatment. Other methods used for tracking the prostate include BeamCath® (Beampoint AB, Kista, Sweden) and Calypso® System (Calypso Medical Technologies, Inc., Seattle, WA).

Stereotactic radiotherapy of prostate may be exclusive or concomitant with standard external-beam radiation as a boost. Because of its assumed accuracy, SBRT is usually delivered in small number of fractions (three to five fractions) with high dose intensity.

11.4 Feasibility and Accuracy of SBRT

Almost all SBRT studies for prostate cancer are relatively recent, attempting to integrate the radiobiological features of prostate cancer with the most developed treatment techniques and technologies to achieve the most convenient treatment. Although these studies are relatively recent, their early results are encouraging.

The feasibility of what its authors called "Stereotactic Hypofractionated Accurate Radiotherapy" or SHARP was evaluated in a phase I/II trial performed for localized prostate cancer using 33.5 Gy in five fractions [18]. Forty patients were treated with an extracranial stereotactic radiotherapy technique suitable for prostate cancer; three fiducial markers were implanted in the gland to help daily treatment positioning. Patients were treated in a flex-prone position on a custom cushion. Treatment was delivered with six stationary noncoplanar fields. Acute and late genitourinary and gastrointestinal toxicity levels were evaluated, in addition to the PSA values and the self-reported sexual function at specific follow-up intervals (all will be discussed later in this chapter). The authors' conclusion was to the effect that "SHARP" was feasible, with minimal acute and late toxicity, for localized prostate cancer.

The technical feasibility of radiotherapy for localized prostate cancer by CyberKnife was demonstrated in the study by C. King [19]. Inverse planning was used to design a radiotherapy course for localized prostate cancer. Conformal isodose lines and dose volume histograms (DVH) were compared with an optimized IMRT plan delivered to the study patient. In this report, DVHs produced by CyberKnife were superior for sparing rectum and bladder, and target coverage, with same degree of dose heterogeneities as the IMRT plan, which could allow further dose escalation while keeping normal tissue doses under current IMRT tolerances.

Not only the efficiency of CyberKnife in delivering conformal therapy with steep gradients have been demonstrated [20, 21], but this feature is also comparable to other established treatments for prostate cancer, e.g., HDR brachytherapy and IMRT.

Dose gradients between the target and the normal tissue interface were compared between two treatment modalities, CyberKnife and IMRT, for prostate cancer [22]. In this study, patients treated with CyberKnife underwent repeat planning for IMRT treatments with nine fixed fields, using the same contours and dose volume constraints. The dose fall-off, conformity index, and homogeneity index were calculated for the two modalities. Dose-volume constraints for the bladder and rectum satisfied the specific planning requirements in all plans, and there was no significant difference observed between the CyberKnife plans and IMRT plans for the average $V_{50\%}$, $V_{60\%}$, $V_{75\%}$, and $V_{80\%}$. For the average $V_{30\%}$ and $V_{40\%}$, there was no significant difference for bladder exposure, but for the rectum, these averages were significantly reduced with CyberKnife plans compared with those with IMRT plans ($p \leq 0.01$). The conformity index (CI) values were 1.18 ± 0.08 and 1.44 ± 0.11 for CyberKnife plans and IMRT plans, respectively, reflecting a significantly better conformity with CyberKnife ($p \leq 0.01$). The homogeneity index (HI) value was 1.45 ± 0.12 for CyberKnife plans and 1.28 ± 0.06 for IMRT plans. The mean HI values were smaller in IMRT plans, and the difference was significant ($p = 0.01$). The dose fall-off was compared between the two plans by the value percentage of dose fall-off per millimeter (PDF/mm), and the result demonstrated that the PDF/mm across the 20-mm expanse of region was similar in the two plans, but posteriorly, the PDF/mm showed a significant difference in the favor of the CyberKnife plans, indicating that the dose fall-off was slightly steeper posteriorly for CyberKnife plans than for IMRT plans. In conclusion, CyberKnife can possess a dose gradient that is equivalent to that of a high-number-of-field (e.g., nine-field) IMRT treatment, and, as mentioned above, SBRT by CyberKnife showed superior bladder and rectal sparing compared with IMRT [19].

Hypofractionation treatment with large doses per fraction can be delivered to the prostate with high-dose-rate (HDR) brachytherapy, which is a precise and powerful technique. It is a demonstrably effective treatment method for prostate cancer [23–26], and is widely used as monotherapy for early-stage prostate cancer [23, 27], or in combination with external-beam radiotherapy (EBRT) for more advanced cases [24–26]. Stereotactic hypofractionated radiotherapy by CyberKnife was also compared with a simulated treatment plan for HDR brachytherapy [28]. PTV coverage by prescribed dose was similar for both plans, whereas the percentage of volume of interest that received a higher-than-prescribed dose ($V_{125\%}$ and $V_{150\%}$) was larger for HDR. Urethral dose was lower for CyberKnife. Bladder maximum doses were higher for HDR, but bladder dose fall-off under the maximum dose was also more rapid with HDR. Maximum rectal wall doses were similar, but the rectal dose fall-off beyond the maximum dose region was sharper with CyberKnife. The obvious advantage of a CyberKnife treatment over an HDR Brachytherapy treatment is the CyberKnife treatment's non-invasive nature. The authors concluded that it was feasible to construct CyberKnife treatment plans that closely recapitulated HDR dosimetry and deliver the treatment noninvasively.

Because of its efficacy in organ motion tracking, its ability of automatic correction of displacement, and its capability of delivering high doses per fraction with conformal target coverage and better sparing of critical organs, CyberKnife has been used in many studies of stereotactic radiotherapy for prostate cancer [28–32].

11.5 Toxicity of SBRT for Prostate Cancer

The toxicity of radiotherapy is caused by the sensitivity of nearby critical structures to radiation. In the case of prostate cancer, likely complications of a radiation therapy are genitourinary (GU) toxicity, gastrointestinal (GI) toxicity, and erectile dysfunction. Several scoring criteria or questionnaires are used in the literature to evaluate these toxicities. Some of the more commonly used are listed below:

- RTOG/EORTC Toxicity Criteria
- Common Toxicity Criteria (CTC) of the National Cancer Institute of Canada

- Common Terminology Criteria for Adverse Events (CTCAE)
- International Prostate Symptom Score (IPSS)
- Expanded Prostate Cancer Index Composite (EPIC)

11.5.1 Bladder and Rectal Toxicity

Radiation-induced toxicities can be either acute or late. These two types of toxicities have distinct features and pathophysiological mechanisms. The post-radiation period during which late effects may start is not precisely defined; however, 3–6 months after radiation is generally accepted.

The α/β value of late bladder and rectal toxicity is estimated to be higher than that of prostate, and is suggested to be somewhere between a typical late effect ratio (typical α/β value: 1–3 Gy) and the classic early-response value (typical α/β value: 8–10 Gy). The estimated α/β value for RTOG grade ≥2 late rectal toxicity is 5.4 ± 1.5 Gy [33]. That means the late-responding tissue of bladder and rectum are sensitive to dose per fraction, but less so than prostate cancer. Therefore, with stereotactic radiotherapy for prostate cancer using extreme hypofractionation with high doses per fraction, late toxicity of bladder and rectum may be expected. At the same time, after such a treatment, the equivalent biological dose at a 2-Gy per fraction rate (EQD2) delivered to the prostate would be remarkably higher than that delivered to the surrounding normal tissue. This fact, along with the small margins used in such highly precise, conformal treatments, makes late toxicity likely remain within the acceptable range.

Unlike acute toxicity, which is evaluated during the radiation therapy or the short period after radiation, late toxicity requires long term follow-up to correctly confirm the safety of any treatment. The clinical data available so far suggests that hypofractionated treatments with doses per fraction in the range of 2.5–10.5 Gy are equivalent in toxicity; however, longer follow-up than currently available is needed to confirm this.

In the SHARP study [18], 40 patients were treated with 33.5 Gy in five fraction of 6.7 Gy in five consecutive days. Median follow-up was 41 months. As far as acute GU toxicity, in about 50% of the patients, Grade 1 or 2 toxicities were noted, with one Grade 3 toxicity (urinary retention requiring catheterization). Regarding GI toxicity, 61% of the patients had no toxicity, 39% had Grade 1 or 2 toxicity, and no Grade 3 or 4 toxicities were noted. As far as late toxicity, no Grade 3 or higher GU or GI toxicities were reported, while 20% and 7.5% of the patients had Grade 2 late GU and GI toxicity, respectively. Therefore, both acute and late GU and GI toxicities could be considered acceptable.

In a prospective Phase II clinical trial by C.R. King [32], 41 low-risk prostate cancer patients received 36.25 Gy in five fractions of 7.25 Gy using the CyberKnife. The first 21 patients were treated in five consecutive days, and the remainder three times per week subsequently. Median follow-up was 33 months (range, 6–45 months), GU and GI toxicity were recorded using the RTOG criteria, and IPSS and EPIC were used to record the quality of life (QOL) data at baseline and during follow-up. No Grade 3 or 4 late GI toxicities were encountered; although two patients experienced Grade 3 late GU toxicity, no patient had a Grade 4 complication. Urinary QOL deteriorated at 3 months, but it recovered to and improved over the baseline at 1 and 2 years, respectively. The rectal QOL deteriorated somewhat at 3 months, but never reached a QOL score of 5. The fact that 89% of the patients had score 1 rectal QOL at baseline, and about half of them still had score 2 or 3 at years 1 and 2, suggests a residual long-term low-level rectal toxicity. There was a significant improvement in late rectal toxicity in patients who received every-other-day treatments compared with those that were treated daily. These encouraging early and late toxicity results need longer follow-up to confirm.

Similar results with similar regimens have been demonstrated in several other studies [28–31].

11.5.2 Sexual Function

The mechanism of radiation-induced erectile dysfunction (ED) is complicated and not well understood. Several factors can contribute to this effect, such as treatment-related toxicity, age, comorbidities, and psychological factors. Sexual function usually is evaluated by self-assessment questionnaire, and EPIC (sexual domain) is commonly used. ED is the most commonly identified measurable endpoint for evaluating sexual function. ED among healthy men is mainly associated with age. In a study among healthy men, the prevalence of complete impotence was 5% and 15% at ages 40 and 70, respectively, and the prevalence of moderate impotence was 17% and 34% at ages 40 and 70, respectively. ED has been evaluated following different radiation treatment modalities. Among men in their late 60s without ED at baseline according to self-assessment questionnaires, ED was noted in 35–54% after EBRT [34–37], in 30% after Iodine-125 brachytherapy [38], and in 40–47% after HDR brachytherapy combined with EBRT [39, 40]. Sexual function after SBRT for prostate cancer has been evaluated in few studies [18, 29, 30].

A separate report of King et al. [32] study analyzing sexual function of 32 consecutive patients has been published [41]. These patients were followed at 3- to 6-month intervals with a validated QOL questionnaire using the EPIC form, for a minimum follow-up of 12 months. None of the patients had prior treatment with androgen deprivation therapy (ADT). The median age of the patients was 67.5 years (range, 57–83 years), and the median follow-up was 35.5 months (range, 12–62 months). One patient (3%) was using ED medication, and at last follow-up, there were eight patients (25%) on medication, with a median time to initiation of ED medication of 18 months after radiation. The data from the questionnaire was analyzed in three categories: Sexual summary score, sexual function sub-domain, and sexual bother sub-domain. All scores declined progressively after treatment. ED (erection not adequate for intercourse) was noted in 38% at baseline, which progressed to 71% at 50-month follow-up ($p=0.024$). For the subset of patients without ED at baseline, 22% developed ED at 1 year and 71% at a median follow-up of 4 years. For patients with age <70 years at follow-up, 60% maintained satisfactory erectile function after treatment compared with only 12% of patients with age ≥70 years ($p=0.008$). The author concluded that the frequency of ED after SBRT for prostate cancer was comparable with the upper end of published reports for other modalities of radiotherapy alone without ADT. Age appears to be a major factor for ED in treated patients.

11.6 Efficacy of SBRT for Prostate Cancer

The main objective of radiotherapy is to deliver a maximum dose to the tumor while sparing the normal tissue as much as possible. This should increase the probability of tumor control and decrease normal tissue complication probability. The principle of SBRT for prostate cancer is to deliver a highly toxic dose to the prostate in a very precise manner that insures maximum sparing of bladder and rectum to match the radiobiological features of the tumor cells and normal tissue to achieve highest tumor control with minimum toxicity, i.e., a high therapeutic ratio.

Tumor control for prostate cancer is usually measured by observation of the level of Prostate Specific Antigen (PSA). After a therapeutic irradiation, the blood levels of PSA decline progressively to reach its lowest level known as the PSA nadir. The biochemical criteria used by the American Society of Therapeutic Radiology and Oncology (ASTRO) to define a biochemical failure mentions three consecutive higher PSA readings following a PSA nadir. A more recent and acceptable definition is the Phoenix definition, which defines a biochemical failure as a rise of PSA by 2 ng/ml or more above the nadir. As all studies of SBRT for prostate cancer are recent, patient follow-up is relatively short to determine the PSA response from the published results. Nevertheless, the results are encouraging.

Katz et al. [29] have published their preliminary results following SBRT treatment for 304 patients with localized prostate cancer. Two regimens, consisting of 36.25 Gy in five fractions (7.25 Gy per fraction) and 35 Gy in five fractions (7 Gy per fraction), were delivered to 354 and 50 patients, respectively. Median follow-up was 30 months (range, 26–37 months). PSA analysis was limited to patients with a minimum 12-month follow-up and who did not receive ADT. The mean PSA decreased progressively after treatment, and the overall PSA response was similar in the two different treatment doses. At 24-month follow-up, 88% and 65% of the patients who received 35 Gy achieved <1 ng/ml and <0.5 ng/ml, respectively; and the 36.25-Gy cohort achieved the corresponding percentages of 81% and 66%. Four biochemical failures occurred, which were treated with the higher dose. No biochemical failures were reported in the group who received 35 Gy. In the study of King et al. [32], the pattern of PSA readings was highly encouraging. At a median follow-up of 33 months (range, 6–45 months), no biochemical failure was noted, and 78% of the patients with a minimum of 12-month follow-up achieved a PSA nadir of 0.4 ng/ml. They also observed that the PSA nadir achieved was progressively lower with the time, up to 3 years. Other studies reported similar encouraging results [18, 28, 30].

11.7 SBRT Boost to the Prostate

Unlike other conformal radiotherapy techniques, e.g., IMRT and Tomotherapy® (Tomotherapy Inc., Madison, WI), SBRT treatment can only be applied to small volumes. In cases that need larger treatment volumes, such as pelvic irradiation in more advanced prostate cancer, or when it is difficult to give the entire treatment dose with SBRT techniques, SBRT can be performed to escalate the dose to the prostate after the standard EBRT. Only limited data is found in the literature about the use of SBRT as a complement to standard EBRT. Similar to the notion of HDR brachytherapy boost for prostate cancer, the use of SBRT techniques to escalate the dose to the prostate seems to be reasonable.

As early as the year 2000, Gleinitz et al. proposed daily CT planning for boost irradiation of prostate cancer, using the BrainLAB ExacTrac positioning system® and found the practice feasible yet time-consuming [42]. In 2002, Fransson et al. added a 4- to 8-Gy boost using the BeamCath® technology (BeamPoint AB, Umea, Sweden) for the treatment of 195 patients with 70-Gy conventional EBRT. Another 168-patient cohort was treated only with the conventional EBRT regimen. It was observed that the boost did not result in an increase in late GI or GU side effects at 1 or 3 years post-therapy [43]. More recently, in a dose escalation study involving fixed-dose conventional fractionation followed by increasing doses of two-fraction boost, the incidence and severity of observed toxicities did not correlate with the dose level.

Miralbell et al. [44] have published their preliminary results for hypofractionated boost to the dominant tumor region with stereotactic IMRT for prostate cancer. Fifty patients received 64–64.4 Gy by conventional fractionation, then treated by hypofractionated IMRT boost under stereotactic conditions using inflated rectal balloons, customized vacuum body casts, and metallic infrared reflecting markers. Twenty-one patients received two fractions of 5, 6, or 7 Gy, corresponding to the normalized total doses in 2-Gy per fraction (NTD2) of <100 Gy (the low-dose group), whereas the remaining 29 patients received two fractions of 8 Gy resulting in an NTD2 of >100 Gy (the high-dose group). The tumor-bearing zone was defined by information gathered from endorectal MRI (erMRI), biopsy, and digital rectal examination (DRE). The authors concluded that this type of dose escalation (82–104 NTD2) delivered as IMRT hypofractionation boost under stereotactic conditions was feasible with excellent outcomes. Urinary toxicity was moderate, but its prevalence was increasing with time. Grade 2 and 3 late rectal toxicities were similar to those typical with 74–79 Gy of conventionally fractionated EBRT.

In another study by Katz et al., 73 intermediate- or high-risk patients were treated with a boost of 18–21 Gy delivered in three fractions following a conventional delivery of 45 Gy. The results were described as safe and feasible with minimal acute toxicity and promising biochemical control [45]. Two more studies employing post-IMRT SBRT boost from Georgetown University Hospital and University of California San Francisco have reported similar results [46, 47].

As shown earlier in this chapter, CyberKnife is capable of delivering radiotherapy plans similar to those of HDR brachytherapy [28], which have also been used in combination with EBRT [24–26]. Therefore, following from this logic, SBRT could also be used as a boost to the prostate after standard EBRT with the added advantages of a non-invasive treatment. A phase II prospective study was proposed by the CLCC Oscar-Lambret Institute to evaluate the benefits of stereotactic hypofractionated boost by CyberKnife for intermediate-risk prostate cancer after conventionally fractionated EBRT to the prostate [48].

11.8 SBRT and Recurrence

The standard treatment for local failure after prostate irradiation is salvage surgery. But if surgery is contraindicated, could SBRT be an alternative treatment? There are only two recently published studies about SBRT in these cases, and several issues should be considered: delay of failure, previous prostate radiotherapy treatment, volume to be re-irradiated, and the dose and fractionation that should be used. All these issues make the answer for this question difficult with little and immature data in the literature [49, 50].

The second of the two studies, which was an update of the first study, concerned 15 patients re-irradiated for local recurrence with CyberKnife with 30 Gy in five fractions. The regimen resulted in a low toxicity profile; yet, five of the patients demonstrated disease progression despite in-field disease control [50].

References

1. Hanks GE, Martz KL, Diamond JJ (1988) The effect of dose on local control of prostate cancer. Int J Radiat Oncol Biol Phys 15:1299–1305
2. Zelefsky MJ, Leibel SA, Gaudin PB et al (1998) Dose escalation with three-dimensional conformal radiation therapy affects the outcome in prostate cancer. Int J Radiat Oncol Biol Phys 41:491–500
3. Vicini FA, Abner A, Baglan KL et al (2001) Defining a dose-response relationship with radiotherapy for prostate cancer: is more really better? Int J Radiat Oncol Biol Phys 51:1200–1208
4. Fiveash JB, Hanks G, Roach M et al (2000) 3D conformal radiation therapy (3DCRT) for high grade prostate cancer: a multi-institutional review. Int J Radiat Oncol Biol Phys 47:335–342
5. Hanks GE, Hanlon AL, Epstein B et al (2002) Dose response in prostate cancer with 8–12 years' follow-up. Int J Radiat Oncol Biol Phys 54:427–435
6. Kupelian P, Kuban D, Thames H et al (2005) Improved biochemical relapse-free survival with increased external radiation doses in patients with localized prostate cancer: the combined experience of nine institutions in patients treated in 1994 and 1995. Int J Radiat Oncol Biol Phys 61:415–419
7. Sathya JR, Davis IR, Julian JA et al (2005) Randomized trial comparing iridium implant plus external-beam radiation therapy with external-beam radiation therapy alone in node-negative locally advanced cancer of the prostate. J Clin Oncol 23:1192–1199
8. Pollack A, Zagars GK, Starkschall G et al (2002) Prostate cancer radiation dose response: results of the M. D. Anderson phase III randomized trial. Int J Radiat Oncol Biol Phys 53:1097–1105
9. Zietman AL, DeSilvio ML, Slater JD et al (2005) Comparison of conventional-dose vs high-dose conformal radiation therapy in clinically localized adenocarcinoma of the prostate: a randomized controlled trial. JAMA 294:1233–1239
10. Brenner DJ, Hall EJ (1999) Fractionation and protraction for radiotherapy of prostate carcinoma. Int J Radiat Oncol Biol Phys 43:1095–1101
11. King CR, Mayo CS (2000) Is the prostrate alpha/beta ratio of 1.5 from Brenner & Hall a modeling artifact. Int J Radiat Oncol Biol Phys 47:536–539
12. Fowler J, Chappell R, Ritter M (2001) Is alpha/beta for prostate tumors really low? Int J Radiat Oncol Biol Phys 50: 1021–1031
13. Brenner DJ, Martinez AA, Edmundson GK et al (2002) Direct evidence that prostate tumors show high sensitivity to fractionation (low alpha/beta ratio), similar to late-responding normal tissue. Int J Radiat Oncol Biol Phys 52:6–13
14. Wang JZ, Guerrero M, Li XA (2003) How low is the alpha/beta ratio for prostate cancer? Int J Radiat Oncol Biol Phys 55:194–203
15. Miles EF, Lee WR (2008) Hypofractionation for prostate cancer: a critical review. Semin Radiat Oncol 18:41–47
16. Ritter M (2008) Rationale, conduct, and outcome using hypofractionated radiotherapy in prostate cancer. Semin Radiat Oncol 18:249–256
17. Macias V, Biete A (2009) Hypofractionated radiotherapy for localised prostate cancer. Review of clinical trials. Clin Transl Oncol 11:437–445
18. Madsen BL, Hsi RA, Pham HT et al (2007) Stereotactic hypofractionated accurate radiotherapy of the prostate (SHARP), 33.5 Gy in five fractions for localized disease: first clinical trial results. Int J Radiat Oncol Biol Phys 67:1099–1105
19. King CR, Lehmann J, Adler JR et al (2003) CyberKnife radiotherapy for localized prostate cancer: rationale and technical feasibility. Technol Cancer Res Treat 2:25–30
20. Webb S (1999) Conformal intensity-modulated radiotherapy (IMRT) delivered by robotic linac-testing IMRT to the limit? Phys Med Biol 44:1639–1654
21. Yu C, Jozsef G, Apuzzo ML et al (2003) Dosimetric comparison of CyberKnife with other radiosurgical modalities for an ellipsoidal target. Neurosurgery 53:1155–1162; discussion 1162–1153
22. Hossain S, Xia P, Huang K et al (2010) Dose gradient near target-normal structure interface for nonisocentric CyberKnife and isocentric intensity-modulated body radiotherapy for prostate cancer. Int J Radiat Oncol Biol Phys 78:58–63
23. Grills IS, Martinez AA, Hollander M et al (2004) High dose rate brachytherapy as prostate cancer monotherapy reduces toxicity compared to low dose rate palladium seeds. J Urol 171:1098–1104
24. Demanes DJ, Rodriguez RR, Schour L et al (2005) High-dose-rate intensity-modulated brachytherapy with external beam radiotherapy for prostate cancer: California endocurietherapy's 10-year results. Int J Radiat Oncol Biol Phys 61:1306–1316
25. Mate TP, Gottesman JE, Hatton J et al (1998) High dose-rate afterloading 192Iridium prostate brachytherapy: feasibility report. Int J Radiat Oncol Biol Phys 41:525–533
26. Vargas CE, Martinez AA, Boike TP et al (2006) High-dose irradiation for prostate cancer via a high-dose-rate brachytherapy boost: results of a phase I to II study. Int J Radiat Oncol Biol Phys 66:416–423
27. Demanes D (2006) High dose rate (HDR) monotherapy is equivalent to combined HDR brachytherapy and external beam radiation therapy (EBRT) for early prostate cancer. Int J Radiat Oncol Biol Phys 66(suppl):S351
28. Fuller DB, Naitoh J, Lee C et al (2008) Virtual HDR CyberKnife treatment for localized prostatic carcinoma: dosimetry comparison with HDR brachytherapy and preliminary clinical observations. Int J Radiat Oncol Biol Phys 70:1588–1597
29. Katz AJ, Santoro M, Ashley R et al (2010) Stereotactic body radiotherapy for organ-confined prostate cancer. BMC Urol 10:1
30. Friedland JL, Freeman DE, Masterson-McGary ME et al (2009) Stereotactic body radiotherapy: an emerging treatment

approach for localized prostate cancer. Technol Cancer Res Treat 8:387–392
31. Townsend NC, Huth BJ, Ding W et al (2010) Acute toxicity after cyberknife-delivered hypofractionated radiotherapy for treatment of prostate cancer. Am J Clin Oncol 34:6–10
32. King CR, Brooks JD, Gill H et al (2009) Stereotactic body radiotherapy for localized prostate cancer: interim results of a prospective phase II clinical trial. Int J Radiat Oncol Biol Phys 73:1043–1048
33. Brenner DJ (2004) Fractionation and late rectal toxicity. Int J Radiat Oncol Biol Phys 60:1013–1015
34. Crook J, Esche B, Futter N (1996) Effect of pelvic radiotherapy for prostate cancer on bowel, bladder, and sexual function: the patient's perspective. Urology 47:387–394
35. Potosky AL, Legler J, Albertsen PC et al (2000) Health outcomes after prostatectomy or radiotherapy for prostate cancer: results from the Prostate Cancer Outcomes Study. J Natl Cancer Inst 92:1582–1592
36. van der Wielen GJ, van Putten WL, Incrocci L (2007) Sexual function after three-dimensional conformal radiotherapy for prostate cancer: results from a dose-escalation trial. Int J Radiat Oncol Biol Phys 68:479–484
37. Lim AJ, Brandon AH, Fiedler J et al (1995) Quality of life: radical prostatectomy versus radiation therapy for prostate cancer. J Urol 154:1420–1425
38. Raina R, Agarwal A, Goyal KK et al (2003) Long-term potency after iodine-125 radiotherapy for prostate cancer and role of sildenafil citrate. Urology 62:1103–1108
39. Duchesne GM, Williams SG, Das R et al (2007) Patterns of toxicity following high-dose-rate brachytherapy boost for prostate cancer: mature prospective phase I/II study results. Radiother Oncol 84:128–134
40. Joly F, Brune D, Couette JE et al (1998) Health-related quality of life and sequelae in patients treated with brachytherapy and external beam irradiation for localized prostate cancer. Ann Oncol 9:751–757
41. Wiegner EA, King CR (2010) Sexual function after stereotactic body radiotherapy for prostate cancer: results of a prospective clinical trial. Int J Radiat Oncol Biol Phys 78: 442–448
42. Geinitz H, Zimmermann FB, Kuzmany A et al (2000) Daily CT planning during boost irradiation of prostate cancer. Feasibility and time requirements. Strahlenther Onkol 176:429–432
43. Fransson P, Bergstrom P, Lofroth PO et al (2002) Prospective evaluation of urinary and intestinal side effects after BeamCath stereotactic dose-escalated radiotherapy of prostate cancer. Radiother Oncol 63:239–248
44. Miralbell R, Molla M, Rouzaud M et al (2010) Hypofractionated boost to the dominant tumor region with intensity modulated stereotactic radiotherapy for prostate cancer: a sequential dose escalation pilot study. Int J Radiat Oncol Biol Phys 78:50–57
45. Katz AJ, Santoro M, Ashley R et al (2010) Stereotactic body radiotherapy as boost for organ-confined prostate cancer. Technol Cancer Res Treat 9:575–582
46. Oermann EK, Slack RS, Hanscom HN et al (2010) A pilot study of intensity modulated radiation therapy with hypofractionated stereotactic body radiation therapy (SBRT) boost in the treatment of intermediate- to high-risk prostate cancer. Technol Cancer Res Treat 9:453–462
47. Jabbari S, Weinberg VK, Kaprealian T et al (2010) Stereotactic body radiotherapy as monotherapy or post-external beam radiotherapy boost for prostate cancer: technique, early toxicity, and PSA response. Int J Radiat Oncol Biol Phys(in press)
48. Thariat J, Li G, Angellier G, Marchal S, Palamini G, Rucka G, Bénézery K, Castelli J, Trimaud R, Mammar H, Marcie S, Gérard JP, Bondiau PY (2009) Current indications and ongoing clinical trials with CyberKnife stereotactic radiotherapy in France in 2009. Bull Cancer 96:853–864
49. Vavassori A, Jereczek-Fossa BA, Beltramo G et al (2010) Image-guided robotic radiosurgery as salvage therapy for locally recurrent prostate cancer after external beam irradiation: retrospective feasibility study on six cases. Tumori 96:71–75
50. Jereczek-Fossa BA, Beltramo G, Fariselli L et al (2011) Robotic image-guided stereotactic radiotherapy, for isolated recurrent primary, lymph node or metastatic prostate cancer. Int J Radiat Oncol Biol Phys(in press)

Stereotactic Body Radiotherapy for Prostate Cancer: Updated Results from a Prospective Trial

12

Christopher R. King

CONTENTS

12.1 Abstract

Hypofractionated radiotherapy has an intrinsically different normal tissue and tumor radiobiology. The results of a prospective trial of stereotactic body radiotherapy (SBRT) for prostate cancer with long-term patient-reported toxicity and tumor control rates are presented. Sixty-seven patients with clinically localized low-risk prostate cancer were enrolled from 2003 to 2009. Treatment consisted of 36.25 Gy in five fractions with CyberKnife®. No patient received hormone therapy. Median follow-up was 2.7 years. Significant late bladder and rectal toxicities were infrequent. There were no Grade 4 toxicities. RTOG Grade 3, 2, and 1 bladder toxicities were seen in 3% (two patients), 5% (three patients), and 23% (13 patients), respectively. Dysuria exacerbated by urologic instrumentation accounted for both patients with Grade 3 toxicity. Urinary incontinence, complete obstruction, or persistent hematuria was not observed. Rectal Grade 3, 2, and 1 toxicities were seen in 0%, 2% (one patient), and 12.5% (seven patients), respectively. Persistent rectal bleeding was not observed. Low-grade toxicities were substantially less frequent with QOD vs. QD dose regimen. There were two, biopsy-proven PSA failures with negative metastatic work-up. Median PSA at follow-up was 0.5 ± 0.72 ng/ml. The 5-year Kaplan–Meier PSA relapse-free survival was 94% (95% CI: 85–102%) and compares favorably with other definitive treatments. The current evidence supports consideration of SBRT among the therapeutic options for localized prostate cancer.

12.2 Introduction

The particular radiobiology of prostate cancer offers a biologic rationale in favor of hypofractionated radiotherapy relative to the standard protracted course using

L.E. Ponsky et al. (eds.), *Treating Prostate Cancer and Related Genitourinary Applications*, Robotic Radiosurgery, DOI 10.1007/978-3-642-11495-3_12, © Springer-Verlag Berlin Heidelberg 2012 conventionally fractionated doses with the potential for improving the therapeutic ratio of radiotherapy, i.e., simultaneous higher rates of tumor control rates and lower incidence of toxicities. Several contemporary clinical series have shown excellent biochemical control rates and low rectal and bladder toxicities with the use of modestly hypofractionated radiotherapy schedules. These clinical programs used external-beam hypofractionated regimens, with dose-per-fraction ranging from 2.5 to 3.1 Gy [1–4] delivered daily over a 4- to 6-week period. A landmark historical series which was run in the UK in the 1980s delivered six fractions of 6 Gy each over a 2-week period, and documented good outcomes and acceptable toxicities [5]. There are two published series using Ir-192 HDR brachytherapy as monotherapy with dose-per-fraction ranging from eight to nine fractions of 6 Gy each [6] and four fractions of 9.5 Gy or six fractions of 7 Gy each [7].

Several factors highlight the relative impact of the current study with regard to newly open and pending analogous trials as well as the eagerness in the community to adopt this novel technique for practical as well as economic reasons. Being among the first of its kind, our study, therefore, has the longest follow-up to date, and given the potential for late effects and late recurrences to appear after any prostate radiotherapy, it provides the basis for comparison with other approaches for the definitive treatment of prostate cancer. In this chapter we discuss some of the treatment planning issues, present our data on the late urinary and bowel toxicities, as well as the PSA response rates.

12.3 Methods and Materials

12.3.1 Patient Eligibility

An IRB-approved phase II clinical trial of stereotactic body radiotherapy (SBRT) for low-risk prostate cancer accrued 67 patients at Stanford between December 2003 and June 2009. While details of this trial were outlined previously [8, 9], the major features are summarized here. Eligible patients were newly diagnosed with biopsy-proven prostate cancer presenting with low- to favorable-intermediate-risk features, including a pre-biopsy PSA of 10 ng/ml or less, a biopsy Gleason score of 3+3 or 3+4, and a clinical stage T1c or T2a/b. All biopsy grading was obtained at our institution. Patients with prior treatment, including hormone therapy or transurethral resection of the prostate (TURP), were excluded. The median age was 66 years.

12.3.2 Treatment Specifics

CyberKnife® (Accuray Incorporated, Sunnyvale, CA) was used to deliver fiducial-based image-guided SBRT. Three gold fiducials were placed in the prostate via trans-rectal ultrasound. A non-contrast CT scan was obtained the same day with the patient in supine position and in an alpha cradle, at 1.25-mm slice thickness and indexing. Anatomical contouring of the prostate, seminal vesicles, rectum, bladder, penile bulb, femoral heads, and testes were done by the same radiation oncologist. Dose was prescribed to the planning target volume (PTV) that consisted of a volumetric expansion of the prostate by 5 mm, except a 3-mm expansion in the posterior direction. The course of radiotherapy consisted of five fractions of 7.25 Gy for a total dose of 36.25 Gy. Dose was normalized to the 90% (±2%) isodose line in order for the prescription dose to cover 95% of the PTV. Dose Volume Histogram (DVH) goals for the rectum were such that the V50% <50% (i.e., the volume receiving 50% of the prescribed dose was <50%), V80% <20%, V90% <10%, and V100% <5%. The bladder DVH goals were V50% <40% and V100% <10%. The femoral head DVH goal was V40% <5%. The treatments were given over five consecutive days (QD) for the first 22 patients and three times a week (on alternating days, QOD) subsequently. No eligible patient needed to be excluded due to anatomical considerations – despite two patients having unilateral hip prosthesis – and there was no gland-size limit.

12.3.3 Treatment Planning Considerations with the CyberKnife

An issue that is rarely considered is the potential for incidental dose to the testes. This is particularly important for those patients treated with CyberKnife, as the device renders a very non-coplanar beam

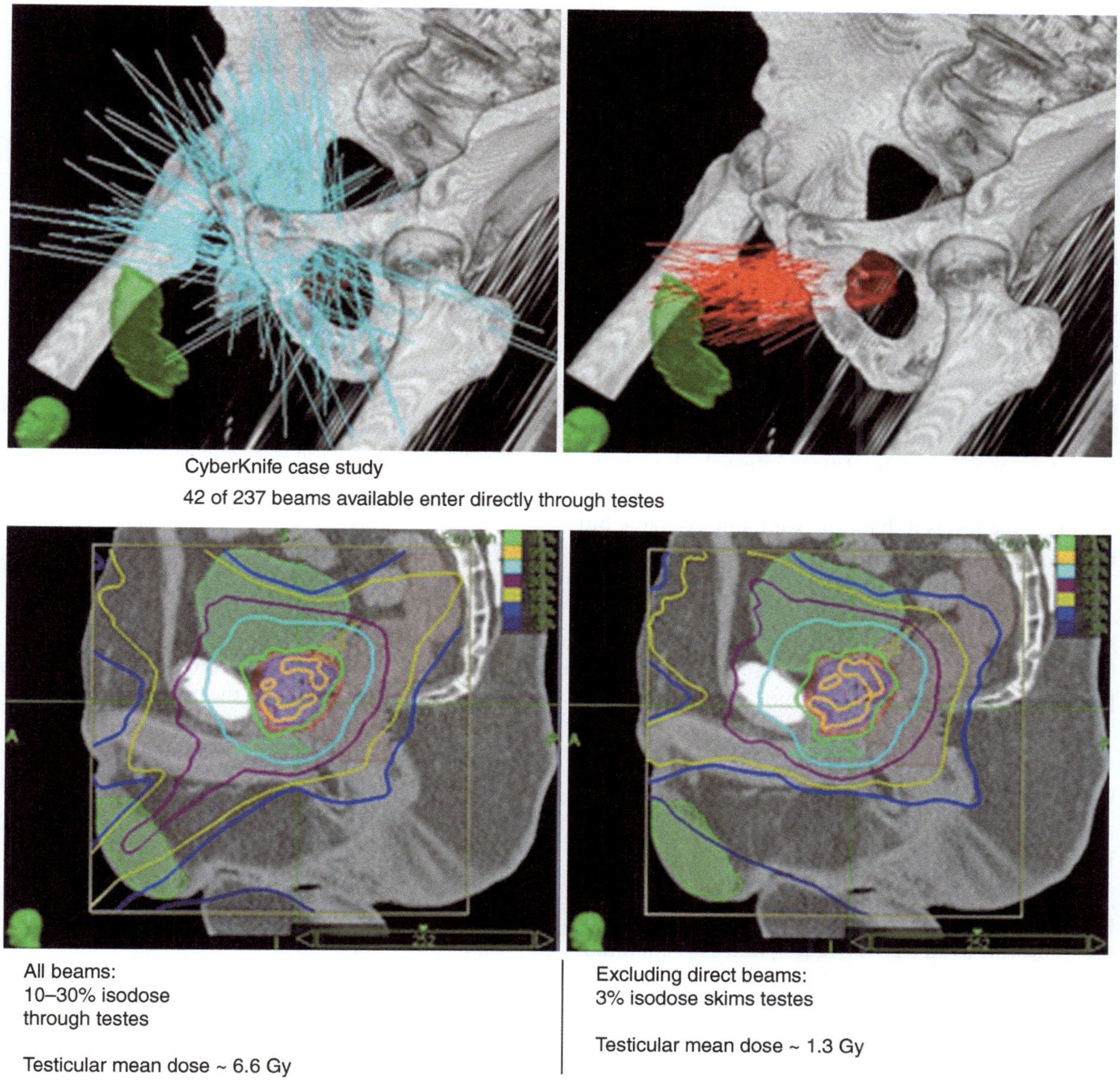

Fig. 12.1 Testicular dose resulting from non-coplanar therapy. *Left*: incident beams and isodose profile resulting from planning without delineating testes as an avoidance region. *Right*: possible dose reduction to testes with testicular avoidance

delivery, although the issue could apply to other approaches as well. Figure 12.1 shows the testes, in green, and the beam entries relative to the organs. As an example, in a plan using all of the available CyberKnife beams, 42 of the available 237 beams would be incident on the testes and are shown highlighted in red. This would result in the 10–30% isodose line being delivered directly through the testis, for a mean testicular dose of 6.6 Gy given in hypofractionated dose. A review of the literature estimates the LD50 of the testicular Leydig cells to be about 10 Gy. Therefore, a dose of 6 Gy would be a significant normal tissue exposure. Not only would it cause hypogonadism, with all of its attendant consequences, but it would also confound any PSA response of treatment for years. Through planning, one can exclude all of the CyberKnife beams incident on the testes and reduce this dose to about 1.3 Gy or less, without significant degradation of the plan quality. Our review shows less than a 1% difference in any of the dose statistics between the two plans.

12.3.4 Follow-up and Toxicity Scoring

Patient-reported toxicity was objectively scored on the Radiation Therapy Oncology Group (RTOG) urinary and rectal toxicity scale [10] at last follow-up in order to allow for comparison with published radiotherapy studies. PSA and validated Quality of Life (QOL) questionnaires pertaining to urinary and bowel function were prospectively obtained at baseline, at 3-month post-treatment intervals during the first 2 years and at 6-month intervals thereafter. Testosterone levels at baseline were not available but were collected for most patients after treatment.

12.4 Results

12.4.1 Urinary and Rectal Toxicities

Median follow-up was 2.7 years (25th–75th percentile: 1.8–4.5 years, max 5.9 years). At baseline, 92% of patients reported no urinary issues (translatable from the QOL scale to an RTOG Grade 0) and 8% with minor issues (translatable to an RTOG Grade between 0 and 1). The corresponding baseline function for bowel was 89% with Grade 0 and 11% with Grade between 0 and 1. In Table 12.1 we summarize the rates of urinary and rectal RTOG toxicity (incidence) at last follow-up.

Table 12.1 Late urinary (GU) and rectal (GI) toxicity on the RTOG scale after prostate SBRT

RTOG grade	GU	GI
0	68% (39/57 pts)	84% (48/57 pts)
1	23% (13/57 pts)	14% (8/57 pts)
2	5% (3/57 pts)	2% (1/57 pts)
3	3.5% (2/57 pts)	0
4	0	0

RTOG Radiation Therapy Oncology Group, *GU* genitourinary, *GI* gastrointestinal

Table 12.2 Late urinary (GU) and late rectal (GI) RTOG toxicity compared between consecutive daily treatments (QD) vs. those delivered three times a week on alternating days (QOD)

	QD	QOD	*p*-Value*
GU toxicity			
RTOG grade 0	37% (6/16 pts)	80% (33/41 pts)	0.003
RTOG grade 1	50% (8/16 pts)	12% (5/41 pts)	0.004
RTOG grade 2	6% (1/16 pts)	5% (2/41 pts)	1
RTOG grade 3	6% (1/16 pts)	2% (1/41 pts)	0.48
GI toxicity			
RTOG grade 0	56% (9/16 pts)	95% (39/41 pts)	0.001
RTOG grade 1	37% (6/16 pts)	5% (2/41 pts)	0.0004
RTOG grade 2	6% (1/16 pts)	0% (0/41 pts)	0.28

RTOG Radiation Therapy Oncology Group, *GU* genitourinary, *GI* gastrointestinal
**p*-Values from Fisher's exact test

There were no Grade 4 toxicities. The only common factor among both patients with Grade 3 GU toxicity was repeated urologic instrumentation (cystoscopies and dilatation procedures) for dysuria. None of the other patients had urologic instrumentation procedures. In these two patients, the urinary symptoms were progressively exacerbated following these interventions. Urinary incontinence, complete obstruction, or persistent hematuria was not observed. Persistent rectal bleeding was not observed. In Table 12.2 we compare toxicity rates between QOD treatments vs. QD treatments. QOD resulted in substantially less frequent Grade 1–2 urinary toxicity and less frequent Grade 1–2 rectal toxicity. There were no rectal Grade 3 toxicities.

12.4.2 PSA Response

The patterns of PSA response after completion of SBRT show a gradual decline to a median PSA of 0.50 ± 0.72 ng/mL (25th–75th percentile: 0.12–0.90 ng/mL) at last follow-up. In Fig. 12.2 we present the Kaplan–Meier relapse-free survival curve. Relapse was defined by progression (biochemical progression based on the "nadir + 2" PSA failure definition) or by a PSA rise with biopsy-proven recurrence. The 5-year biochemical relapse-free survival was 94% (95% CI: 85–102%). There were two patients with PSA recurrence who underwent prostate biopsy which revealed pathologic persistence within the prostate gland, occurring at 2.8 and 3.2 years after treatment. Both had

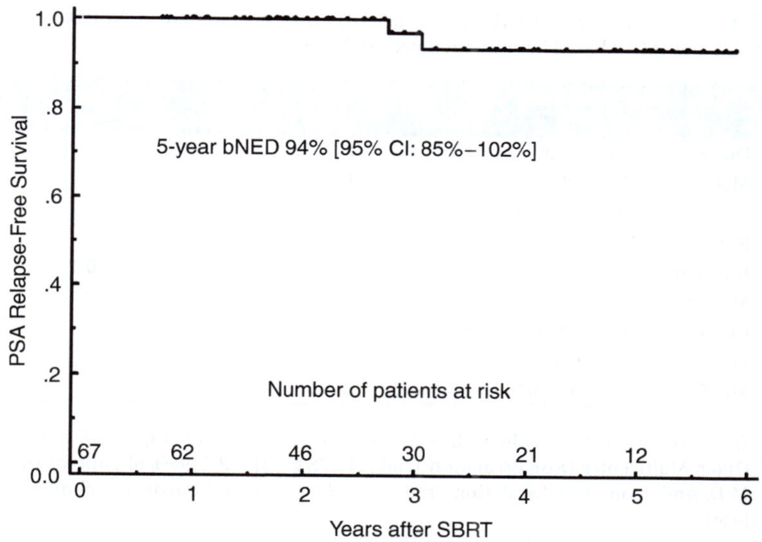

Fig. 12.2 PSA relapse-free survival Kaplan-Meier curve. *Tick marks* indicate censoring. Number of patients at risk for each year is indicated. There were two events (biochemical and biopsy-proven failures) within a median follow-up of 2.7 years (25th–75th percentile: 1.8–4.5 years). The 5-year actuarial PSA relapse-free survival rate is 94% (95% confidence interval is 85–102%)

a negative work-up for metastatic disease that included a bone scan, CT scan, and MRI. All other patients continue to have declining PSA levels at last follow-up.

12.5 Discussion

12.5.1 Urinary and Rectal Toxicities

The outcomes from this clinical trial demonstrate that a hypofractionated course using stereotactic body radiotherapy for localized prostate cancer is associated with infrequent rates of clinically significant urinary and rectal toxicities. With a median follow-up of 2.7 years, there has been no Grade 3 or higher rectal toxicity, no Grade 4 urinary toxicity, and 3.5% Grade 3 urinary toxicity. No patients experienced complete urinary obstruction, persistent urinary bleeding, or incontinence, and no patients experienced persistent rectal bleeding, or fecal incontinence.

We compared our toxicity rates on the same RTOG scale with those published in the four randomized-controlled trials using dose-escalation [11–14] and with hypofractionated IMRT studies [3, 15–17]. These data are summarized in Table 12.3. Our study demonstrates that the rates of urinary and rectal toxicities are equal to or lower than those observed in the dose-escalated trials as well as in the hypofractionated studies. In comparing these data, it is important to keep in mind that not only is the dose-per-fraction in our study different from these conventionally fractionated or hypofractionated courses, but the radiotherapy technique is also substantially different. It is impossible to entirely disentangle the interaction between technique and dose-per-fraction. It is well established that a proportional reduction in both the volume and dose of irradiated normal tissues will result in diminished acute and late effects. With the benefit of image guidance, our SBRT technique is able to safely minimize the expansion margins treated around the prostate (5 mm overall, reduced to 3 mm posteriorly) whereas the simpler radiotherapy techniques used in the dose-escalation trials, for example, typically required margin expansions of 10–15 mm generally and 5–7.5 mm posteriorly.

Equally complex is the interaction between the dose-per-fraction to normal tissues and the total cumulative dose delivered. While classic radiobiology teaches us that a larger dose-per-fraction will lead to an increase in the rate of late normal tissue complications, this effect has to be tempered when there is a reduction in the total dose delivered. As an illustration of these points, we note that the rate of Grade 2 rectal toxicity for the Dutch [11] and MGH dose-escalation trials [12] are several-fold higher than those of the other two dose-escalation trials [13, 14], while the total dose and dose-per-fraction are equal. One of the main differences between these two pairs of studies is

Table 12.3 Late urinary (GU) and rectal (GI) toxicity compared on the RTOG scale from the dose-escalation arm of randomized trials and IMRT-based hypofractionated studies

Series	*n*	Dose/fx	FU median (years)	GI grade 2 (%)	GI grade 3 (%)	GI grade 4 (%)	GU grade 2 (%)	GU grade 3 (%)	GU grade 4 (%)
Dutch[a]	333	78/39	4.2	27	5	0	26	13	0
MDA[b]	151	78/39	8.7	19	7	0	7	3	0
MGH[c]	196	79.2/44	8.9	24	1	0	27	2	0
RT01[d]	422	74/37	5.2	20	6	0	4	4	0
Kupelian[e]	770	70/28	3.7	3.1	1.3	0.1	5.1	0.1	0
Martin[f]	92	60/20	3.2	4	NR	0	3	NR	0
Coote[g]	60	60/20	2[j]	4	NR	0	4.2	1.6	0
Lock[h]	66	63.2/20	3	25	3.1	1.5	14.1	4.7	0
SBRT[i]	67	36.25/5	2.7	2	0	0	5	3.5	0

NR not reported, *3DCRT* three-dimensional conformal radiotherapy, *CGE* cobalt gray equivalent (dose equivalent to Gy)
[a]Dutch Multicenter Dose Escalation Trial [11], 78 Gy 3DCRT (90% of patients treated with three-field technique)
[b]M.D. Anderson Dose Escalation Trial [12], 78 Gy 3DCRT (four-field technique 46 Gy followed by six-field technique for boost dose)
[c]Proton Radiation Oncology Group [13], 79.2 CGE (50.4 Gy 3DCRT with four-field technique + 28.8 Gy with one- or two-field technique for proton boost)
[d]UK MRC RT01 Dose Escalation Trial [14], 74 Gy 3DCRT (four-field technique)
[e]Kupelian et al. [3]; IMRT with daily transabdominal ultrasound image guidance (bat)
[f]Martin et al. [15]; IMRT with fiducial-based daily image guidance
[g]Coote et al. [16]; IMRT with 2D portal imaging set-up
[h]Lock et al. [17]; IMRT with daily fiducial-based image guidance
[i]Current study
[j]Reported at exactly 2-year follow-up

their technique. The Dutch trial used a much simpler three-field technique in 90% of their patients, and the MGH trial used a simpler one- to two-field technique for their proton-boost dose (although a rectal balloon was used to ensure anatomical stability). These technical considerations alone will result in proportionally more rectal wall receiving larger doses than with the more conformal techniques such as four-field or IMRT used in the other two trials.

12.5.2 Possible Association of High-Grade GU Toxicity with Instrumentation

We had only two patients (3.5%) that experienced Grade 3 urinary toxicity. They both had severe dysuria and frequency but did not suffer from complete obstruction. These two patients had in common the fact that they were followed by outside Urologists who performed multiple (two or more) cystoscopies and urethral dilatation procedures. The timeline of symptoms for both these patients suggests that these symptoms were not alleviated by, but in fact appear to have been further exacerbated by these procedures. To date, dysuria persists in these two patients, but appears to be stable and very slowly resolving. We have urged them to limit any further urethral instrumentation unless absolutely necessary and that is our medical advice for all radiotherapy patients. Neither of these patients has progressed to Grade 4. Urethral strictures after external-beam radiotherapy can occur but are relatively uncommon. In two large studies, Grade 3 urethral strictures occurred in 3% and in 2% of patients, respectively [18, 19]. They are more common with brachytherapy when combined with external beam, 5%, and after surgery, 8% [19].

12.5.3 Comparing Treatment Regimens: QD Versus QOD

Toxicities between patients treated over 5 consecutive days (QD) and those treated every other day (QOD) were compared. A fourfold reduction in Grade 1 urinary toxicity and a sevenfold reduction in Grade 1 rectal toxicity were observed in favor of the QOD dose schedule. Low-grade toxicities, even Grade 1, are not to be overlooked as clinically insignificant, in part because they may be predictors of potential for very late toxicities, in part because they can lead patients to unnecessary interventions and in part because of their impact on quality of life. Although the radio-pathology is not completely understood, given our observations, we recommend treating with a QOD regimen for SBRT to minimize normal tissue late effects.

12.5.4 PSA Response

The 5-year actuarial PSA relapse-free survival in our study is 94% (95% CI: 85–102%). A comparison between all definitive therapies for localized prostate cancer (i.e., radical prostatectomy, conventional external-beam radiotherapy, permanent low-dose-rate brachytherapy, high-dose-rate brachytherapy) is well beyond the scope of this chapter. As a surrogate for this comparison, we used a validated nomogram [20] that in essence comprises a synthesis of all modern surgical and radiotherapy outcome studies. Using our individual patient characteristics as upper and lower bounds of risk features based on PSA, Gleason Grade, clinical T-stage, percent of positive cores, we calculate using the nomogram the following 5-year range in predicted biochemical relapse-free survival rates after radical prostatectomy as 95–98%, after 78 Gy external-beam radiotherapy as 91–94%, and after permanent brachytherapy as 80–90%. Nomograms are of course susceptible to all of the caveats of retrospective studies. We consider outcomes of >90% among all of the therapeutic options for low-risk prostate cancer to be essentially equivalent.

12.5.5 Radiobiological Concerns

Standard linear-quadratic radiobiologic models can be used to estimate the equivalent dose from hypofractionated radiotherapy in terms of conventional 2 Gy per fraction (known as the EQD2). This standard model yields $EQD2 = D \times [(\alpha/\beta + d)/(\alpha/\beta + 2)]$, where D is the total dose given, d is the dose-per-fraction and α/β is a measure of sensitivity to dose-per-fraction. The hypofractionated dose regimen in our trial (36.25 Gy in five fractions) corresponds to a tumor EQD2 of 91 Gy, a normal tissue late effect EQD2 of 74 Gy, and an acute toxicity EQD2 of 52 Gy (assuming prostate cancer α/β of 1.5 Gy, normal tissue late effect α/β of 3 Gy, and normal tissue acute effect α/β of 10 Gy). Thus, compared with conventional radiotherapy (where dose is 78 Gy), it is predicted that tumor-control rates will potentially be higher (equivalent dose of 91 Gy), late effects will be the same or lower (equivalent dose of 74 Gy), and acute effects will be lower (equivalent dose of 52 Gy).

What if our radiobiological hypothesis for prostate cancer is wrong? What if prostate cancer possesses in fact an α/β ratio (i.e., a sensitivity to dose-per-fraction) that is similar to other tumors (i.e., ~10 Gy instead of the hypothesized value of ~1.5 Gy)? In that case the equivalent dose (EQD2) from our hypofractionated regimen would be a seriously inadequate dose of 52 Gy. Based on the known dose–response curve for low-risk prostate cancer [2], a dose of 52 Gy would yield only a ~40% rate of biochemical control at 5 years. With conventional doses of 78 Gy the 5-year biochemical control rate are predicted (and observed) to be ~90–95%. Our current PSA relapse-free survival rates of >90% are consistent with other studies and support hypofractionated radiotherapy as a biologically effective dose regimen for prostate cancer.

12.6 Conclusions

This study shows that clinically significant late bladder and rectal toxicities from SBRT for prostate cancer are infrequent. Due to its possible association with late urethral toxicity, we recommend avoiding urologic instrumentation after SBRT unless absolutely necessary. PSA relapse-free survival at 5 years compares favorably with those for radical prostatectomy, conventional external-beam RT, or permanent brachytherapy. These findings, consistent with others, support the radiobiological basis for prostate cancer hypofractionation and the consideration of SBRT among the treatment options for patients with low-risk localized prostate cancer.

References

1. Yeoh EE, Holloway RH, Fraser RJ et al (2006) Hypofractionated versus conventionally fractionated radiation therapy for prostate carcinoma: updated results of a phase III randomized trial. Int J Radiat Oncol Biol Phys 66:1072–1083
2. Lukka H, Hayter C, Julian JA et al (2005) Randomized trial comparing two fractionation schedules for patients with localized prostate cancer. J Clin Oncol 23:6132–6138
3. Kupelian PA, Willoughby TR, Reddy CA et al (2007) Hypofractionated intensity-modulated radiotherapy (70 Gy at 2.5 Gy per fraction) for localized prostate cancer: Cleveland Clinic experience. Int J Radiat Oncol Biol Phys 68:1424–1430
4. Livsey JE, Cowan RA, Wylie JP et al (2003) Hypofractionated conformal radiotherapy in carcinoma of the prostate: five-year outcome analysis. Int J Radiat Oncol Biol Phys 57:1254–1259
5. Lloyd-Davies RW, Collins CD, Swan AV (1990) Carcinoma of prostate treated by radical external beam radiotherapy using hypofractionation. Twenty-two years' experience (1962–1984). Urology 36:107–111
6. Yoshioka Y, Konishi K, Sumida I et al (2011) Monotherapeutic high-dose-rate brachytherapy for prostate cancer: five-year results of an extreme hypofractionation regimen with 54 Gy in nine fractions. Int J Radiat Oncol Biol Phys 80(2):469–475, Epub 2010 Jun 18
7. Martinez AA, Demanes J, Vargas C et al (2009) High-dose-rate prostate brachytherapy: an excellent accelerated-hypofractionated treatment for favorable prostate cancer. Am J Clin Oncol 33:481–488
8. King CR, Brooks JD, Gill H et al (2009) Stereotactic body radiotherapy for localized prostate cancer: interim results of a prospective phase II clinical trial. Int J Radiat Oncol Biol Phys 73:1043–1048
9. King CR, Brooks JD, Gill H et al (2011) Long-term outcomes from a prospective trial of stereotactic body radiotherapy for low-risk prostate cancer. Int J Radiat Oncol Biol Phys 78(3):S336
10. Common toxicity criteria (1998) National Institutes of Health publication (Version 2.0)
11. Peeters ST, Heemsbergen WD, Koper PC et al (2006) Dose-response in radiotherapy for localized prostate cancer: results of the Dutch multicenter randomized phase III trial comparing 68 Gy of radiotherapy with 78 Gy. J Clin Oncol 24:1990–1996
12. Kuban DA, Tucker SL, Dong L et al (2008) Long-term results of the M. D. Anderson randomized dose-escalation trial for prostate cancer. Int J Radiat Oncol Biol Phys 70:67–74
13. Zietman AL, Bae K, Slater JD et al (2010) Randomized trial comparing conventional-dose with high-dose conformal radiation therapy in early-stage adenocarcinoma of the prostate: long-term results from proton radiation oncology group/American college of radiology 95-09. J Clin Oncol 28:1106–1111
14. Dearnaley DP, Sydes MR, Graham JD et al (2007) Escalated-dose versus standard-dose conformal radiotherapy in prostate cancer: first results from the MRC RT01 randomised controlled trial. Lancet Oncol 8:475–487
15. Martin JM, Rosewall T, Bayley A et al (2007) Phase II trial of hypofractionated image-guided intensity-modulated radiotherapy for localized prostate adenocarcinoma. Int J Radiat Oncol Biol Phys 69:1084–1089
16. Coote JH, Wylie JP, Cowan RA et al (2009) Hypofractionated intensity-modulated radiotherapy for carcinoma of the prostate: analysis of toxicity. Int J Radiat Oncol Biol Phys 74:1121–1127
17. Lock M, Best L, Wong E et al (2011) A phase II trial of Arc-based hypofractionated intensity-modulated radiotherapy in localized prostate cancer. Int J Radiat Oncol Biol Phys 80(5):1306–1315, Epub 2010 Aug 12
18. Zelefsky MJ, Chan H, Hunt M et al (2006) Long-term outcome of high dose intensity modulated radiation therapy for patients with clinically localized prostate cancer. J Urol 176:1415–1419
19. Elliott SP, Meng MV, Elkin EP et al (2007) Incidence of urethral stricture after primary treatment for prostate cancer: data From CaPSURE. J Urol 178:529–534; discussion 534
20. Katz MS, Efstathiou JA, D'Amico AV et al (2010) The 'CaP Calculator': an online decision support tool for clinically localized prostate cancer. BJU Int 105:1417–1422

Prostate Radiosurgery with Homogeneous Dose Distribution: A Summary of Outcomes So Far

Debra Freeman and Mary Ellen Masterson-McGary

CONTENTS

13.1 Abstract

This chapter will focus on hypofractionated, stereotactic body radiation treatment (SBRT) of localized prostate cancer using a homogeneous dose distribution. The biologic rationale for hypofractionation in the management of prostate cancer has been addressed in a previous chapter. Patient selection, treatment planning, dose specification, treatment delivery, outcome measures, and published experience using the CyberKnife® Radiosurgery System for prostate cancer will be reviewed.

13.2 Introduction

The goal of radiation for localized prostate cancer is to deliver a prescribed dose of radiation to the prostate gland while minimizing dose to adjacent normal structures. This can be accomplished through a variety of treatment techniques, including 3D conformal therapy, intensity-modulated radiotherapy, image-guided radiation therapy, and stereotactic body radiotherapy. However, technical limitations in external-beam radiation delivery, including target motion during treatment and variation in patient position, generally necessitate inclusion of a margin of normal tissue beyond the prostate to avoid a "geographic miss." The risk of normal tissue injury is mitigated by fractionation, delivering the intended radiation dose over multiple sessions.

Image-guided stereotactic radiation systems utilize recent technological advances to minimize targeting "errors" during treatment delivery, resulting in more accurate treatment of the intended target volume and avoidance of adjacent normal tissues. For prostate cancer treatment, these include implantation of fiducials for organ-motion tracking, real-time image guidance, and automatic correction of patient position during treatment. In addition, the use of multiple, non-coplanar beams can achieve dose gradients superior to conventional linear accelerators, further differentiating adjacent structures from the target volume and facilitating dose escalation. If the radiobiology of prostate cancer cells favors hypofractionation, treatment systems that optimally spare

L.E. Ponsky et al. (eds.), *Treating Prostate Cancer and Related Genitourinary Applications*, Robotic Radiosurgery,
DOI 10.1007/978-3-642-11495-3_13,

normal tissues while delivering the dose to the target tissues would be best suited to minimize the risk of injury with this fractionation scheme.

13.3 Methods and Materials

13.3.1 Patient Selection

In December 2003, King et al. treated, for the first time, a patient with localized prostate cancer using robotic radiosurgery at Stanford University. Since that time, over 5,000 men with prostate cancer have been successfully treated with stereotactic body radiotherapy (SBRT), which is the general term referring to high-dose radiation delivered in a minimal number of fractions to an extracranial area. The initial experience with SBRT "monotherapy" has been limited to risk groups with the lowest probability of extraprostatic disease. These include "low-risk" patients (clinical stage T1c–T2a, Gleason score ≤6, PSA < 10) or patients with only one "intermediate-risk" feature (clinical stage T2b, Gleason score = 7 or PSA = 10–20). Patients with T3 or N1 disease, Gleason score > 7, and/or PSA > 20 are not currently considered candidates for SBRT alone. SBRT as a "boost" following external-beam treatment is addressed in a separate chapter. Other eligibility criteria include: no prior pelvic radiation, ultrasound therapy (HIFU) or cryotherapy; and no implanted hardware (e.g., bilateral hip prostheses) that could impair treatment planning or treatment delivery. In addition, patients with markedly enlarged prostate glands (>100 cc volume) or significant urinary obstructive symptoms prior to treatment (IPSS score > 20) are not ideal candidates for SBRT monotherapy.

13.3.2 Treatment Planning

Prior to initiation of treatment, all patients must have fiducial markers implanted in the prostate for tracking during treatment. For CyberKnife® (Accuray Incorporated, Sunnyvale, CA) treatment, these markers are 18-carat gold, measuring 5 mm in length and 1.2 mm in diameter. A minimum of three fiducial markers are required, but typically four to six of them are implanted in the prostate, using either a transperineal or transrectal approach, with local anesthesia or sedation, as needed. Fiducials must be visible on orthogonal imaging, ideally separated by at least 2 cm in all directions. Once fiducial markers are placed, 5–10 days should elapse before imaging studies are obtained for planning purposes to allow for fiducial stabilization and resolution of prostate edema.

Whenever possible, both CT and MRI scans are utilized for treatment planning. In preparation for simulation, patients are asked to "prep" their bowel and bladder by evacuating the rectum using a Fleets enema and emptying the bladder approximately 1 h prior to scanning. At scanning, patients are positioned supine, arms across chest, with either a custom Alpha cradle or head support as needed for patient comfort. Scans are obtained feet-first and should include the entire body surface contour in the field of view. If MRI is available, CT can be a non-contrast study. If MRI is not available or permitted for a given patient, a contrast-enhanced CT may be preferable. CT slices should be 1.25–1.5 mm, contiguous, centered on the prostate, 300 slices total. MRI slice thickness should be equivalent to or a multiple of CT slice thickness, contiguous, with no slice variability permitted. Preferred MRI sequences are T2*FGRE and T2 fat sat. Catheter placement is not required prior to imaging for a homogeneous dosing protocol, but urethral anatomy is generally discernable on MRI without a catheter in place. Ideally, scans should be completed at one location and in one session to minimize variations in bladder and rectal positioning between studies.

Once scanning is completed, CT and MRI data sets are transferred to a MultiPlan® (Accuray) workstation for fusion and contouring. Initially, scans are fused on the implanted fiducial markers identifiable in each data set. Fusion is then fine-tuned manually so prostate, rectum, and bladder volumes overlie as closely as possible between data sets. If significant differences in organ position are noted between the studies, the treating physician must decide whether to repeat the planning scans or develop "modified" contours, best reflecting organ position in relation to the prostate. All contours must be finalized on CT, as this is the data set used for dose calculations.

Normal structures to be contoured for DVH analysis should include the rectum, bladder, penile bulb, bowel within 2 cm of target, and prostatic urethra and neurovascular bundle (NVB) from prostatic apex to the base. "Rectum" should include the rectal lumen and rectal wall from ischial tuberosities to sigmoid colon; "bladder," the bladder lumen and wall; "urethra," the lumen extending from bladder neck to urogenital diaphragm; and "penile bulb," the bulbous spongiosum inferior to the urogenital diaphragm. Dose calculation grids for DVH analysis should be sufficiently large to include the entire structure contoured.

The GTV (gross tumor volume) for the homogeneous protocol is defined as the prostate alone, with no more than 0.5 cm of adjacent seminal vesicles included. The CTV (clinical target volume) for low-risk patients equals the GTV, meaning only the prostate gland is included in the high-dose volume. For patients with one intermediate-risk feature, the CTV is defined as the prostate and proximal 2 cm of the seminal vesicles. Pelvic lymph nodes are not included in the CTV for either risk group. The prescription dose is delivered to the PTV (planning target volume), defined for the homogeneous protocol as the CTV plus a 5-mm expansion anteriorly and laterally, and a 3-mm expansion posteriorly. This PTV expansion allows for targeting uncertainty due to deformation of the prostate with motion and prostate movement that might occur after imaging but before or during dose delivery. In addition, microscopic extracapsular disease should lie within 3–5 mm of the prostate.

13.3.3 Dose Specification

The prescription dose to the PTV for a homogeneous dose distribution using SBRT is 36.25 Gy in five fractions, 7.25 Gy per fraction. Per protocol, the prescription isodose should cover at least 95% of the PTV and, ideally, should be within 75–85% of D_{max}. An optimal plan will deliver a "secondary dose" of 40 Gy to the GTV. Given the steep dose gradient achievable with radiosurgical technique, it is possible to deliver these prescription doses to the PTV and GTV while applying reasonable normal tissue constraints to surrounding structures. The recommended rectal constraint is $V_{36\,Gy} < 1$ cc, derived from HDR and IMRT dose-escalation studies. For bladder, recommendation is $V_{37\,Gy} < 10$ cc. For urethra, $V_{47\,Gy} < 20\%$ of contoured volume; and for penile bulb, $V_{29.5\,Gy} < 50\%$ are recommended. If possible, <50% of the contoured NVB should receive 38 Gy.

13.3.4 Treatment Delivery

As mentioned above, patients are asked to complete a brief bowel and bladder "prep" prior to simulation. This prep is repeated prior to each treatment to ensure that rectal and bladder positions, relative to the prostate, will be reasonably reproducible. In addition, patients are asked to follow a low-residue diet during their course of therapy to minimize gas and stool production. Variations in bladder fill or significant stool/gas in the rectal vault can lead to marked deformation of prostate position, making treatment delivery quite challenging.

Systems capable of automatic, 6-D couch corrections, such as CyberKnife, have set tolerance limits and will not accept prostate movement >0.5 cm in any direction. Variations in bladder and rectal position most often result in problems with "pitch," and differences up to 45° have been observed. Radiosurgery systems that rely only on translational movement corrections risk significant geographic miss.

Optimally, patients should complete their course of therapy within 11 days. Every-other-day treatment delivery can reduce rectal complaints during therapy but is not mandatory. If daily treatments are preferred, a minimum of 12 h between fractions is recommended. Imaging frequency during treatment delivery will depend on degree of prostate motion noted during each session and often varies between sessions. At a minimum, imaging should occur every three beams, or every 45 s.

13.3.5 Outcome Measures

Whether or not a patient is participating in a clinical research study, certain baseline measures are necessary to assess the outcome of the prostate radiosurgery. These include pretreatment PSA (expressed in ng/ml), some measure of pretreatment urinary function (AUA score; IPSS score), bowel function, and baseline erectile function. Many men will report difficulty in one or all of these areas prior to receiving treatment, so it is important to record objective values that can be monitored at regular intervals once treatment is completed.

13.4 Results and Discussion

Stereotactic body radiotherapy (SBRT) has recently emerged as an alternative technique to deliver hypofractionated radiotherapy to the prostate, comparable in many respects to HDR brachytherapy, but using a non-invasive approach. In the 1980s, prostate cancer patients were treated in the United Kingdom with six fractions of 6 Gy each, delivered over three weeks, which resulted in good disease control with no major early or late morbidity [1–3]. In August 2000, Virginia Mason initiated their "SHARP" trial (Stereotactic Hypofractionated Accurate Radiotherapy of the Prostate). Using six non-coplanar beams and "daily stereotactic localization," they delivered 33.5 Gy in five fractions to 40 low-risk prostate patients. Five-year outcome results were reported at ASTRO 2010. According to this, biochemical relapse-free survival was 93% using a nadir + 2 definition, but only 71% using the ASTRO definition. Median PSA nadir was 0.65 ng/ml. Late GU toxicity was 33% and late GI toxicity was 30%. Reportedly, all toxicities eventually resolved [4, 5].

Delivering hypofractionated radiation to the prostate, particularly doses of 5 Gy or more per fraction, demands precision in both treatment planning and treatment delivery. This was emphasized in a report on prostate SBRT released by ASTRO's Emerging Technologies committee in 2010 [6].

Most important is the ability to track and correct for the unpredictable motion of the prostate that occurs during treatment set-up and delivery. Positional changes of up to 7 mm have been recorded, with most marked differences noted in pitch [7]. At present, only the CyberKnife System is able to detect and correct for prostate positional variation in six dimensions.

The first results of robotic radiosurgery for localized prostate cancer have been published by King and colleagues [8]. In that study, 41 patients received a dose of 36.25 Gy in five equal fractions, using homogeneous delivery. Approximately half received treatment on consecutive days, the remainder every other day. At a median follow-up of 33 months, no patient had experienced biochemical failure. Toxicity was generally limited to mild to moderate (grade 1–2) urinary symptoms and moderate rectal complaints. Two patients did develop grade 3 urinary toxicity. No patient developed significant rectal toxicity. Erectile function was preserved in approximately 50% of the patients.

Friedland et al. have reported on 112 patients with localized prostate cancer treated with SBRT, also using a homogeneous dose distribution [9]. Most patients received 35 Gy in five fractions delivered on consecutive days. At a median 24-month follow-up, two patients had developed biopsy-confirmed local relapse. One patient developed distant failure with no evidence of local recurrence. Urinary and rectal toxicities were generally mild to moderate and self-limiting. One patient developed a grade 3 rectal complication. Erectile function was preserved in 82% of the patients.

Katz et al. have published results on 304 patients treated with SBRT for localized prostate cancer. Fifty patients received 35 Gy in five fractions and the remaining 254 patients received 36.25 Gy. At a median follow-up of 30 months, no biochemical failures were noted in the 35-Gy group, but four biochemical progressions were observed in the 36.25-Gy group. Only one had local recurrence documented on repeat prostate biopsy. Toxicity was limited to moderate (grade 2) urinary symptoms in 4.7% and rectal symptoms in 3.6%. Only one grade 3 urinary complication was reported. Erectile function was preserved in 87% at 18 months [10].

King et al. have updated their previously published experience, reporting on 67 patients with a median 33-month follow-up. All patients received 36.25 Gy in five fractions using a homogeneous dose distribution. Only two patients developed PSA, biopsy-proven local failures. Median PSA nadir was 0.5 ng/ml. There were no grade 4 toxicities. Two patients did experience grade 3 GU toxicity, exacerbated in both cases by urological instrumentation. No grade 3 rectal toxicities were reported [11].

Meier and coworkers have recently reported results from a multi-institutional study of SBRT for low- to intermediate-risk prostate cancer using homogeneous

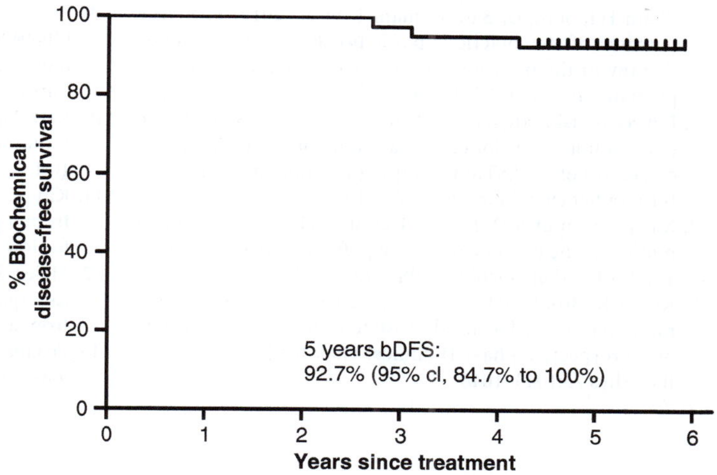

Fig. 13.1 Kaplan–Meier biochemical disease-free survival curve after SBRT for prostate cancer. Median follow-up is 5 years. Three of the forty-one patients recurred, at 33, 37, and 42 months post-treatment

dosing. With a minimum follow-up of three months, no acute grade 3 toxicities developed in the 211 patients included in the study. Grade 2 GU toxicity developed in 20%, and three patients required temporary catheter placement for acute urinary retention. Only one late grade 3 GU toxicity was reported (bladder neck necrosis). Acute GI toxicity occurred in <10% of patients. The 12-month median PSA was 0.9 ng/ml (n=73) [12].

Most recently, Freeman and King have published five year outcome data on 41 low-risk patients treated with 35–36.25 Gy in five fractions using a homogeneous dose distribution. The five year median biochemical disease-free survival was 92.7% (Fig. 13.1). No patient experienced grade 3 or 4 rectal toxicity. One patient did develop grade 3 urinary toxicity following repeated instrumentation. Most patients experienced mild to moderate acute symptoms that resolved within three months of treatment completion. No patient developed regional or distant metastases [13].

13.5 Conclusions

Five years ago, fewer than 20 patients with prostate cancer had been treated with "hypofractionated stereotactic radiotherapy (SBRT)" using the CyberKnife system. Today, over 5,000 men with localized prostate cancer have received CyberKnife SBRT, and that number is growing. As data from the early cohorts of patients matures, we are gaining a better understanding of the potential long-term benefits of this form of therapy. Biochemical disease control appears comparable to other available therapies, with no increased toxicity. In addition, the treatment can be completed in a time period that is notably shorter (one to two weeks) than conventional radiotherapy (about seven weeks) or moderately hypofractionated radiotherapy (about four to five weeks), and neither hospitalization nor surgical recovery are involved. By shortening overall treatment times, SBRT for prostate cancer has the potential to improve patients' quality of life, reduce time commitment to treatment, and reduce health-care costs.

References

1. Brenner DJ (2003) Hypofractionation for prostate cancer radiotherapy – what are the issues? Int J Radiat Oncol Biol Phys 57:912–914
2. Collins CD, Lloyd-Davies RW, Swan AV (1991) Radical external beam radiotherapy for localised carcinoma of the prostate using a hypofractionation technique. Clin Oncol (R Coll Radiol) 3:127–132
3. Lloyd-Davies RW, Collins CD, Swan AV (1990) Carcinoma of prostate treated by radical external beam radiotherapy using hypofractionation. Twenty-two years' experience (1962–1984). Urology 36:107–111
4. Madsen BL, Hsi RA, Pham HT et al (2007) Stereotactic hypofractionated accurate radiotherapy of the prostate (SHARP), 33.5 Gy in five fractions for localized disease: first clinical trial results. Int J Radiat Oncol Biol Phys 67:1099–1105

5. Phẫm HT, Song G, Badiozamani K et al (2010) Five-year outcome of stereotactic hypofractionated accurate radiotherapy of the prostate (sharp) for patients with low-risk prostate cancer. In: ASTRO Annual Meeting, vol. 78, S58pp
6. Buyyounouski MK, Balter P, Lewis B et al (2010) Stereotactic body radiotherapy for early-stage non-small-cell lung cancer: report of the ASTRO Emerging Technology Committee. Int J Radiat Oncol Biol Phys 78:3–10
7. Xie Y, Djajaputra D, King CR et al (2008) Intrafractional motion of the prostate during hypofractionated radiotherapy. Int J Radiat Oncol Biol Phys 72:236–246
8. King CR, Brooks JD, Gill H et al (2009) Stereotactic body radiotherapy for localized prostate cancer: interim results of a prospective phase II clinical trial. Int J Radiat Oncol Biol Phys 73:1043–1048
9. Friedland JL, Freeman DE, Masterson-McGary ME et al (2009) Stereotactic body radiotherapy: an emerging treatment approach for localized prostate cancer. Technol Cancer Res Treat 8:387–392
10. Katz AJ, Santoro M, Ashley R et al (2010) Stereotactic body radiotherapy for organ-confined prostate cancer. BMC Urol 10:1
11. King CR, Brooks JD, Gill H et al (2011) Long-term outcomes from a prospective trial of stereotactic body radiotherapy for low-risk prostate cancer. Int J Radiat Oncol Biol Phys
12. Meier R, Sanda M, Kaplan I (2010) Robotic radiosurgery for organ-confined prostate cancer: early toxicity outcomes from a multi-institutional trial. J Urol 183:E785
13. Freeman DE, King CR (2011) Stereotactic body radiotherapy for low-risk prostate cancer: five-year outcomes. Radiat Oncol 6:3

Virtual HDR® CyberKnife Treatment for Localized Prostatic Carcinoma: Principles and Clinical Update

14

Donald B. Fuller

CONTENTS

14.1 Abstract

CyberKnife® (CK) robotic stereotactic body radiotherapy (SBRT) is a noninvasive method to deliver radiation dose distributions that very closely resemble those delivered by high-dose-rate (HDR) brachytherapy. We have applied "Virtual HDR" CK SBRT as an "HDR surrogate," using comparable dose fractionation schedules in all settings where HDR brachytherapy has been applied, including as monotherapy for favorable to intermediate-risk cases, as a boost for high risk cases and as a salvage method for post-radiotherapeutic relapse cases.

Clinical results are encouraging in all three settings, suggesting at least comparable safety and efficacy. Our Virtual HDR CyberKnife monotherapy pilot series to test the equivalence to HDR brachytherapy and other methods of radiation delivery continues, as does a significantly larger multi-institutional series, to confirm our pilot series findings in a larger number of patients, treated across a wider variety of CyberKnife practices.

14.2 Heterogeneous Dose Distribution CyberKnife SBRT for Prostate Cancer Rationale

Our CyberKnife prostate treatment method is based on high dose rate (HDR) brachytherapy, a precise and powerful hypofractionated radiation delivery mechanism, with established efficacy for prostate cancer [1–4]. HDR brachytherapy allows flexible radiation dose sculpting, with increased dose in the peripheral zone of the prostate, so that the highest radiation dose matches the cancer-cell distribution in this region (Fig. 14.1) [3, 5]. The dose fractionation delivered by this method also appears well suited to prostate cancer, due to the purported low α/β ratio, which indicates a high sensitivity to hypofractionation [1, 6, 7]. HDR brachytherapy is used as monotherapy for early prostate cancer [1, 8] and in combination with external beam radiotherapy in the treatment of

L.E. Ponsky et al. (eds.), *Treating Prostate Cancer and Related Genitourinary Applications*, Robotic Radiosurgery, DOI 10.1007/978-3-642-11495-3_14,

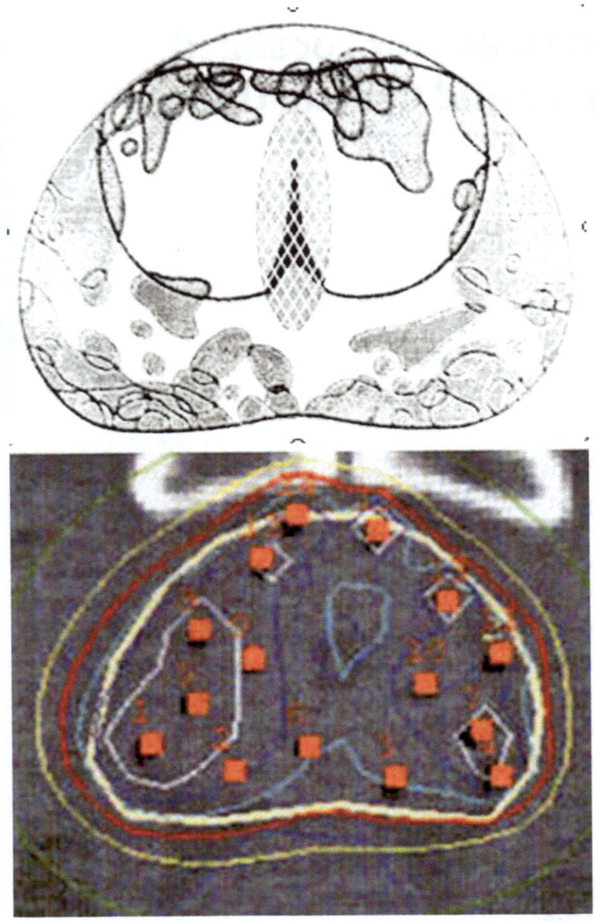

Fig. 14.1 Illustration of typical peripheral zone prostate cancer distribution (*dark gray shaded regions; top panel*) versus typical peripheral HDR dose-escalation pattern (*white and light blue isodose lines, bottom panel*)

intermediate-to-advanced prostate cancer [2–4]. The primary drawback of HDR brachytherapy is that it is an invasive procedure, requiring hospital admission, anesthesia, nursing support, and narcotic analgesia to place and manage the indwelling transperineal HDR catheters and deals with their attendant pain and risk of infection and thromboembolism.

CyberKnife® (CK; Accuray Incorporated, Sunnyvale, CA) stereotactic body radiotherapy (SBRT) is an image-guided method for accurately delivering a quantitative radiation distribution to a precisely defined three-dimensional target volume, and is capable of creating very steep dose gradients within and beyond the planning target volume (PTV). This facilitates the safe use of biologically potent, large dose-per-fraction, hypofractionated radiation dose schedules to the prostate similar to those delivered by HDR brachytherapy. CK SBRT treatment plans for the prostate have shown superior bladder and rectal tissue sparing compared with intensity-modulated radiotherapy (IMRT), although as yet there is no clinical documentation of clinical superiority [7].

Our founding project, published in 2008, evaluated ten patients treated with a CK SBRT treatment method that we entitled "Virtual HDR" to describe the core philosophy of emulating HDR brachytherapy dose distribution, using CK as the SBRT delivery platform. We compared the CK SBRT dose distributions with simulated actual HDR brachytherapy on the same 10 CK SBRT treatment plans, replanning all of them using simulated idealized HDR catheter placements on the Varisource® (Varian Medical Systems, Palo Alto, CA) HDR brachytherapy treatment planning system [9]. In addition to delivering a published HDR brachytherapy dose fractionation regimen of 38 Gy/4 fractions, our study demonstrated substantial equivalence in intraprostatic dose morphology patterns between Virtual HDR CK SBRT treatment plans and simulated actual HDR treatment plans. Significant dose escalation was obtained within the peripheral zone of the prostate, with relative sparing of bladder, urethra, and rectum that also appeared at least as favorable with CK Virtual HDR treatment plans as with simulated actual HDR treatment plans [9]. This ability of CK SBRT to substantially mimic HDR brachytherapy dose distribution has subsequently been confirmed by other investigators [10]. These authors found this method feasible to deliver to their patients, with a suggestion of lower urinary tract toxicity versus their historical actual HDR patients. This was postulated by them as possibly due to the removal of HDR catheter trauma from the equation in their CK SBRT cases.

A comparison of our original Virtual HDR® CK SBRT with simulated actual HDR brachytherapy dose distribution is illustrated in Fig. 14.2. The flexibility of the virtual HDR® CK SBRT approach in the creation of "HDR-like" dosimetry morphology in a variety of prostate cancer presentations is illustrated in Fig. 14.3.

In addition to duplicating HDR dosimetry and accurate plan delivery, the Virtual HDR® CK SBRT method offers several practical advantages over actual HDR brachytherapy, the most obvious being the avoidance of the surgical placement of HDR catheters, with attendant HDR catheter-induced trauma,

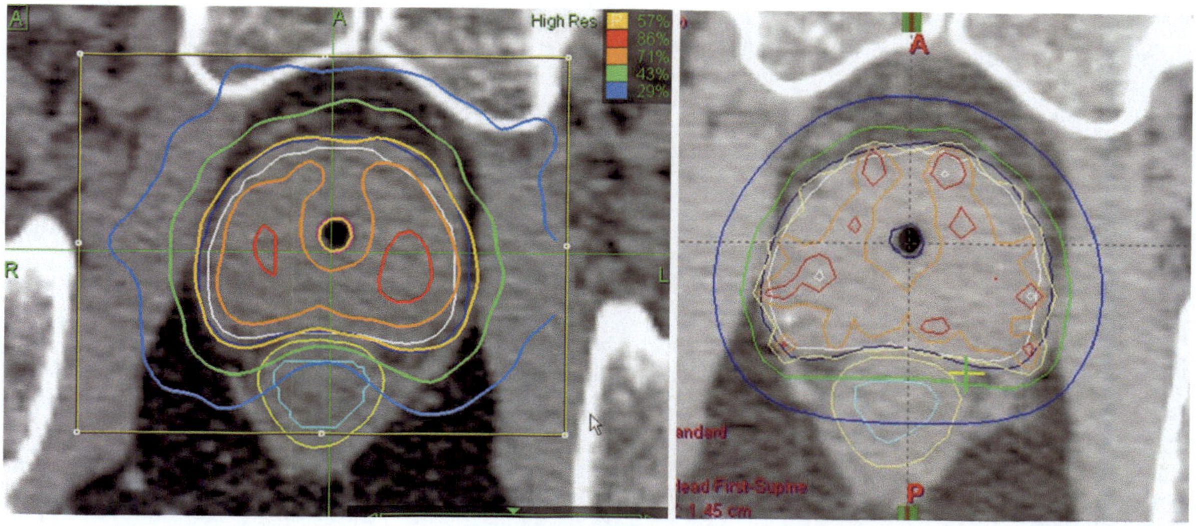

Fig. 14.2 Comparative coverage and dose-escalation morphology between Virtual HDR® CyberKnife SBRT (MultiPlan® image; *left panel*) and simulated actual HDR (Varisource® image; *right panel*). *Blue* = 50%; *Green* = 75%; *Yellow* = 100%; *Orange* = 125% and *red* = 150% isodose coverage

associated hospitalization, and pain management issues [9–11]. By comparison, the delivery of CK SBRT is a noninvasive outpatient procedure. Additionally, the delivery of a "HDR-like" CK SBRT pattern is possible in virtually all anatomic situations, while the delivery of actual HDR brachytherapy may be compromised by issues such as a large or inaccessible prostate or pubic arch interference altering the planned trajectory of HDR brachytherapy catheters. Finally, CK SBRT is capable of delivering the dose pattern with at least comparable accuracy versus actual HDR brachytherapy, due to the continuously updated image-guidance robotic tracking feature intrinsic to the CyberKnife device [12, 13].

14.3 Clinical Results of Heterogeneous CyberKnife SBRT Treatment for Prostate Cancer

We began treating patients using the Virtual HDR® CK SBRT method under IRB-approved clinical trial protocol in 2006, open to favorable prognosis patients (DRE stage T1–T2b, Gleason Score ≤ 6, PSA level ≤ 10 ng/mL), and selected intermediate prognosis patients (Gleason Score 7 or PSA level 10.1–20 ng/mL if other favorable characteristics still present), first reporting preliminary results in 2008, describing typically self-limited acute toxicity and a favorable short-term PSA response [9].

All patients received 38 Gy in four fractions, a schedule that has been shown efficacious with HDR brachytherapy, using "HDR-like" dosimetry molding within and around the prostate [9]. Our CK SBRT treatment plans have had a specific set of objectives and constraints, including a minimum PTV prescription dose coverage requirement of 95% (V100 ≥ 95%), a minimum intraprostatic D_{max} dose escalation level of 150% (57 Gy), and a maximum intraprostatic D_{max} dose of 200% (76 Gy). A higher intraprostatic dose was considered only a minor protocol deviation as long as other normal tissue dosimetry requirements are met. Other constraints included a maximum rectal wall dose of 100% of the prescription dose (38 Gy), a maximum rectal mucosa dose of 75% (28.5 Gy), a maximum urethra dose of 120% (45.6 Gy), and a maximum bladder dose of 120% (45.6 Gy). These normal tissue dose limitation objectives are designed to resemble those commonly prescribed in the application of HDR brachytherapy. The rectal mucosa is defined as a solid structure formed by a 3-mm contraction of the MRI/CT determined rectal wall, which we believe coincides with the ultrasound-based HDR brachytherapy "rectum" structure (outer rectal wall is typically *not* visible on ultrasound imaging). The

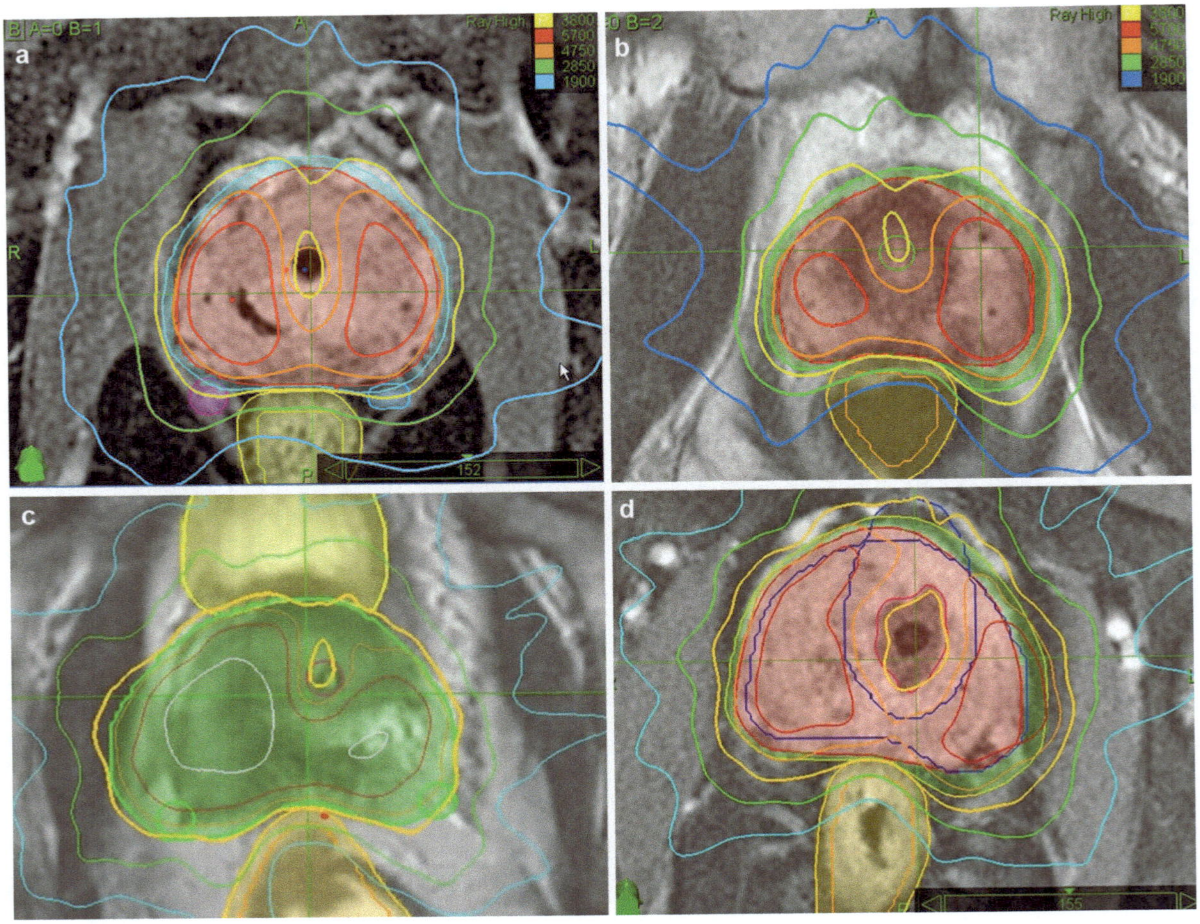

Fig. 14.3 The Virtual HDR® dose pattern may accommodate a variety of clinical presentations, including: (**a**) Classic narrow margin coverage for a favorable prognosis case (*upper left image*); (**b**) Extended extracapsular coverage for an intermediate prognosis lesion (*upper right hand image*, showing asymmetrically larger margin coverage of the left lobe to accommodate high-risk pathology features on that side; note that this plan also concentrates hyperdosage within the prostate ipsilaterally, as indicated by the red 150% isodose line); (**c**) Extreme dose escalation applied to a CK SBRT boost for a right-sided T4 lesion (*lower left image*; *red* = 150% and *white* = 200% isodose coverage); (**d**) Exaggerated Central Sparing in a patient with a pre-existing TURP defect (*lower right image*). In each image, regardless of the magnitude of internal prostate dosimetry escalation and extracapsular coverage, note that the *yellow prescription yellow isodose line* touches, but does not encroach upon, the outer rectal wall. There is no specific prostate volume limit to this approach

interested reader is referred to our 2008 manuscript for a more detailed description of the dosimetry morphology of Virtual HDR® CK SBRT versus that produced by simulated actual HDR brachytherapy [9].

14.3.1 Clinical Outcomes: 2010 Update

Our Virtual HDR CK SBRT study has continued and enlarged to 54 patients, with a current median follow-up of 30 months and a maximum follow-up of 4 years. Our series includes 33 favorable and 21 intermediate prognosis patients; with a median presenting PSA level of 6.33 ng/mL (range 1.0–14.1 ng/mL). Thirty-eight patients presented with a Gleason score of 5–6 and 16 presented with a Gleason score of 7.

14.3.1.1 PSA Response

Our most recent PSA response data are displayed in Fig. 14.4. Compared with the baseline median PSA

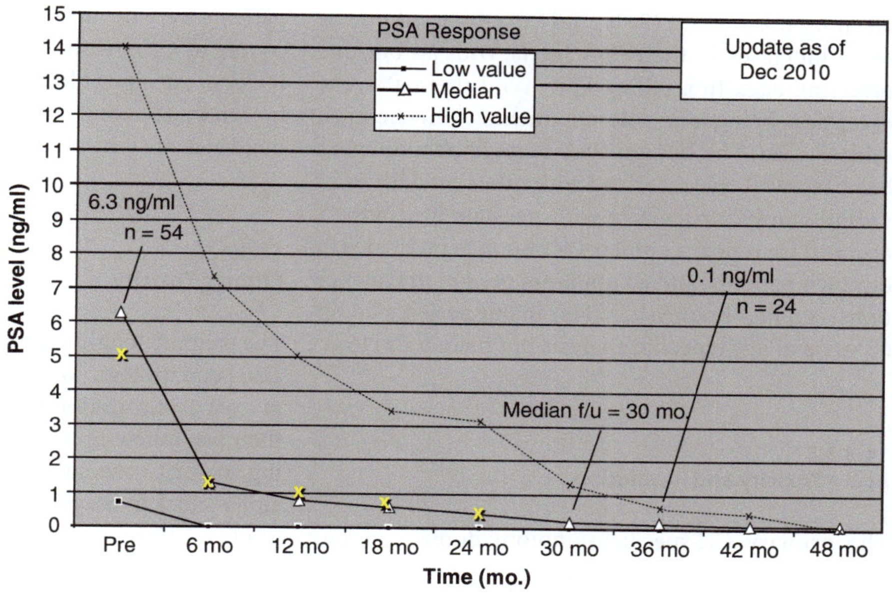

Fig. 14.4 PSA Response to 4 years for our Virtual HDR® Clinical trial patient cohort. Median follow-up is 2.5 years. *Yellow* "X" marks denote corresponding values for the Multi-institutional "Emulating HDR" CyberKnife SBRT Study, which has a significantly larger patient sample size, but shorter maximum follow-up

value of 6.33 ng/mL, the median 1-year ($n=41$), 2-year ($n=40$), 3-year ($n=24$), and 4-year ($n=8$) PSA levels measure 0.8 ng/mL, 0.4 ng/mL, 0.1 ng/mL, and 0.1 ng/mL, respectively. In particular, out to 4 years, the PSA-response graph in our cohort bears a striking resemblance to that reported with ^{103}palladium prostate brachytherapy, described by Blasko et al. [14]. Although our CK SBRT approach is modeled more directly after HDR brachytherapy than ^{103}palladium brachytherapy, we were unable to locate a specific published HDR-monotherapy-based 4-year PSA kinetic analysis with which we could directly compare our biochemical response result.

As demonstrated by the multi-institutional PSA nadir analysis reported by Ray et al., a lower PSA nadir and longer time to PSA nadir constitute powerful predictors (surrogates) for long-term success in the treatment of prostate cancer, with respect to 10-year PSA-based disease-free survival and 10-year freedom from distant metastatic disease [15]. In their study, an absolute PSA nadir <0.5 ng/mL and a time to PSA nadir >24 months were the strongest predictors of subsequent 10-year freedom from biochemical relapse and distant-metastases. In our series, the median 3- and 4-year PSA values each measure 0.1 ng/mL, with 88% of patients achieving a PSA-nadir ≤ 0.5 ng/mL by 3 years ($n=24$) and 100% reaching this level by 4 years ($n=8$). In our 36 patients followed 30 months or greater, a PSA nadir has not yet been reached in 34 of them (94%), indicating that the typical time to PSA nadir in our series is well beyond the 24-month favorable prognosis benchmark. As such, by both PSA endpoints reported in the Ray et al. analysis, our series displays PSA kinetics that are strongly predictive of a long-term freedom from biochemical relapse and freedom from distant metastases rates that will compare favorably with other contemporary methods of radiotherapy. At the time of this writing, only one of our protocol patients has relapsed, and this was a distant relapse (para-aortic lymph nodes) that occurred at 24 months, also accompanied by biochemical relapse. This leads to an absolute 98% freedom from biochemical and clinical relapse rate in our series, which is comparable to the 98% HDR brachytherapy monotherapy freedom from relapse result, with an identical dose fractionation (38 Gy/4 fractions), reported by Grills et al. [1]. Of note, our own series contains a higher percentage of intermediate prognosis patients, while the Grills' series has a slightly longer median follow-up period. This comparison may be further complicated by unknown differences and biases in selection criteria, prognostic factors, pathologic grading differences, etc., but there is at least a suggestion of comparable efficacy between our respective patient series.

Finally, we also report a substantial incidence of benign PSA bounces in our Virtual HDR® protocol patient series. Of our 41 protocol patients followed for at least a year, 14 (33%) have experienced one or more increases in their PSA levels, with all but one reverting back to a falling PSA trend thereafter, the exception being our sole-documented biochemical relapse case. The benign PSA bounce phenomenon has been well characterized with other modalities of radiotherapy, particularly with prostate brachytherapy, and we report a similar PSA bounce incidence in our own patients, and an apparent greater prevalence of benign PSA bounce behavior in our patients under 60 years of age (specific analysis not included) [16].

14.3.1.2 Acute Toxicity and Resolution

The primary CK-specific symptom domain in our patients has been urologic; 98% of patients developed grade 1–2 GU symptoms within 3 months of treatment, with a median 10-point I-PSS score increase 14 days post-treatment, frequently accompanied by dysuria. Partial resolution was observed at 1 month and a complete return to their I-PSS baseline was observed at 2 months post-treatment (Fig. 14.5). All patients have been placed on alpha blockade medication immediately prior to the initiation of their CK SBRT treatment, with a median time to alpha blockade withdrawal of 8 weeks, with some patients requiring a longer course of alpha blockade medication for persistent obstructive symptoms. It should be noted that 34% of our patients were on alpha blocker medicines before their course of CyberKnife treatment, and a return to this incidence of alpha blocker medicine use in our patients is seen by 18-months post-treatment, with an elevated incidence of alpha blocker usage in the interim.

14.3.1.3 Chronic Toxicity

The primary long-term post-CK symptom domain has also been urologic, with 15/41 (37%) patients followed at least 1 year presenting grade 1–2 GU symptoms at their last follow-up (13/15 = grade 1). The overwhelming majority are so classified because of protracted alpha blocker usage, with 2/41 (5%) displaying late grade 3 GU toxicity (catheter-dependent late obstruction), one improving to grade 0 status following successful TURP at 16 months, and the other continuing to require self-catheterization 42 months out. Both patients with delayed grade 3 GU toxicity presented significant obstructive issues before their CK treatment, including a combination of double digit I-PSS scores, a prominent median lobe on imaging, and pre-existing alpha blocker usage at baseline. Excluding patients with this pre-CK profile yields a chronic grade 3 or higher GU toxicity incidence of zero. Long-term grade 1–2 rectal toxicity has been seen in 5/41 patients followed greater than a year, including three patients with grade 1 hematochezia, a single patient with grade

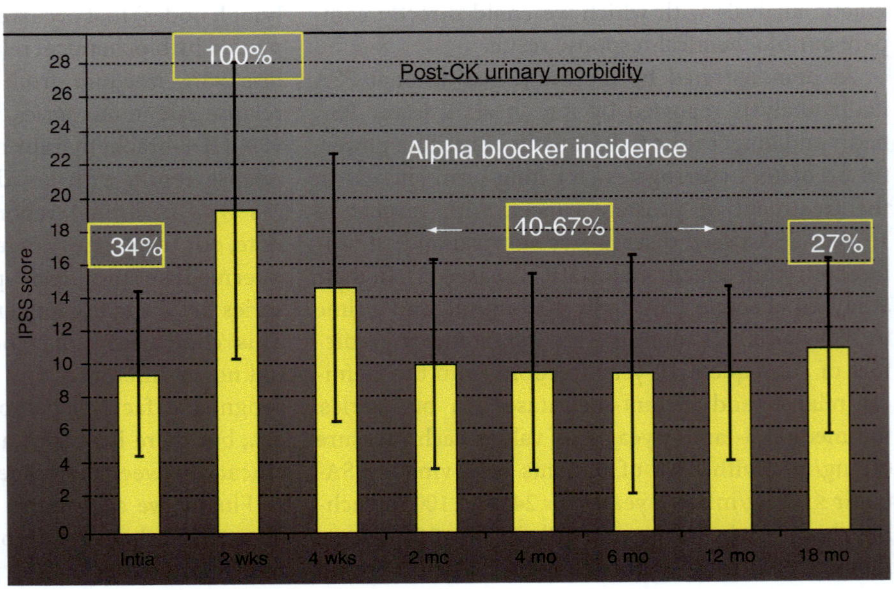

Fig. 14.5 I-PSS Score progression pre- and post-Virtual HDR® CyberKnife SBRT. Note peak at 2 weeks, with return to baseline by 2 months, with elevated incidence of alpha blocker usage to 12–18 months

2 hematochezia that responded completely to laser photocoagulation, and one patient with proctalgia at his last follow-up. Of the four cases of delayed hematochezia, two have resolved completely, and the remaining two persist but are mild and nonprogressive. There has been no long-term grade 3 or higher GI toxicity. Regarding potency preservation, 18% of our patients followed a year or longer have developed erectile dysfunction, defined as a ≥7 point drop in their Sexual Health Inventory Matrix (SHIM) score at their last follow-up, compared with their pre-CK baseline SHIM function. This compares favorably with the potency preservation rates using other radiotherapeutic and surgical treatment methods.

14.4 Conclusions

14.4.1 CyberKnife Monotherapy Using "HDR-Like" Dose Molding

It is our hypothesis that the CyberKnife SBRT may be used to deliver HDR-like dosimetry to the prostate noninvasively. Our comparative dosimetry evaluation project revealed this to be true in terms of prostate-dose escalation and adjacent tissue sparing capability on respective CK versus HDR treatment plans [9]. Clinically, with a median 30-month follow-up period, we are seeing biochemical tumor control rates comparable to HDR and seed brachytherapy, with a 98% absolute biochemical disease-free survival rate and a median 4-year PSA nadir of 0.1 ng/mL. Long-term GU and GI delayed toxicity rates appear no higher than those reported with HDR and permanent source brachytherapy [1, 14]. A modicum of "brachytherapy wisdom" may also be appropriate when considering CK monotherapy in prostate cancer patients with pre-existing severe obstructive uropathy, as our few cases with grade 3 delayed GU toxicity appear limited to that group. Patients with this presenting profile may benefit from the judicious use of urethral opening interventions followed by a suitable recovery period pre-CK treatment, or alternatively, may be more seriously considered for other methods of local treatment instead.

14.4.2 Other Uses of "HDR-Like" CK SBRT for Prostate Cancer

Although we most commonly use CK SBRT as monotherapy, this treatment method has also been used as a boost in conjunction with conventionally fractionated wide-field radiotherapy, or as local salvage therapy in patients who have failed following prior prostate radiotherapy [2, 4, 17]. We have used CK SBRT as a "HDR surrogate" in each of these clinical situations.

14.4.2.1 "HDR-Like" CK SBRT Boosting

We have done this for a select group of patients with clinically localized high-risk lesions, typically having at least one of the following features: T3 primary lesion, Gleason score ≥8, iPSA ≥ 20 ng/mL, or multiple non-favorable prognostic features (e.g., – Gleason 7 *and* iPSA > 10 ng/mL). In these cases, where both central tumor burden *and* the potential for substantial tumor spread beyond the prostate are each major concerns, we have used a CK SBRT boost schedule described by the William Beaumont Hospital HDR brachytherapy group to maximize the radiobiologic dose centrally, delivering a "HDR-like" CK SBRT boost dose of 21 Gy/2 fractions [17]. This has been done in conjunction with whole pelvis IMRT to address the potential for subclinical disease spread beyond the prostate, using a dose of 41.4 Gy/23 fractions, which is a slight reduction compared with the William Beaumont external beam protocol of 45 Gy/25 fractions. This reduction applied out of respect for a somewhat larger "low isodose spillover" to the lower pelvis tissues with CK SBRT relative to HDR brachytherapy, effectively adding the equivalent of about two IMRT fractions to first echelon pelvic lymph nodes. This treatment approach has been used in 20 of our patients, and in spite of its more aggressive nature compared with CK monotherapy, the curative result appears inferior, with an absolute biochemical control rate of 75% (versus 98% for our CK SBRT monotherapy group). Although we have not routinely rebiopsied biochemical relapse cases, we have followed their prostates serially post-treatment, through the use of multiple sequential Dynamic Contrast Enhanced (DCE) MRI studies, and all biochemical relapse cases evaluated by this methodology appear to have persistently controlled prostate primary lesions, suggesting that their relapses are more likely distant, reflecting the more advanced nature of their disease at presentation.

14.4.2.2 "HDR-Like" Salvage of Post-Radiotherapeutic Local Recurrence

This has been performed in a very limited number of patients at our center, under its own IRB-approved clinical trial [18], based on successful HDR brachytherapy salvage results reported by the UCSF group [18]. Our dose fractionation schedule in this group is 34 Gy/5 fractions, which is of similar calculated biologic potency compared with the UCSF series [18], and biologically less aggressive than our CK monotherapy regimen for radiation-naïve cases. This dose de-escalation is applied to reduce the risk of complications in this pre-treated group, which undoubtedly presents a significantly higher risk of significant radiation injury, due to the likely existence of preexisting subclinical radiation injury from their initial prostate radiotherapy course.

Our selection criteria for treatment under this protocol include a period of at least 2 years following the initial radiation course, biopsy proof of post-radiotherapeutic local recurrence, absence of disease beyond the prostate/seminal vesicle region, and absence of preexisting injury greater than grade 1 from their initial course of radiotherapy.

At this juncture only five patients have been treated under this protocol; at a maximum follow-up period of 18 months, with 4/5 patients displaying a major PSA decrease by 12 months, with our only "non-responder" lost to follow-up after 6 months. None of them have experienced severe complications from retreatment. Interestingly, the responders have shown identical PSA decline kinetics out to 12–18 months, versus our de novo Virtual HDR cases, which were treated to a substantially more aggressive dose and larger PTV. Obviously these results are preliminary, yet they do seem encouraging, and provocatively, suggest that the next modification using this technique could well be a de-escalation of dose for the substantially larger population of radiation naïve cases.

References

1. Grills IS, Martinez AA, Hollander M et al (2004) High dose rate brachytherapy as prostate cancer monotherapy reduces toxicity compared to low dose rate palladium seeds. J Urol 171:1098–1104
2. Demanes DJ, Rodriguez RR, Schour L et al (2005) High-dose-rate intensity-modulated brachytherapy with external beam radiotherapy for prostate cancer: California endocurietherapy's 10-year results. Int J Radiat Oncol Biol Phys 61:1306–1316
3. Mate TP, Gottesman JE, Hatton J et al (1998) High dose-rate afterloading 192Iridium prostate brachytherapy: feasibility report. Int J Radiat Oncol Biol Phys 41:525–533
4. Vargas CE, Martinez AA, Boike TP et al (2006) High-dose irradiation for prostate cancer via a high-dose-rate brachytherapy boost: results of a phase I to II study. Int J Radiat Oncol Biol Phys 66:416–423
5. McNeal JE, Redwine EA, Freiha FS et al (1988) Zonal distribution of prostatic adenocarcinoma. Correlation with histologic pattern and direction of spread. Am J Surg Pathol 12:897–906
6. Williams SG, Taylor JM, Liu N et al (2007) Use of individual fraction size data from 3756 patients to directly determine the alpha/beta ratio of prostate cancer. Int J Radiat Oncol Biol Phys 68:24–33
7. King CR, Lehmann J, Adler JR et al (2003) CyberKnife radiotherapy for localized prostate cancer: rationale and technical feasibility. Technol Cancer Res Treat 2:25–30
8. Demanes D, Altieri G, Barnaba M et al (2006) High dose rate (HDR) monotherapy is equivalent to combined HDR brachytherapy and external beam radiation therapy (EBRT) for early prostate cancer. Int J Radiat Oncol Biol Phys 66:S351
9. Fuller DB, Naitoh J, Lee C et al (2008) Virtual HDR CyberKnife treatment for localized prostatic carcinoma: dosimetry comparison with HDR brachytherapy and preliminary clinical observations. Int J Radiat Oncol Biol Phys 70:1588–1597
10. Aluwini S, van Rooij P, Hoogeman M et al (2010) CyberKnife stereotactic radiotherapy as monotherapy for low- to intermediate-stage prostate cancer: early experience, feasibility, and tolerance. J Endourol 24:865–869
11. Chang SD, Main W, Martin DP et al (2003) An analysis of the accuracy of the CyberKnife: a robotic frameless stereotactic radiosurgical system. Neurosurgery 52:140–146, discussion 146–147
12. Ho AK, Fu D, Cotrutz C et al (2007) A study of the accuracy of cyberknife spinal radiosurgery using skeletal structure tracking. Neurosurgery 60:ONS147–ONS156, discussion ONS156
13. Xie Y, Djajaputra D, King CR et al (2008) Intrafractional motion of the prostate during hypofractionated radiotherapy. Int J Radiat Oncol Biol Phys 72:236–246
14. Blasko JC, Grimm PD, Sylvester JE et al (2000) Palladium-103 brachytherapy for prostate carcinoma. Int J Radiat Oncol Biol Phys 46:839–850
15. Ray ME, Thames HD, Levy LB et al (2006) PSA nadir predicts biochemical and distant failures after external beam radiotherapy for prostate cancer: a multi-institutional analysis. Int J Radiat Oncol Biol Phys 64: 1140–1150

16. Caloglu M, Ciezki JP, Reddy CA et al (2011) PSA bounce and biochemical failure after brachytherapy for prostate cancer: a study of 820 patients with a minimum of 3 years of follow-Up. Int J Radiat Oncol Biol Phys 80(3):735–741, Epub 2010 Jun 18
17. Lee B, Shinohara K, Weinberg V et al (2007) Feasibility of high-dose-rate brachytherapy salvage for local prostate cancer recurrence after radiotherapy: the University of California-San Francisco experience. Int J Radiat Oncol Biol Phys 67:1106–1112
18. Fuller D, et al. Virtual HDR CyberKnife Radiosurgery for locally recurrent Prostatic Carcinoma: A phase II Study. http://clinicaltrials.gov/. Accessed Sept, 2011

15

Patient Selection for Robotic Radiosurgery for Clinically Localized Prostate Cancer: Come One, Come All

Sean P. Collins, Simeng Suy, Eric Oermann, Siyan Lie, Xia Yu, Heather Hanscom, Joy Kim, Benjamin Sherer, Hyeon U. Park, Brian T. Collins, Kevin McGeagh, Nancy Dawson, John H. Lynch, and Anatoly Dritschilo

CONTENTS

15.1 Abstract

Optimal treatment of prostate cancer patients is provided by a multidisciplinary team comprised of urologists, radiation oncologists, and medical oncologists, working together to stratify patients based upon their life expectancy, extent of disease, acceptance of risks and benefits, and consideration of potential changes in quality of life. Available treatment options range from radical prostatectomy to various forms of radiation therapy including intensity-modulated radiation therapy (IMRT), low dose rate (LDR) brachytherapy, high dose rate (HDR) brachytherapy, proton beam therapy, and robotic radiosurgery. Robotic radiosurgery is the most recent addition to the treatment arsenal for clinically localized prostate cancer that builds upon developments in enhanced precision of radiation delivery and the use of imaging guidance throughout treatment. Given the variety of available treatment options, the clinical considerations and patient selection criteria for each of these treatment options will be reviewed with a focus on applications of robotic radiosurgery for patients with disease confined to the prostate and adjacent tissues.

15.2 Radical Prostatectomy

Prostate-specific antigen (PSA) screening has led to earlier diagnosis of prostate cancer in men at stages in which the tumor is organ-confined and potentially curable by radical surgery or radiation therapy [1, 2]. Radical prostatectomy is an effective treatment for younger men presenting with organ-confined disease and low- to intermediate-risk factors [3–6]. Radical prostatectomy reduces the risk of local progression, metastasis development, prostate cancer-specific mortality and overall mortality as compared to watchful waiting [7]. Patients with limited life expectancy

L.E. Ponsky et al. (eds.), *Treating Prostate Cancer and Related Genitourinary Applications*, Robotic Radiosurgery, DOI 10.1007/978-3-642-11495-3_15,

and/or pre-existing medical conditions such as obesity or cardiovascular diseases generally are not candidates for radical prostatectomy. Furthermore, the risks of surgery include higher incidences of incontinence and impotence, leading some men in surgical age groups to select radiation therapy, based on quality of life considerations [8, 9].

Unfortunately, there are no definitive randomized-clinical trials that directly compare surgery to radiation therapy treatment options. Data from retrospectively reviewed series support radical prostatectomy for long-term local tumor control [3–6], while radiation therapy provides comparable intermediate-term local control with improved quality of life [8, 9]. Local tumor-control impacts cancer cure and failure to achieve local control in the treatment of prostate cancer has been correlated with the development of metastases and death [10–12].

15.3 Radiation Dose Escalation

Local tumor control with radiation is dose-dependent, following a sigmoid dose–response relationship. Results of early clinical applications of conventional external beam radiation treatment (60–70 Gy in 2 Gy fractions) yielded 10-year disease-free survivals ranging from 40% to 70% prompting investigations of dose escalation [13–18]. The randomized-dose escalation trial performed at the M. D. Anderson Cancer Center compared 70–78 Gy [19]. As expected, the 78 Gy arm resulted in improved local control, but, at the price of increased rectal complications. Similar results have been obtained in other reported randomized trials [20, 21]. The risk of rectal bleeding appears to be dependent upon both, the radiation dose and the volume of the rectum subjected to high doses [22, 23]. Although attempts have been made to limit rectal dose, the incidence of rectal bleeding becomes unacceptable as doses exceed 75–80 Gy using conventional radiation therapy technology. It has become clear that increases in the total dose delivered to the prostate enhance local tumor control, offering a therapeutic benefit as long as normal tissue tolerances are respected. Current techniques to achieve dose-escalation include IMRT with image-guided radiation therapy (IGRT), LDR brachytherapy, HDR brachytherapy, proton beam therapy, and robotic radiosurgery.

15.4 Intensity Modulated and Image Guided Radiation Therapy

Intensity modulation of the radiation beam was developed to escalate the radiation dose while minimizing the dose to normal tissues. Dosimetric comparisons of conventional treatment plans with IMRT plans have revealed that IMRT is capable of sparing adjacent normal tissues [24, 25]. Use of IMRT for prostate cancer treatment allows for high levels of clinical and biochemical local control with lower complication rates as compared to conventional external beam techniques [25, 26]. This technique has been reported to permit dose-escalation within the prostate to greater than 80 Gy with acceptable risks of radiation-related morbidity [27].

Image guidance has been employed to assure reproducibility in matching the delivered dose distribution to the tumor volume as it is positioned in the patient. The prostate gland has been shown to move to various extents, both from day-to-day (inter-fraction motion) and during treatment (intra-fraction motion) [28, 29]. To adjust for these uncertainties in IMRT treatment, a 10-mm margin is commonly added to the clinical treatment volume (the prostate and seminal vesicles) to generate the planning treatment volume (PTV). Unfortunately, this relatively large margin limits the clinician's ability to escalate the radiation dose to the prostate and accelerate treatment while sparing normal tissues. Recently, the use of intraprostatic metallic fiducials and X-ray detection has been implemented [30]. Daily isocenter localization and set-up offers to reduce the required PTV margin required by inter-fraction motion [31]. Further improvements in IMRT treatment delivery require continuous tracking to minimize the required PTV margin for intra-fraction motion.

15.5 Proton Beam Radiation Therapy

Much recent attention has been directed to the application of proton beam radiation therapy for the treatment of prostate cancer. This approach utilizes charged particles to deliver the radiation dose to a target volume, with the potential benefits of improved physical radiation dose distribution attributable to the Bragg peak associated with particle energy deposition [32]. Proton therapy is not a new modality; protons have been used to treat prostate cancer patients for more than 20 years [33, 34]. However, the technical hurdles associated with clinical applications of proton technology have proven substantial, and there is no clinical evidence of superiority of this approach to linear accelerator generated radiations using IMRT technology [35].

15.6 Low Dose Rate (LDR) Brachytherapy

LDR prostate brachytherapy is performed by interstitial placement of permanent radioactive sources into the prostate in a pre-planned dose distribution using transrectal ultrasound (TRUS) guidance for accurate placement of the needle applicators. The ability to place the radioactive seeds under visual guidance negates the effect of prostate motion. In general, low-risk patients (PSA $\leq$ 10 ng/mL, Gleason score $<$ 7 and clinical stage $<$ T2b) [36] can be effectively treated with LDR brachytherapy as monotherapy with the expectation of PSA relapse-free survival rates exceeding 70% at 8 years [37–43]. Indeed, brachytherapy may be the optimal radiation treatment for select patients including those who are morbidly obese [44]. The treatment of obese patients using external beam techniques is challenged by equipment weight limitations and increased depth of the prostate leading to diminished dose at depth and reproducibly of daily set-up, thereby increasing risks of marginal misses [45]. Obesity does not adversely affect oncologic [46] or quality of life outcomes [47] in brachytherapy series.

The efficacy [37, 48–52] and morbidity [53–57] of LDR brachytherapy as monotherapy are highly dependent on accurate seed placement and reported excellent results may not be reproducible in patients with anatomic limitations or when performed at centers with insufficient patient volumes for the procedure [58, 59]. Not all patients are ideal candidates for LDR brachytherapy. Patients with very small or very large prostates, benign prostatic hyperplasia (large transitional zones and median lobes), pretreatment obstructive urinary symptoms [60–62], and/or prior transurethral resection of the prostate (TURP) are factors recognized to limit patient suitability as optimal candidates for LDR brachytherapy. Patients with large prostates ($>$ 60 cm^3) present technical difficulties such as pubic arch interference [63] and the possible increased risk of urinary morbidity. While prostate volume reduction with neoadjuvant androgen deprivation therapy (ADT) may result in down-sizing of some patients to become LDR brachytherapy candidates [64, 65], patients with poorly responsive benign prostatic hyperplasia are less likely to benefit from ADT [66–69] and the morbidity of ADT may be unacceptable in low-risk patients [70]. Likewise, patients with very small ($<$20 cm^3) prostates [71, 72] or large TURP defects [73, 74] may experience high rates of biochemical failure due to poor dosimetry and increased urinary toxicity due to high urethral doses.

The limited ability of LDR brachytherapy monotherapy to reproducibly cover the areas of extracapsular extension (ECE) [75] and proximal seminal vesicle involvement [76, 77], has provided the rationale to treat patients presenting with intermediate- to high-risk features with external radiation techniques and LDR brachytherapy boost [78–80]. The combination of external radiation to a dose sufficient for treatment of microscopic disease followed by prostatic LDR brachytherapy boost offers the opportunity to dose escalate and limit the dose to the rectal mucosa.

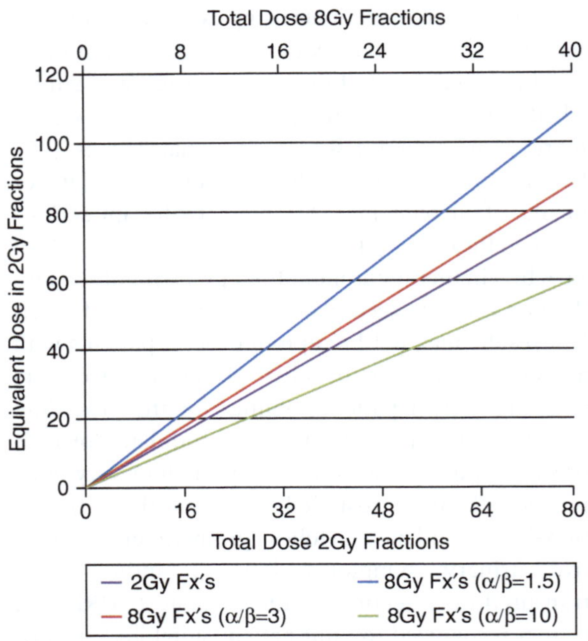

Fig. 15.1 Plot showing the relationship between total dose and equivalent dose in 2 Gy fractions for various α/β ratio values

Intermediate-risk patients can be effectively treated in this manner with a 10-year disease-free survival rate of 70–80% [78–80].

15.7 Rationale for Hypofractionation

The optimal radiation schedule for the treatment of prostate cancer is an area of active scientific inquiry. The alpha–beta ratio (α/β) is a radiobiologic measure of the sensitivity of a tumor or normal tissue to fraction size with values typically ranging between 1 and 10 Gy. The slower the proliferating normal tissue or tumor the lower is the α/β ratio [81, 82]. In general, tumors have α/β values around 10 Gy. Thus, the α/β value for prostate cancer was originally thought to be close to 10 Gy. The α/β value for the major dose-limiting structure, the rectum, is about 3–4 Gy [82]. In this scenario, large fraction sizes would be expected to proportionally damage the rectum more than the tumor (Fig. 15.1). This led clinicians to employ long-treatment courses of low dose per fraction radiation.

Radiobiological interpretation of clinical outcomes has suggested that the α/β for prostate cancer is less than 10 Gy, actually as low as 1–3 Gy. This is consistent with biological data that shows that prostate cancer cells proliferate slowly [83]. If tumor and late responding tissues have similar α/β ratios, there is no clinical rationale for hyperfractionation. If the α/β ratio for the tumor is indeed lower than normal tissues, hypofractionated regimens could allow radiobiological dose escalation with lower acute morbidity and similar late normal tissue toxicity (Fig. 15.1). If the α/β ratio for the tumor is indeed lower than normal tissues, conventional fractionation may be preferentially sparing the cancer [84]. These observations have supported hypofractionated radiation therapy regimens as offering improvements in the therapeutic ratio for prostate cancer treatment by improving tumor control with less harm to normal tissue.

15.8 High Dose Rate (HDR) Brachytherapy

Large radiation fraction sizes have been clinically utilized in the treatment of prostate cancer for many years. HDR brachytherapy as a boost to external-beam radiation therapy (EBRT) has shown promise in this regard [85–91]. HDR brachytherapy was employed to escalate the dose to gross disease within the prostate and seminal vesicles with 3–11.5 Gy fractions over two to four sessions. HDR brachytherapy allows greater flexibility in dose delivery which provides for intra-prostatic dose escalation and optimization of peri-prostatic doses. The supplemental EBRT was designed to treat the prostate and seminal vesicles with a margin to encompass adjacent microscopic disease.

Several studies have reported 5-year biochemical control rates in excess of 85% and 70% for intermediate- and high-risk prostate cancer, respectively with acceptable toxicities [85–91]. More recently, HDR monotherapy has been explored with favorable early results [92–94]. HDR brachytherapy is generally delivered using remote after loading technology. This procedure requires patient hospitalization, with the patient confined to bed and remaining supine for 24–48 h to accommodate applicator positioning and treatment. Even so, catheter migration between treatments is common and must be corrected for [95–97]. Unfortunately, not all prostate cancer patients are eligible for such therapy based on age and co-morbidities.

15.9 Hypofractionated Robotic Radiosurgery

Patients receiving conventional, fractionated radiation therapy are treated daily for approximately 7–9 weeks. Based on logistics and life responsibilities, such prolonged treatment courses present unnecessary hardship for many patients [98]. Early experience with investigations of limited hypofractionation (fraction sizes from 2.5 to 3.5 Gy) has revealed that such regimens were effective without undue toxicity [99–102]. Early investigations of hypofractionated stereotactic body radiation therapy (fraction sizes > 3.5 Gy) were performed with radiation delivery systems that did not allow continuous tracking of the prostate with intrafractional adjustment [103]. Initially, the goal was to maintain a similar level of local control while sparing normal tissue using fairly low fractionated doses. This resulted in relatively low biochemical equivalent dose and inadequate biochemical control [104]. Highly accurate radiation delivery systems able to detect prostate movement and adjust the radiation beam accordingly have allowed other investigators to administer higher doses with excellent biochemical disease-free survivals and toxicities similar to conventional treatments [105–109] (Table 15.1).

The CyberKnife® (Accuray Incorporated, Sunnyvale, CA) is a robotic radiosurgical device with a targeting error of less than 1 mm [110]. Hundreds of individual beams are delivered by a linear accelerator mounted on a flexible robotic arm. The CyberKnife can deliver a highly conformal, uniform dose with steep dose gradients [111, 112] similar to HDR brachytherapy [108]. Unlike standard IGRT, the CyberKnife system incorporates a real-time tracking system that provides updated position information to the robot to correct the targeting of the therapeutic beam during treatment allowing for correction of intra-fraction motion [103]. These features allow for a reduction in the planning target volume (PTV) and therefore limit the dose to surrounding critical organs.

The Stanford protocol used the CyberKnife to treat low-risk patients with 36.25 Gy in five fractions of 7.25 Gy [105]. This dose and fractionation was selected to escalate the biological effective dose while keeping a constant predicted normal tissue late effect (Fig. 15.1). The PTV included the prostate with 3–5 mm margins. The mean PSA at a median of 33 months after treatment was 0.44 ng/mL with no biochemical failures suggesting a high rate of long-term control with this dose and fractionation (Table 15.1). No patient experienced grade 4 toxicity, and only two patients experienced grade 3 late urinary morbidity (Table 15.1) [105].

Due to difficulties in reproducibly treating ECE and the proximal seminal vesicles, LDR brachytherapy monotherapy is not commonly offered to intermediate- to high-risk patients [75–77]. Supplemental EBRT can be added but may increase the risk of bowel/bladder toxicity and sexual dysfunction in this group of patients with a relatively favorable prognosis [113]. In addition, supplemental EBRT could unnecessarily increase the cost of such treatments [114]. Given the excellent results with low-risk patients, hypofractionated robotic radiosurgery monotherapy has been suggested for treatment of intermediate-risk patients [106, 107]. Unlike LDR brachytherapy, hypofractionated robotic radiosurgery reproducibly treats the prostate with 3–5 mm margins (Fig. 15.2) which should be adequate to treat areas of ECE in this patient population [115–117]. For example, as shown in Fig. 15.2 delivery of 36.25 Gy to the isodose line that covers at least 95% of the PTV results in a 30 Gy isodose line (equivalent dose of approximately 60 Gy in 2 Gy fractions) extending on average 14 mm from the prostate covering both areas of microscopic ECE and the proximal seminal vesicles. The addition of the proximal seminal vesicles to the clinical target volume (CTV) does not appear to increase the toxicity of hypofractionated stereotactic body radiation therapy and initial results suggest that this treatment is effective in this patient population (Table 15.1) [106, 107]. Likewise, the addition of ADT may not be required in this patient population

Table 15.1 Hypofractionated radiosurgery results

Group	Number of patients	Dose and fractionation	Biochemical disease-free survival	Grade 3 GU complications (%)	Grade 3 GI complications (%)	Preserved sexual function (%)
Stanford [105]	41	7.25 Gy × 5	100% (2.8 years)	5	0	40
Naples [106]	112	7 Gy × 5	94% (2 years)	0	1	81
Winthrop [107]	50	7 Gy × 5	100% (2.5 years)	0	0	87
	254	7.25 Gy × 5	98% (1.5 years)	0.5	1	

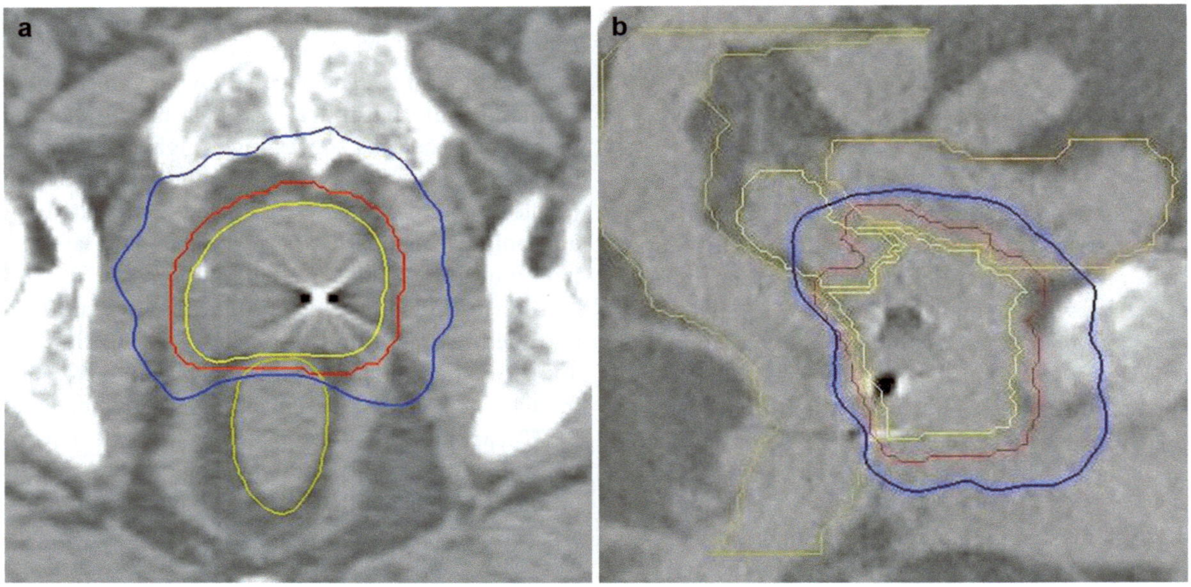

Fig. 15.2 Treatment planning axial (**a**) and sagittal (**b**) computed tomography scan demonstrating the prostate and seminal vesicles (*yellow*), PTV expansion (*red*), bladder (*orange*), and rectum (*green*). In this treatment plan, the prescribed dose of 36.25 Gy is delivered to the isodose line that covers at least 95% of the PTV. This results in a 30 Gy isodose line (*blue*), with a equivalent dose of approximately 60 Gy in 2 Gy fractions that extends on average 14 mm from the prostate and covers both areas of microscopic ECE and the proximal seminal vesicles

because of the high biochemically equivalent radiation dose given (>90 Gy) [118].

Treatment planning MRIs are a standard component of hypofractionated robotic radiosurgery protocols [106, 107] that allow for treatment volume reduction [119, 120] and the discrimination of the prostatic peripheral zone and apex from adjacent critical structures such as the rectum, bladder, neurovascular bundles, urethra, and penile bulb [121, 122]. In addition, the treatment planning MRI gives additional information on the extent of disease [123] and could guide the selective use of supplemental EBRT [124, 125]. At our institution, patients with gross ECE, seminal vesicle, and/or peri-prostatic lymph node involvement on their treatment planning MRIs are encouraged to complete a course of supplemental external beam irradiation. Future research will determine if this treatment modification affects outcomes.

Supplemental external beam irradiation and ADT may be necessary for patients with extensive ECE or at high risk of seminal vesicle and/or pelvic lymph node involvement. In high-risk patients, the risk of ECE beyond 3 mm and seminal vesicle involvement is approximately 30% [126, 127]. In many cases, the seminal vesicle involvement extends beyond the proximal seminal vesicles [127]. Over time, the seminal vesicle volumes can change dramatically [128] and this change is not accounted for in standard treatment planning. In addition, the seminal vesicles move more than the prostate and this motion cannot be accounted for by intraprostatic fiducials [129]. In the opinion of the authors, the large PTV margins required to take seminal vesicle volume changes and motion into account are not safely integrated into hypofractionation protocols. A high percentage of patients with seminal vesicle involvement also have lymph node involvement [127]. Currently, it is not clear if first echelon nodes are included in conventional radiation therapy plans. It should be noted that due to the presence of distant disease at presentation, there is a high rate of relapse independent of the treatment approach in this patient population explaining the benefit of ADT [123, 130].

15.10 Conclusions

A multidisciplinary team of urologists, radiation oncologists, and medical oncologists, combined with an educated patient, participate in the selection of the appropriate patient treatment options for clinically localized prostate cancer. Treatment approaches include radical prostatectomy, IMRT, LDR, HDR, and robotic radiosurgery. Currently, patients with low- to intermediate-risk prostate cancers are offered hypofractionated robotic radiosurgery alone. The ability to perform robotic radiosurgery as an outpatient procedure, with a short recovery time, leading to minimal disruption of the patient's schedule is an important factor, assuming similar intermediate and perhaps improved long-term local control. Patients are not excluded from hypofractionated robotic radiosurgery based on prostate anatomy or prior TURP. Clinical trials will determine the role of supplemental irradiation to robotic radiosurgery for intermediate- and high-risk patients.

References

1. Jemal A, Siegel R, Ward E et al (2009) Cancer statistics, 2009. CA Cancer J Clin 59:225–249
2. Caso JR, Mouraviev V, Tsivian M et al (2010) Prostate cancer: an evolving paradigm. J Endourol 24:805–809
3. Catalona WJ, Smith DS (1998) Cancer recurrence and survival rates after anatomic radical retropubic prostatectomy for prostate cancer: intermediate-term results. J Urol 160:2428–2434
4. Pound CR, Partin AW, Epstein JI et al (1997) Prostate-specific antigen after anatomic radical retropubic prostatectomy. Patterns of recurrence and cancer control. Urol Clin North Am 24:395–406
5. Zincke H, Oesterling JE, Blute ML et al (1994) Long-term (15 years) results after radical prostatectomy for clinically localized (stage T2c or lower) prostate cancer. J Urol 152:1850–1857
6. Swanson GP, Riggs MW, Earle JD et al (2002) Long-term follow-up of radical retropubic prostatectomy for prostate cancer. Eur Urol 42:212–216
7. Bill-Axelson A, Holmberg L, Ruutu M et al (2005) Radical prostatectomy versus watchful waiting in early prostate cancer. N Engl J Med 352:1977–1984
8. Potosky AL, Davis WW, Hoffman RM et al (2004) Five-year outcomes after prostatectomy or radiotherapy for prostate cancer: the prostate cancer outcomes study. J Natl Cancer Inst 96:1358–1367
9. Sanda MG, Dunn RL, Michalski J et al (2008) Quality of life and satisfaction with outcome among prostate-cancer survivors. N Engl J Med 358:1250–1261
10. Kuban DA, el-Mahdi AM, Schellhammer PF (1987) Effect of local tumor control on distant metastasis and survival in prostatic adenocarcinoma. Urology 30:420–426
11. Fuks Z, Leibel SA, Wallner KE et al (1991) The effect of local control on metastatic dissemination in carcinoma of the prostate: long-term results in patients treated with 125I implantation. Int J Radiat Oncol Biol Phys 21:537–547
12. Swanson GP, Riggs MW, Earle JD (2004) Long-term follow-up of radiotherapy for prostate cancer. Int J Radiat Oncol Biol Phys 59:406–411
13. Bagshaw MA, Cox RS, Ramback JE (1990) Radiation therapy for localized prostate cancer. Justification by long-term follow-up. Urol Clin North Am 17:787–802
14. Perez CA, Lee HK, Georgiou A et al (1993) Technical and tumor-related factors affecting outcome of definitive irradiation for localized carcinoma of the prostate. Int J Radiat Oncol Biol Phys 26:581–591
15. Shipley WU, Thames HD, Sandler HM et al (1999) Radiation therapy for clinically localized prostate cancer: a multi-institutional pooled analysis. JAMA 281:1598–1604
16. del Regato JA, Trailins AH, Pittman DD (1993) Twenty years follow-up of patients with inoperable cancer of the prostate (stage C) treated by radiotherapy: report of a national cooperative study. Int J Radiat Oncol Biol Phys 26:197–201
17. Zagars GK, von Eschenbach AC, Johnson DE et al (1987) Stage C adenocarcinoma of the prostate. An analysis of 551 patients treated with external beam radiation. Cancer 60:1489–1499
18. Collins S, McRae D, Gagnon G et al (2008) New directions in radiation therapy of prostate cancer: brachytherapy and intensity-modulated radiation therapy. In: Pestell R, Nevalainen M (eds) Prostate cancer signaling networks, genetics and New treatment strategies. Humana Press, Totowa
19. Kuban DA, Tucker SL, Dong L et al (2008) Long-term results of the M. D. Anderson randomized dose-escalation trial for prostate cancer. Int J Radiat Oncol Biol Phys 70:67–74
20. Zietman AL, DeSilvio ML, Slater JD et al (2005) Comparison of conventional-dose vs high-dose conformal radiation

therapy in clinically localized adenocarcinoma of the prostate: a randomized controlled trial. JAMA 294:1233–1239
21. Peeters ST, Heemsbergen WD, Koper PC et al (2006) Dose-response in radiotherapy for localized prostate cancer: results of the Dutch multicenter randomized phase III trial comparing 68 Gy of radiotherapy with 78 Gy. J Clin Oncol 24:1990–1996
22. Huang EH, Pollack A, Levy L et al (2002) Late rectal toxicity: dose-volume effects of conformal radiotherapy for prostate cancer. Int J Radiat Oncol Biol Phys 54:1314–1321
23. Boersma LJ, van den Brink M, Bruce AM et al (1998) Estimation of the incidence of late bladder and rectum complications after high-dose (70–78 GY) conformal radiotherapy for prostate cancer, using dose-volume histograms. Int J Radiat Oncol Biol Phys 41:83–92
24. Ling CC, Burman C, Chui CS et al (1996) Conformal radiation treatment of prostate cancer using inversely-planned intensity-modulated photon beams produced with dynamic multileaf collimation. Int J Radiat Oncol Biol Phys 35:721–730
25. Zelefsky MJ, Fuks Z, Happersett L et al (2000) Clinical experience with intensity modulated radiation therapy (IMRT) in prostate cancer. Radiother Oncol 55:241–249
26. Zelefsky MJ, Fuks Z, Hunt M et al (2002) High-dose intensity modulated radiation therapy for prostate cancer: early toxicity and biochemical outcome in 772 patients. Int J Radiat Oncol Biol Phys 53:1111–1116
27. Cahlon O, Zelefsky MJ, Shippy A et al (2008) Ultra-high dose (86.4 Gy) IMRT for localized prostate cancer: toxicity and biochemical outcomes. Int J Radiat Oncol Biol Phys 71:330–337
28. Crook JM, Raymond Y, Salhani D et al (1995) Prostate motion during standard radiotherapy as assessed by fiducial markers. Radiother Oncol 37:35–42
29. Dawson LA, Mah K, Franssen E et al (1998) Target position variability throughout prostate radiotherapy. Int J Radiat Oncol Biol Phys 42:1155–1161
30. Litzenberg DW, Balter JM, Hadley SW et al (2006) Influence of intrafraction motion on margins for prostate radiotherapy. Int J Radiat Oncol Biol Phys 65:548–553
31. Kupelian PA, Langen KM, Willoughby TR et al (2008) Image-guided radiotherapy for localized prostate cancer: treating a moving target. Semin Radiat Oncol 18:58–66
32. Loeffler JS, Smith AR, Suit HD (1997) The potential role of proton beams in radiation oncology. Semin Oncol 24: 686–695
33. Talcott JA, Rossi C, Shipley WU et al (2010) Patient-reported long-term outcomes after conventional and high-dose combined proton and photon radiation for early prostate cancer. JAMA 303:1046–1053
34. Zietman AL, Bae K, Slater JD et al (2010) Randomized trial comparing conventional-dose with high-dose conformal radiation therapy in early-stage adenocarcinoma of the prostate: long-term results from proton radiation oncology group/American college of radiology 95-09. J Clin Oncol 28:1106–1111
35. Coen JJ, Zietman AL (2009) Proton radiation for localized prostate cancer. Nat Rev Urol 6:324–330
36. D'Amico AV, Whittington R, Malkowicz SB et al (1998) Biochemical outcome after radical prostatectomy, external beam radiation therapy, or interstitial radiation therapy for clinically localized prostate cancer. JAMA 280:969–974
37. Zelefsky MJ, Kuban DA, Levy LB et al (2007) Multi-institutional analysis of long-term outcome for stages T1-T2 prostate cancer treated with permanent seed implantation. Int J Radiat Oncol Biol Phys 67:327–333
38. Grimm PD, Blasko JC, Sylvester JE et al (2001) 10-Year biochemical (prostate-specific antigen) control of prostate cancer with (125)I brachytherapy. Int J Radiat Oncol Biol Phys 51:31–40
39. Kollmeier MA, Stock RG, Stone N (2003) Biochemical outcomes after prostate brachytherapy with 5-year minimal follow-up: importance of patient selection and implant quality. Int J Radiat Oncol Biol Phys 57:645–653
40. Merrick GS, Butler WM, Wallner KE et al (2005) Monotherapeutic brachytherapy for clinically organ-confined prostate cancer. W V Med J 101:168–171
41. Zelefsky MJ, Hollister T, Raben A et al (2000) Five-year biochemical outcome and toxicity with transperineal CT-planned permanent I-125 prostate implantation for patients with localized prostate cancer. Int J Radiat Oncol Biol Phys 47:1261–1266
42. Brachman DG, Thomas T, Hilbe J et al (2000) Failure-free survival following brachytherapy alone or external beam irradiation alone for T1–2 prostate tumors in 2222 patients: results from a single practice. Int J Radiat Oncol Biol Phys 48:111–117
43. Potters L, Morgenstern C, Calugaru E et al (2005) 12-Year outcomes following permanent prostate brachytherapy in patients with clinically localized prostate cancer. J Urol 173:1562–1566
44. Mitsuyama H, Wallner KE, Merrick GS (2006) Treatment of prostate cancer in obese patients. Oncology (Williston Park) 20:1191–1197, discussion 1198, 1206, 1208
45. Millender LE, Aubin M, Pouliot J et al (2004) Daily electronic portal imaging for morbidly obese men undergoing radiotherapy for localized prostate cancer. Int J Radiat Oncol Biol Phys 59:6–10
46. Merrick GS, Butler WM, Wallner KE et al (2005) Influence of body mass index on biochemical outcome after permanent prostate brachytherapy. Urology 65:95–100
47. Merrick GS, Butler WM, Wallner K et al (2002) Permanent prostate brachytherapy-induced morbidity in patients with grade II and III obesity. Urology 60:104–108
48. Stock RG, Stone NN, Tabert A et al (1998) A dose-response study for I-125 prostate implants. Int J Radiat Oncol Biol Phys 41:101–108
49. Potters L, Cao Y, Calugaru E et al (2001) A comprehensive review of CT-based dosimetry parameters and biochemical control in patients treated with permanent prostate brachytherapy. Int J Radiat Oncol Biol Phys 50:605–614
50. Wallner K, Merrick G, Sutlief S et al (2005) High-dose regions versus likelihood of cure after prostate brachytherapy. Int J Radiat Oncol Biol Phys 62:170–174
51. Stone NN, Stock RG, Unger P (2005) Intermediate term biochemical-free progression and local control following 125iodine brachytherapy for prostate cancer. J Urol 173: 803–807

52. Urbanic JJ, Lee WR (2006) Update on brachytherapy in localized prostate cancer: the importance of dosimetry. Curr Opin Urol 16:157–161
53. Merrick GS, Butler WM, Tollenaar BG et al (2002) The dosimetry of prostate brachytherapy-induced urethral strictures. Int J Radiat Oncol Biol Phys 52:461–468
54. Allen ZA, Merrick GS, Butler WM et al (2005) Detailed urethral dosimetry in the evaluation of prostate brachytherapy-related urinary morbidity. Int J Radiat Oncol Biol Phys 62:981–987
55. Snyder KM, Stock RG, Hong SM et al (2001) Defining the risk of developing grade 2 proctitis following 125I prostate brachytherapy using a rectal dose-volume histogram analysis. Int J Radiat Oncol Biol Phys 50:335–341
56. Mueller A, Wallner K, Merrick G et al (2004) Perirectal seeds as a risk factor for prostate brachytherapy-related rectal bleeding. Int J Radiat Oncol Biol Phys 59:1047–1052
57. Tran A, Wallner K, Merrick G et al (2005) Rectal fistulas after prostate brachytherapy. Int J Radiat Oncol Biol Phys 63:150–154
58. Chen AB, D'Amico AV, Neville BA et al (2009) Provider case volume and outcomes following prostate brachytherapy. J Urol 181:113–118, discussion 118
59. Lee WR, de Guzman AF, Bare RL et al (2000) Postimplant analysis of transperineal interstitial permanent prostate brachytherapy: evidence for a learning curve in the first year at a single institution. Int J Radiat Oncol Biol Phys 46:83–88
60. Merrick GS, Butler WM, Lief JH et al (2000) Temporal resolution of urinary morbidity following prostate brachytherapy. Int J Radiat Oncol Biol Phys 47:121–128
61. Terk MD, Stock RG, Stone NN (1998) Identification of patients at increased risk for prolonged urinary retention following radioactive seed implantation of the prostate. J Urol 160:1379–1382
62. Bucci J, Morris WJ, Keyes M et al (2002) Predictive factors of urinary retention following prostate brachytherapy. Int J Radiat Oncol Biol Phys 53:91–98
63. Bellon J, Wallner K, Ellis W et al (1999) Use of pelvic CT scanning to evaluate pubic arch interference of transperineal prostate brachytherapy. Int J Radiat Oncol Biol Phys 43:579–581
64. Kucway R, Vicini F, Huang R et al (2002) Prostate volume reduction with androgen deprivation therapy before interstitial brachytherapy. J Urol 167:2443–2447
65. Stone NN, Marshall DT, Stone JJ et al (2010) Does neoadjuvant hormonal therapy improve urinary function when given to men with large prostates undergoing prostate brachytherapy? J Urol 183:634–639
66. Thomas MD, Cormack R, Tempany CM et al (2000) Identifying the predictors of acute urinary retention following magnetic-resonance-guided prostate brachytherapy. Int J Radiat Oncol Biol Phys 47:905–908
67. Merrick GS, Butler WM, Galbreath RW et al (2001) Relationship between the transition zone index of the prostate gland and urinary morbidity after brachytherapy. Urology 57:524–529
68. Crook J, Toi A, McLean M et al (2002) The utility of transition zone index in predicting acute urinary morbidity after 125I prostate brachytherapy. Brachytherapy 1:131–137
69. Hinerman-Mulroy A, Merrick GS, Butler WM et al (2004) Androgen deprivation-induced changes in prostate anatomy predict urinary morbidity after permanent interstitial brachytherapy. Int J Radiat Oncol Biol Phys 59:1367–1382
70. Levine GN, D'Amico AV, Berger P et al (2010) Androgen-deprivation therapy in prostate cancer and cardiovascular risk: a science advisory from the American Heart Association, American Cancer Society, and American Urological Association: endorsed by the American Society for Radiation Oncology. Circulation 121: 833–840
71. Badiozamani KR, Wallner K, Sutlief S et al (1999) Anticipating prostatic volume changes due to prostate brachytherapy. Radiat Oncol Investig 7:360–364
72. McNeely LK, Stone NN, Presser J et al (2004) Influence of prostate volume on dosimetry results in real-time 125I seed implantation. Int J Radiat Oncol Biol Phys 58:292–299
73. Cesaretti JA, Stone NN, Stock RG (2004) Does prior transurethral resection of prostate compromise brachytherapy quality: a dosimetric analysis. Int J Radiat Oncol Biol Phys 60:648–653
74. Moran BJ, Stutz MA, Gurel MH (2004) Prostate brachytherapy can be performed in selected patients after transurethral resection of the prostate. Int J Radiat Oncol Biol Phys 59:392–396
75. Patel AB, Waterman FM, Dicker AP (2003) A detailed examination of the difference between planned and treated margins in 125I permanent prostate brachytherapy. Brachytherapy 2:223–228
76. Stock RG, Lo YC, Gaildon M et al (1999) Does prostate brachytherapy treat the seminal vesicles? a dose-volume histogram analysis of seminal vesicles in patients undergoing combined PD-103 prostate implantation and external beam irradiation. Int J Radiat Oncol Biol Phys 45:385–389
77. Ho AY, Burri RJ, Jennings GT et al (2007) Is seminal vesicle implantation with permanent sources possible? a dose-volume histogram analysis in patients undergoing combined 103Pd implantation and external beam radiation for T3c prostate cancer. Brachytherapy 6:38–43
78. Sylvester JE, Grimm PD, Blasko JC et al (2007) 15-Year biochemical relapse free survival in clinical stage T1-T3 prostate cancer following combined external beam radiotherapy and brachytherapy; Seattle experience. Int J Radiat Oncol Biol Phys 67:57–64
79. Dattoli M, Wallner K, True L et al (2007) Long-term prostate cancer control using palladium-103 brachytherapy and external beam radiotherapy in patients with a high likelihood of extracapsular cancer extension. Urology 69:334–337
80. Dattoli M, Wallner K, True L et al (2007) Long-term outcomes after treatment with brachytherapy and supplemental conformal radiation for prostate cancer patients having intermediate and high-risk features. Cancer 110:551–555
81. Brenner DJ, Hall EJ (1999) Fractionation and protraction for radiotherapy of prostate carcinoma. Int J Radiat Oncol Biol Phys 43:1095–1101
82. Fowler JF (2005) The radiobiology of prostate cancer including new aspects of fractionated radiotherapy. Acta Oncol 44:265–276

83. Haustermans KM, Hofland I, Van Poppel H et al (1997) Cell kinetic measurements in prostate cancer. Int J Radiat Oncol Biol Phys 37:1067–1070
84. Brenner DJ (2000) Toward optimal external-beam fractionation for prostate cancer. Int J Radiat Oncol Biol Phys 48:315–316
85. Mate TP, Gottesman JE, Hatton J et al (1998) High dose-rate afterloading 192Iridium prostate brachytherapy: feasibility report. Int J Radiat Oncol Biol Phys 41:525–533
86. Martinez AA, Gustafson G, Gonzalez J et al (2002) Dose escalation using conformal high-dose-rate brachytherapy improves outcome in unfavorable prostate cancer. Int J Radiat Oncol Biol Phys 53:316–327
87. Galalae RM, Kovacs G, Schultze J et al (2002) Long-term outcome after elective irradiation of the pelvic lymphatics and local dose escalation using high-dose-rate brachytherapy for locally advanced prostate cancer. Int J Radiat Oncol Biol Phys 52:81–90
88. Demanes DJ, Rodriguez RR, Altieri GA (2000) High dose rate prostate brachytherapy: the California Endocurietherapy (CET) method. Radiother Oncol 57: 289–296
89. Syed AM, Puthawala A, Sharma A et al (2001) High-dose-rate brachytherapy in the treatment of carcinoma of the prostate. Cancer Control 8:511–521
90. Deger S, Boehmer D, Roigas J et al (2005) High dose rate (HDR) brachytherapy with conformal radiation therapy for localized prostate cancer. Eur Urol 47:441–448
91. Hsu IC, Kyounghwa B, Shinohara K et al (2010) Phase II trial of combined high-dose-rate brachytherapy and external beam radiotherapy for adenocarcinoma of the prostate: preliminary results of RTOG 0321. Int J Radiat Oncol Biol Phys 78(3):751–758, Epub 2010 Mar 6
92. Martinez AA, Demanes J, Vargas C et al (2010) High-dose-rate prostate brachytherapy: an excellent accelerated-hypofractionated treatment for favorable prostate cancer. Am J Clin Oncol 33(5):481–488
93. Konishi K, Yoshioka Y, Isohashi F et al (2009) Correlation between dosimetric parameters and late rectal and urinary toxicities in patients treated with high-dose-rate brachytherapy used as monotherapy for prostate cancer. Int J Radiat Oncol Biol Phys 75:1003–1007
94. Corner C, Rojas AM, Bryant L et al (2008) A phase II study of high-dose-rate afterloading brachytherapy as monotherapy for the treatment of localized prostate cancer. Int J Radiat Oncol Biol Phys 72:441–446
95. Hoskin PJ, Bownes PJ, Ostler P et al (2003) High dose rate afterloading brachytherapy for prostate cancer: catheter and gland movement between fractions. Radiother Oncol 68:285–288
96. Simnor T, Li S, Lowe G et al (2009) Justification for inter-fraction correction of catheter movement in fractionated high dose-rate brachytherapy treatment of prostate cancer. Radiother Oncol 93:253–258
97. Tiong A, Bydder S, Ebert M et al (2010) A small tolerance for catheter displacement in high-dose rate prostate brachytherapy is necessary and feasible. Int J Radiat Oncol Biol Phys 76:1066–1072
98. Krupski TL, Kwan L, Afifi AA et al (2005) Geographic and socioeconomic variation in the treatment of prostate cancer. J Clin Oncol 23:7881–7888
99. Livsey JE, Cowan RA, Wylie JP et al (2003) Hypofractionated conformal radiotherapy in carcinoma of the prostate: five-year outcome analysis. Int J Radiat Oncol Biol Phys 57:1254–1259
100. Higgins GS, McLaren DB, Kerr GR et al (2006) Outcome analysis of 300 prostate cancer patients treated with neoadjuvant androgen deprivation and hypofractionated radiotherapy. Int J Radiat Oncol Biol Phys 65:982–989
101. Lukka H, Hayter C, Julian JA et al (2005) Randomized trial comparing two fractionation schedules for patients with localized prostate cancer. J Clin Oncol 23:6132–6138
102. Kupelian PA, Willoughby TR, Reddy CA et al (2007) Hypofractionated intensity-modulated radiotherapy (70 Gy at 2.5 Gy per fraction) for localized prostate cancer: Cleveland clinic experience. Int J Radiat Oncol Biol Phys 68:1424–1430
103. Xie Y, Djajaputra D, King CR et al (2008) Intrafractional motion of the prostate during hypofractionated radiotherapy. Int J Radiat Oncol Biol Phys 72:236–246
104. Madsen BL, Hsi RA, Pham HT et al (2007) Stereotactic hypofractionated accurate radiotherapy of the prostate (SHARP), 33.5 Gy in five fractions for localized disease: first clinical trial results. Int J Radiat Oncol Biol Phys 67:1099–1105
105. King CR, Brooks JD, Gill H et al (2009) Stereotactic body radiotherapy for localized prostate cancer: interim results of a prospective phase II clinical trial. Int J Radiat Oncol Biol Phys 73:1043–1048
106. Friedland JL, Freeman DE, Masterson-McGary ME et al (2009) Stereotactic body radiotherapy: an emerging treatment approach for localized prostate cancer. Technol Cancer Res Treat 8:387–392
107. Katz AJ, Santoro M, Ashley R et al (2010) Stereotactic body radiotherapy for organ-confined prostate cancer. BMC Urol 10:1
108. Fuller DB, Naitoh J, Lee C et al (2008) Virtual HDR CyberKnife treatment for localized prostatic carcinoma: dosimetry comparison with HDR brachytherapy and preliminary clinical observations. Int J Radiat Oncol Biol Phys 70:1588–1597
109. Townsend NC, Huth BJ, Ding W et al (2011) Acute toxicity after CyberKnife-delivered hypofractionated radiotherapy for treatment of prostate cancer. Am J Clin Oncol 34(1):6–10
110. Kilby W, Dooley J, Kuduvalli G et al (2010) The CyberKnife robotic radiosurgery system in 2010. Technol Cancer Res Treat 9(5):433–452
111. Webb S (1999) Conformal intensity-modulated radiotherapy (IMRT) delivered by robotic linac–testing IMRT to the limit? Phys Med Biol 44:1639–1654
112. Hossain S, Xia P, Huang K et al (2010) Dose gradient near target-normal structure interface for nonisocentric CyberKnife and isocentric intensity-modulated body radiotherapy for prostate cancer. Int J Radiat Oncol Biol Phys 78(1):58–63
113. Merrick GS, Wallner KE, Butler WM (2003) Minimizing prostate brachytherapy-related morbidity. Urology 62: 786–792
114. Brandeis J, Pashos CL, Henning JM et al (2000) A nationwide charge comparison of the principal treatments for early stage prostate carcinoma. Cancer 89:1792–1799

115. Davis BJ, Pisansky TM, Wilson TM et al (1999) The radial distance of extraprostatic extension of prostate carcinoma: implications for prostate brachytherapy. Cancer 85:2630–2637
116. Sohayda C, Kupelian PA, Levin HS et al (2000) Extent of extracapsular extension in localized prostate cancer. Urology 55:382–386
117. Teh BS, Bastasch MD, Mai WY et al (2003) Predictors of extracapsular extension and its radial distance in prostate cancer: implications for prostate IMRT, brachytherapy, and surgery. Cancer J 9:454–460
118. Krauss D, Kestin L, Ye H et al (2011) Lack of benefit for the addition of androgen deprivation therapy to dose-escalated radiotherapy in the treatment of intermediate- and high-risk prostate cancer. Int J Radiat Oncol Biol Phys 80(4):1064–1071
119. Roach M 3rd, Faillace-Akazawa P, Malfatti C et al (1996) Prostate volumes defined by magnetic resonance imaging and computerized tomographic scans for three-dimensional conformal radiotherapy. Int J Radiat Oncol Biol Phys 35: 1011–1018
120. Kagawa K, Lee WR, Schultheiss TE et al (1997) Initial clinical assessment of CT-MRI image fusion software in localization of the prostate for 3D conformal radiation therapy. Int J Radiat Oncol Biol Phys 38:319–325
121. McLaughlin PW, Troyer S, Berri S et al (2005) Functional anatomy of the prostate: implications for treatment planning. Int J Radiat Oncol Biol Phys 63:479–491
122. Villeirs GM KLV, De Neve WJ et al (2005) Magnetic resonance imaging anatomy of the prostate and periprostatic area: a guide for radiotherapists. Radiother Oncol 76:99–106
123. D'Amico AV (1996) The role of MR imaging in the selection of therapy for prostate cancer. Magn Reson Imaging Clin N Am 4:471–479
124. D'Amico AV, Schnall M, Whittington R et al (1998) Endorectal coil magnetic resonance imaging identifies locally advanced prostate cancer in select patients with clinically localized disease. Urology 51:449–454
125. Clarke DH, Banks SJ, Wiederhorn AR et al (2002) The role of endorectal coil MRI in patient selection and treatment planning for prostate seed implants. Int J Radiat Oncol Biol Phys 52:903–910
126. Chao KK, Goldstein NS, Yan D et al (2006) Clinicopathologic analysis of extracapsular extension in prostate cancer: should the clinical target volume be expanded posterolaterally to account for microscopic extension? Int J Radiat Oncol Biol Phys 65:999–1007
127. Kestin L, Goldstein N, Vicini F et al (2002) Treatment of prostate cancer with radiotherapy: should the entire seminal vesicles be included in the clinical target volume? Int J Radiat Oncol Biol Phys 54:686–697
128. Roeske JC, Forman JD, Mesina CF et al (1995) Evaluation of changes in the size and location of the prostate, seminal vesicles, bladder, and rectum during a course of external beam radiation therapy. Int J Radiat Oncol Biol Phys 33:1321–1329
129. Liang J, Wu Q, Yan D (2009) The role of seminal vesicle motion in target margin assessment for online image-guided radiotherapy for prostate cancer. Int J Radiat Oncol Biol Phys 73:935–943
130. Bolla M, Collette L, Blank L et al (2002) Long-term results with immediate androgen suppression and external irradiation in patients with locally advanced prostate cancer (an EORTC study): a phase III randomised trial. Lancet 360:103–106

Part V

Emerging Applications

Radiosurgery for Renal Tumors

16

Lee E. Ponsky and Gino Vricella

CONTENTS

16.1 Abstract

Although conventional EBRT has a limited role in the treatment of renal lesions, the story may be very different for stereotactic radiosurgery (SRS), or stereotactic body radiotherapy (SBRT). These approaches involve the stereotactic delivery, in one or a few fractions, of high radiation doses to limited treatment volumes, with a steep dose fall-off outside the treated region. The goal is the complete ablation of tissue. In this chapter we describe this approach to noninvasive in situ ablation of renal and adrenal lesions and review clinical findings to date. The chapter follows from and expands upon a recent review published by the authors (Vricella et al. [1]).

16.2 Introduction

The incidence of kidney cancer in the United States has risen over the last several years at an accelerated rate. According to the American Cancer Society, an estimated 58,240 cases of newly diagnosed renal cancer will occur in 2010 [2]. The recent rise in the incidence of renal cancer is thought to be a result of the increase in incidental detection of small renal lesions due to the widespread use of cross-sectional abdominal imaging such as CT and MRI [3]. In addition to the increased incidence of renal cell carcinoma (RCC), smaller, more favorable grade and stage lesions are being detected. Most of these small renal masses (SRMs), typically defined as less than 4.0 cm in diameter on cross-sectional imaging, behave in an indolent manner, with a slow growth rate and a low rate of metastasis [4]. Despite the low-risk behavior of SRMs, both patients and physicians typically favor their treatment over surveillance, especially in patients with a long life expectancy [5].

Along with increases in the SRM incidence, has come a growing interest in minimally invasive nephron-sparing surgery and other focal therapies. Nephron-sparing techniques have emerged as a particularly valuable approach to SRMs [6, 7]. Renal ablative technologies, whether completely extracorporeal or needle-based approaches, are intended to preserve normal renal parenchyma and decrease morbidity

L.E. Ponsky et al. (eds.), *Treating Prostate Cancer and Related Genitourinary Applications*, Robotic Radiosurgery,
DOI 10.1007/978-3-642-11495-3_16,

while obtaining long-term oncologic results that are comparable to radical nephrectomy. Energy-based techniques such as cryoablation and radiofrequency ablation (RFA), in which a probe or probes are placed directly into the renal lesion, were originally used to decrease the risk of hemorrhage upon partial nephrectomy. Cryotherapy and RFA have emerged as highly effective RCC therapies, with reported local control rates of 90% or better [8–11].

Conventional external-beam radiation therapy (EBRT), which destroys dividing tumor cells by necrosis and programmed cell death (apoptosis), is often seen as an alternative to surgery for certain types of tumors in patients who are medically inoperable or whose lesions are unresectable. Most urologists and radiation oncologists still accept the traditional teaching that RCC is a relatively "radioresistant" tumor, rendering the role of radiation therapy in the management of these tumors unclear and controversial at best. An early report of one surgeon's case series challenged these previously held notions by demonstrating that neoadjuvant EBRT did produce an improved rate of disease-specific survival [12]. Subsequent clinical trials, however, have failed to demonstrate any increase in survival associated with EBRT in either a neoadjuvant or adjuvant setting [13–15]. Currently, the role of EBRT for RCC is typically limited, possibly to patients in high risk of local tumor recurrence [16].

16.3 Stereotactic Radiosurgery

Prior to the introduction of the Gamma Knife® (Elekta AB, Stockholm, Sweden) for brain tumors, the life expectancy of patients with RCC metastatic to the brain was 1–2 months [17]. Radiosurgical therapy has since been shown to provide excellent local control of these lesions and significantly extends survival [18–21]. A study by Brown et al. [18] produced a median overall survival of nearly 18 months after stereotactic radiosurgery for metastatic brain tumors due to RCC. These outcomes support the contention that even the most aggressive and advanced RCC respond to the appropriate dose of radiation therapy and warrant treatment.

New radiosurgical technologies, such as the CyberKnife® System (Accuray Incorporated, Sunnyvale, CA), Novalis® System (BrainLab AG, Heimstetten, Germany), and Tomotherapy® (Tomotherapy Inc., Madison, WI), can allow for stereotactic radiosurgery to be delivered to organs that move with respiration, such as the kidney. The CyberKnife, favored by the authors, utilizes a lightweight 6-MV linear accelerator mounted to a highly maneuverable robotic manipulator. The manipulator can position and point the accelerator with 0.12 mm precision. An image-guidance system, in which "live" orthogonal X-rays are registered automatically to synthetic radiographs derived from the treatment-planning CT volume, is used to detect the location of the targeted lesion throughout treatment and adjust the aim of the treatment beam automatically when movement is detected. The total system error for stationary targets has been reported to be about 0.5 mm [22, 23]. The total radiation dose is delivered using, typically, more than 100 individual low-dose beams in a session. As a result, the dose of each beam is relatively benign to skin and the tissue surrounding the target; however, at the focal point of the beams (the target tumor), the dose is additive and the desired ablative dose is attained [24, 25].

A major limitation to extracorporeal ablation of renal tumors is the significant movement of the kidney due to respiration. Unlike the treatment of brain lesions (which are unaffected by respiratory movement), the inherent back-and-forth movement of the kidney associated with the respiratory cycle makes precise delivery of traditional EBRT to a lesion a near impossibility. This limitation is circumvented with radiosurgery by a highly advanced radiosurgical image-guidance system that allows the radiation beam to follow and "correct" for the respiratory motion of a target in real time. The Synchrony® respiratory tracking system (Accuray) is a tracking and compensation system that correlates external "fiducial" markers (LEDs on the patient's chest, sampled continuously by an optical tracking system) to radiopaque internal markers placed near the lesion, as sampled frequently during a session by orthogonal diagnostic X-rays. The correlation model is used to guide the robotic arm so that the beam remains aligned with its target. With the aid of Synchrony, renal tumor motion can be tracked in three-dimensional space in real-time, allowing for precise dose placement (overall tracking error less than 1.5 mm; [26, 27]). This capability may be particularly important for kidney, which, studies have shown, can move over a range of about 6–18 mm in the superior–inferior direction [28–31], and for which abdominal compression, a common mode of motion management in SBRT, has not been shown to significantly reduce organ motion [31].

16.4 Renal Radiosurgery

Still in its relative infancy and mostly investigational, the field of radiosurgical ablation for renal tumors is devoid of any long-term studies; however, short-term analysis has been promising. In 2003, Ponsky et al. [32] were the first to report their initial evaluation with CyberKnife technology in eight swine. In each pig, bilateral kidneys were treated at predetermined sites (each approximately 2 cm in diameter) using a single fraction dose escalated up to 48 Gy followed by organ harvest and histological examination 4–8 weeks later. Targeted sites treated with 48 Gy revealed complete tissue ablation at 8 weeks surrounded by a small zone of partial fibrosis. Perhaps just as important, the remainder of the surrounding renal parenchyma demonstrated no evidence of histological damage, and gross inspection at the time of kidney procurement failed to reveal any evidence of radiation injury to the body wall or surrounding organs and no significant change in renal function.

Following this initial animal study, a clinical protocol was initiated to address the safety of renal radiosurgery in humans. Ponsky et al. [33] described their initial three patients with a mean tumor size of 2.03 cm using 16 Gy divided into four fractions over two consecutive days. Each patient underwent a partial nephrectomy for their renal mass 8-weeks post-radiosurgery. Histopathology of the excised specimens demonstrated a cavity without evidence of viable tumor in one patient, whereas the remaining two showed evidence of residual RCC. This trial confirmed the safety of renal radiosurgery, as there were no acute or chronic toxicities using this low dose with a follow-up time of over 1 year. Although the primary end-point of this study was toxicity-related outcomes, the result of complete tumor ablation in one patient was not anticipated at this initial low dose (in comparison to the 48 Gy dose threshold for complete ablation in the animal studies described above). This result underscores the therapeutic potential for complete tissue ablation using radiosurgical technology. At present, our group has an active clinical protocol in place for a gradual dose-escalation study to further confirm safety. Currently, patients are receiving a treatment dose of 48 Gy divided over four fractions (unpublished data). Patients undergo serial cross-sectional imaging at 6-month intervals, with repeat renal biopsies performed 6-months post-radiosurgery to assess for residual tumor cells. There have been no acute toxicities noted to date.

Several other small series have been published as well. Beitler et al. [34] treated nine patients who refused nephrectomy for localized renal tumors using a stereotactic radiotherapy approach. They received a dose of 40 Gy delivered in five fractions over 15 days with a 1-cm circumferential tumor margin. Four of the nine patients were alive at a median follow-up of 26.7 months. The surviving patients all had tumors less than 3.5 cm in maximum diameter with a minimum follow-up of 48 months. The authors concluded that this hypofractionated approach may play a role in the treatment of SRMs; however, the accuracy of the treatment was too low to safely and consistently deliver radiation sufficient for tumor ablation. Svedman et al. [35] treated 30 patients with metastatic renal cell carcinoma (RCC) or inoperable primary RCC; 15 lesions were located in the kidney or adrenal gland. A wide range of doses/fractions was delivered, from five 5-Gy fractions to three 15-Gy fractions, and from the report it is not clear what dose was delivered to the kidney/adrenal. Nevertheless, a high rate of tumor control (98% in the 24 evaluable patients) and low rate of side effects (96% of them Grade I-II), and a median overall survival of 32 months were reported. Two patients whose kidney lesions progressed locally were retreated successfully. More recently this group reported on the successful treatment of a single remaining kidney in seven patients (six metastases and one primary), using doses/fraction ranging from 10 Gy/3 to 10 Gy/4 [36]. Six of the seven lesions were controlled after the initial treatment, and the remaining patient was successfully retreated after local progression. Kidney function of the treated was largely unaffected, with creatinine levels rising but stabilizing at around 150–160 μmol/L at 2-year follow-up. No patient has required dialysis.

In a recent retrospective review of 30 patients treated for adrenal metastases [37], either to achieve disease control or for palliation of bulky lesions, a range of dose schemes, from 16 Gy in four fractions to 50 Gy in 10 fractions, was delivered. Local control at 1-year follow-up was 55%, and overall survival was 44%. No patient developed RTOG grade 2 or greater toxicity. Complete pain relief was achieved in three patients treated primarily to control pain. Poorer local control in this cohort was attributed to the extensive metastatic disease, including bulky lesions, in these patients.

In addition to the ongoing work from our group, promising work has also been reported by Hong et al. [38]. Their initial evaluation included 14 patients with a mean renal tumor diameter of 4.1 cm treated with 21 Gy divided into three fractions. Patients were then imaged every 3 months with serial CT scans. Their data showed that tumor volume decreased by a mean of 44% with no signs of disease progression at 12-month follow-up. These data are reassuring, as it mirrors the type of results our group has witnessed. More recently Kaplan et al. presented results of their phase I study [39]. Twelve medically inoperable patients were treated for SRMs using Synchrony respiratory motion tracking. Dose levels where 21 Gy, 28 Gy, 32 Gy, or 39 Gy delivered in three fractions. The planning tumor volume (PTV) was the tumor plus 3 mm (median PTV, 18.0 cm^3). No RTOG grade I or higher toxicity was observed; renal function worsened in two patients with chronic pre-treatment renal failure. A single local recurrence was observed in a patient treated at the lowest dose (21 Gy). Based on excellent toxicity findings the authors have included a final dose level of 48 Gy in three fractions, and a phase II multi-institutional study is planned.

In summary, several small retrospective studies have shown clearly that SRS/SBRT is safe in patients with kidney and adrenal lesions, even in patients with a single remaining kidney. Two phase I dose-escalation studies (by our group at Case Medical Center and by Kaplan et al. at Beth Israel) have shown safe dose-escalation up to 48 Gy delivered in three or four fractions. The very low rates of toxicity, even at this early stage of investigation, encourage us to pursue rigorous future phase II and perhaps phase III trials of this promising treatment modality.

16.5 Conclusions

With the increasing use of cross-sectional imaging resulting in an increased incidence of SRMs, more minimally invasive, or preferably noninvasive, ablative options need to be considered for their management. Given the relatively good prognosis for SRMs, ablative technologies strive to provide tumor control with minimal morbidity. Radiosurgery is at the forefront of offering completely noninvasive methods for tumor destruction. As leaders in the development and evaluation of new surgical and treatment technologies, urologists must partner with their radiation oncology colleagues to drive the new patterns emerging in minimally invasive treatment modalities. As the perceived eras of surgical evolution have transitioned from maximally to minimally invasive surgery, the next apparent progression would be to noninvasive surgery, in the form of extracorporeal ablation. With the ongoing developments and advances in imaging and tracking technologies, we believe our ability to utilize noninvasive extracorporeal ablation will likely develop into a standard therapy in the future. Urologists have previously witnessed such a transition for the treatment of kidney stones with the introduction of shock wave lithotripsy. The shock wave lithotripter revolutionized the treatment of kidney stones and redefined the standard of care from a major open surgical procedure with significant morbidity to an outpatient procedure with minimal morbidity and excellent efficacy for the majority of patients. Extracorporeal noninvasive ablation of renal tumors is on the near horizon and will certainly become a part of the armamentarium of the multidisciplinary team of surgeons and radiation oncologists.

References

1. Vricella GJ, Boncher NA, Ponsky LE (2010) Extracorporeal stereotactic radiosurgery for small renal masses. Curr Urol Rep 11:33–37
2. Jemal A, Siegel R, Xu J et al (2010) Cancer statistics, 2010. CA Cancer J Clin 60:277–300
3. Jayson M, Sanders H (1998) Increased incidence of serendipitously discovered renal cell carcinoma. Urology 51:203–205
4. Chawla SN, Crispen PL, Hanlon AL et al (2006) The natural history of observed enhancing renal masses: Meta-analysis and review of the world literature. J Urol 175:425–431
5. Van Poppel H (2004) Conservative vs radical surgery for renal cell carcinoma. BJU Int 94:766–768
6. Hsieh TC, Jarrett TW, Pinto PA (2010) Current status of nephron-sparing robotic partial nephrectomy. Curr Opin Urol 20:65–69
7. Heuer R, Gill IS, Guazzoni G et al (2010) A critical analysis of the actual role of minimally invasive surgery and active surveillance for kidney cancer. Eur Urol 57:223–232
8. Ahrar K, Matin S, Wood CG et al (2005) Percutaneous radiofrequency ablation of renal tumors: technique, complications, and outcomes. J Vasc Interv Radiol 16:679–688
9. Anderson JK, Matsumoto E, Cadeddu JA (2005) Renal radiofrequency ablation: technique and results. Urol Oncol 23:355–360
10. Gervais DA, Arellano RS, Mueller PR (2005) Percutaneous radiofrequency ablation of renal cell carcinoma. Eur Radiol 15:960–967
11. Gill IS (2005) Renal cryotherapy: pro. Urology 65:415–418
12. Riches E (1966) The place of radiotherapy in the management of parenchymal carcinoma of the kidney. J Urol 95:313–317
13. Juusela H, Malmio K, Alfthan O et al (1977) Preoperative irradiation in the treatment of renal adenocarcinoma. Scand J Urol Nephrol 11:277–281
14. Kjaer M, Frederiksen PL, Engelholm SA (1987) Postoperative radiotherapy in stage II and III renal adenocarcinoma. A randomized trial by the Copenhagen Renal Cancer Study Group. Int J Radiat Oncol Biol Phys 13:665–672
15. Kjaer M, Iversen P, Hvidt V et al (1987) A randomized trial of postoperative radiotherapy versus observation in stage II and III renal adenocarcinoma. A study by the Copenhagen Renal Cancer Study Group. Scand J Urol Nephrol 21: 285–289
16. Michalski JM (2008) Kidney, renal pelvis, ureter. In: Halperin EC, Perez CA, Brady LW (eds) Principles Perez & Brady's and practice of radiation oncology, 5th edn. Lippincott, Williams & Wilkins, Philadelphia, pp 1397–1411
17. Leksell L (1951) The stereotaxic method and radiosurgery of the brain. Acta Chir Scand 102:316–319
18. Brown PD, Brown CA, Pollock BE et al (2008) Stereotactic radiosurgery for patients with "radioresistant" brain metastases. Neurosurgery 62(Suppl 2):790–801
19. Chang EL, Selek U, Hassenbusch SJ 3rd et al (2005) Outcome variation among "radioresistant" brain metastases treated with stereotactic radiosurgery. Neurosurgery 56:936–945, discussion 936–945
20. Manon R, O'Neill A, Knisely J et al (2005) Phase II trial of radiosurgery for one to three newly diagnosed brain metastases from renal cell carcinoma, melanoma, and sarcoma: an Eastern Cooperative Oncology Group study (E 6397). J Clin Oncol 23:8870–8876
21. Noel G, Valery CA, Boisserie G et al (2004) LINAC radiosurgery for brain metastasis of renal cell carcinoma. Urol Oncol 22:25–31
22. Antypas C, Pantelis E (2008) Performance evaluation of a CyberKnife G4 image-guided robotic stereotactic radiosurgery system. Phys Med Biol 53:4697–4718
23. Muacevic A, Staehler M, Drexler C et al (2006) Technical description, phantom accuracy, and clinical feasibility for fiducial-free frameless real-time image-guided spinal radiosurgery. J Neurosurg Spine 5:303–312
24. Adler JR Jr, Murphy MJ, Chang SD et al (1999) Image-guided robotic radiosurgery. Neurosurgery 44:1299–1306, discussion 1306–1297
25. Lunsford LD, Coffey RJ, Cojocaru T et al (1990) Image-guided stereotactic surgery: a 10-year evolutionary experience. Stereotact Funct Neurosurg 54–55:375–387
26. Hoogeman M, Prevost JB, Nuyttens J et al (2009) Clinical accuracy of the respiratory tumor tracking system of the cyberknife: assessment by analysis of log files. Int J Radiat Oncol Biol Phys 74:297–303
27. Muacevic A, Drexler C, Wowra B et al (2007) Technical description, phantom accuracy, and clinical feasibility for single-session lung radiosurgery using robotic image-guided real-time respiratory tumor tracking. Technol Cancer Res Treat 6:321–328
28. Balter JM, Ten Haken RK, Lawrence TS et al (1996) Uncertainties in CT-based radiation therapy treatment planning associated with patient breathing. Int J Radiat Oncol Biol Phys 36:167–174
29. Brandner ED, Heron D, Wu A et al (2006) Localizing moving targets and organs using motion-managed CTs. Med Dosim 31:134–140
30. Davies SC, Hill AL, Holmes RB et al (1994) Ultrasound quantitation of respiratory organ motion in the upper abdomen. Br J Radiol 67:1096–1102
31. Heinzerling JH, Anderson JF, Papiez L et al (2008) Four-dimensional computed tomography scan analysis of tumor and organ motion at varying levels of abdominal compression during stereotactic treatment of lung and liver. Int J Radiat Oncol Biol Phys 70:1571–1578
32. Ponsky LE, Crownover RL, Rosen MJ et al (2003) Initial evaluation of cyberknife technology for extracorporeal renal tissue ablation. Urology 61:498–501
33. Ponsky LE, Mahadevan A, Gill IS et al (2007) Renal radiosurgery: initial clinical experience with histological evaluation. Surg Innov 14:265–269
34. Beitler JJ, Makara D, Silverman P et al (2004) Definitive, high-dose-per-fraction, conformal, stereotactic external radiation for renal cell carcinoma. Am J Clin Oncol 27:646–648
35. Svedman C, Sandstrom P, Pisa P et al (2006) A prospective phase II trial of using extracranial stereotactic radiotherapy in primary and metastatic renal cell carcinoma. Acta Oncol 45:870–875
36. Svedman C, Karlsson K, Rutkowska E et al (2008) Stereotactic body radiotherapy of primary and metastatic renal lesions for patients with only one functioning kidney. Acta Oncol 47:1578–1583

37. Chawla S, Chen Y, Katz AW et al (2009) Stereotactic body radiotherapy for treatment of adrenal metastases. Int J Radiat Oncol Biol Phys 75:71–75
38. Hong YM, Shanmugham L, La Rosa S (2008) CyberKnife radiosurgical ablation of primary renal tumors. 26th World Congress of Endourology. Shanghai, China
39. Kaplan ID, Redrosa I, Martin C et al (2010) Results of a phase I dose escalation study of stereotactic radiosurgery for primary renal tumors. Annual Meeting of the American Society of Radiation Oncology (ASTRO). San Diego, CA

Adaptive Partial-Boost Stereotactic Radiation Therapy for Muscle-Invasive Carcinoma of the Urinary Bladder

17

Juliette Thariat, Shafak Aluwini, and Martin Housset

CONTENTS

17.1 Abstract

While older external-beam radiation therapy protocols included a full dose to the whole bladder, more recently, protocols have been developed to boost the tumor bed only, using partial-bladder irradiation after a 40–45 Gy of whole-bladder radiotherapy. Due to bladder-filling rate and bladder-volume changes, there is growing evidence that image guidance is essential in order to appropriately treat bladder cancer. Compared with three-dimensional radiotherapy, the CyberKnife® system holds the potential for excellent dose distributions in bladder cancer. There is yet no example of a CyberKnife application for bladder cancer in the literature except a case report with positive outcome. Because each fraction duration is quite long (1–1.5 h), bladder surface deformations and volume changes may occur during fractions and must be taken into account. Data on prostate cancer has demonstrated the feasibility and reliability of ultrasound (US) guidance and voiding protocols in assuring consistent bladder volume for hypofractionated CyberKnife treatments.

17.2 Introduction

17.2.1 Epidemiology of Bladder Cancer

Bladder cancer is the fifth most common cancer in most Western countries including France and the United States. Its incidence is increasing while its mortality rate has declined only slightly in the last 10 years. Yet, although it presents a major health threat, studies of this disease have lagged behind that of other cancers.

L.E. Ponsky et al. (eds.), *Treating Prostate Cancer and Related Genitourinary Applications*, Robotic Radiosurgery,
DOI 10.1007/978-3-642-11495-3_17, © Springer-Verlag Berlin Heidelberg 2012

More than 90% of bladder cancers are transitional-cell carcinomas. The histopathological grading of transitional-cell carcinoma of the bladder has historically been Grade 1 to 3 according to the 1973 WHO classification system, but in 1998, a WHO and International Society of Urological Pathology consensus classified urothelial tumors into four categories: papilloma, papillary urothelial neoplasm of low malignant potential, low-grade carcinoma, and high-grade carcinoma. Histological staging is based on the tumor-node-metastasis (TNM) staging system, in which the T category of the primary tumor is based on the extent of penetration or invasion into the bladder-wall. Of all newly diagnosed cases of transitional-cell carcinomas, about 70% present as superficial tumors of categories Ta, T1, or tumors in situ, but as many as 50–70% of these superficial tumors will recur, and roughly 10–20% will progress to muscularis propria invasive disease (T2–T4). This chapter will only deal with available therapies for muscle-invasive bladder cancer.

17.2.2 Anatomy of the Bladder

Bladder is a musculo-membranous sac that acts as a reservoir for urine. Its size, position, and relation to other organs vary according to the amount of urine it happens to contain at a given time and with rectal filling [1, 2]. An empty bladder forms a flattened tetrahedron. It consists of a triangular fundus, a vertex, and superior and inferior surfaces. The fundus is separated from the rectum by the recto-vesical fascia, the seminal vesicles, and the terminal portions of the ductus deferens. The superior surface is covered by peritoneum. It is in contact with sigmoid colon and some small intestine. The inferior surface may be divided into a posterior area and two infero-lateral surfaces. The posterior area is in direct continuity with the prostate base in men, and from it, the urethra emerges. The infero-lateral portions are separated from the symphysis pubis by a fatty retropubic pad. Behind, they are in contact with the fascia which covers the levatores ani and obturatores interni. An empty bladder is located entirely within the pelvis, below the level of the obliterated hypogastric arteries, and underneath the corresponding portions of the ductus deferens. A moderately full bladder contains 0.5 l. It has a postero-superior, an antero-inferior, and two lateral surfaces: a fundus and a summit. The fundus undergoes little change in position, except being slightly lowered. The line of reflection of the peritoneum from the rectum to the bladder undergoes little or no change with bladder distension; it is situated at about 10 cm from the anus. The orifices of the ureters are connected to the postero-lateral side of the trigone. In a contracted bladder, they are about 2.5 cm apart and at about the same distance from the internal urethral orifice. This distance may increase to about 5 cm in a distended bladder. The internal urethral orifice is at the apex of the trigone.

17.3 Treatment of Bladder Cancer

Although surgery is the frontline treatment for bladder cancer, radiation treatment does have a role in selected patients. Simultaneous radiation and chemotherapy may be used instead of surgery in an effort to save the bladder. Organ preservation strategies for muscle-invasive, clinically node-negative bladder cancer have been described elsewhere [3–6]. Organ preservation is based on external beam radiation therapy (using different fractionation schedules and treatment volumes) and concurrent chemotherapy or partial cystectomy with or without brachytherapy mostly for tumors of the mobile portion depending on the institution [3–6].

17.3.1 Radiation Response

Unlike prostate cancer, bladder cancer has an estimated alpha–beta ratio of 6 [7] which does not justify hypofractionation by itself. Conversely, slightly accelerated treatments without a treatment gap may be interesting. For a TCD50 of 63 Gy, protraction of overall treatment time from 40 to 55 days gives a decrease in local control rate from 50% to about 5%. This likely reflects accelerated tumor repopulation during treatment. From an analysis of the literature, on average tumor clonogen repopulation in transitional cell cancer of the bladder seems to accelerate after a lag period of about 5–6 weeks after the start of treatment. A dose increment of 0.4 Gy per day may be required to compensate for this repopulation and is consistent with about 5–8 day clonogen doubling time. It suggests that overall treatment time is an important factor in the dose fractionation and protraction of time may have a significant impact on treatment outcome [8].

17.3.2 Chemoradiation

The risk-benefit ratio has been in favor of surgery in view of the higher local control rates and of limited small bowel and bladder tolerance to irradiation. For patients with muscle-invasive bladder cancer, who are unwilling or unable to have radical cystectomy, concurrent chemoradiotherapy offers a curative bladder-conserving alternative [9–11]. Because the median age at diagnosis is 65, medical comorbidities are a frequent consideration in patient management. High rates of local control and bladder preservation have been reported with transurethral resection of the bladder (TURB) followed by chemotherapy used concurrently with external beam radiation therapy (EBRT).

Despite advances in bladder reconstructive surgery, orthotopic neobladder after radical cystectomy is not possible for all and some patients undergo cutaneous diversion with a deleterious impact on the quality of life. Furthermore, survival rates are roughly around 60% at 5 years with both surgery and conservative TURB followed by chemoradiation. Although local control rates appear better with surgery, it should be noted that the pathological stage is underestimated in 40–50% of cases in radiation series (staging based on TURB) compared to cystectomy series (staging based on operative specimen). Therefore, local control rates of 70% for T2–T4a with chemoradiation, and rates of 90% with surgery cannot be strictly compared. Moreover, chemoradiation series usually include elderly patients, patients with more advanced disease, and patients unfit for surgery. Randomized trials have been impossible in the modern era. In that context, it is likely that showing a benefit from new chemoradiation schemes on local control in early stages, such as T2a, would require considerable number of patients and might fail to complete accrual [12]. Yet, the conservative chemoradiation approach appears particularly attractive to optimize local control and limit toxicity in the sub-group of patients with incomplete or uncertain transurethral resection, and for patients with muscle-invasive bladder cancer who are medically unfit for radical surgery.

17.3.2.1 Summary of Survival and Organ Preservation Results with Standard Chemoradiation Protocols

Pilot studies of chemoradiation in the 1960s were designed as a preoperative measure and involved radiotherapy and 5-FU or cisplatin. Most phase II studies implemented in the 1990s included selected T2–4 N0 M0 bladder cancer patients. Conventionally fractionated 40–50 Gy radiation therapy with concurrent cisplatin (or carboplatin) ± 5-FU was delivered following TURB performed as completely as possible within limits of safety. Control cystoscopy was performed 4–6 weeks after the induction chemoradiation. Patients with complete histological response were eligible for definitive chemoradiation up to a dose of 55–65 Gy, while non-responders underwent cystectomy. Toxicity profiles were acceptable even in elderly patients and complete response rates were 60–90%, i.e., twice the rate with chemo- or radiation therapy alone, indicating a likely synergistic association. Moreover, local relapse rate was 5–25%, 5-year survival was not inferior to that of cystectomy series with matching T category, and the bladder preservation rate with a functional bladder was 40% with very few late complications. These results have since been confirmed in prospective studies, which are summarized in Table 17.1.

It is worth noting that, patients eligible for bladder preservation strategies must comply with at least twice-yearly cystoscopic follow-up assessments for efficient salvage treatment in case of a local relapse. Such protocols are feasible even in elderly people, who are often contraindicated for surgery. Acute severe toxicities are in the order of 5% and late toxicities of 7% including 5.7% GU and 1.9% GI Grade 3 toxicities in RTOG trials 8903, 9506, 9706, and 9906 (no Grade 4 nor 5) [24]. Yet, these toxicity rates may have been somewhat underreported due to relatively short follow-up of most studies. Quality of life and quality of bladder function were satisfactory in more than two thirds of the patients in a French prospective multicenter study [25]. Prognostic factors are similar among surgical and chemoradiation series as far as staging categories T and N, ureterohydronephrosis, TURB

Table 17.1 Main series of chemoradiation

Author	Patient number	T category	Chemotherapy	CR (%)	% 5-year survival	% 5-year BP
Tester et al. [13]	91	T1–T4a	cis-Pt	75	62	44
Chauvet et al. [14]	109	T2–T4a	cis-Pt	70	36	
Rodel et al. [15]	415	T1–T4a	cis-Pt /CPt ± 5-FU	72	51	42
Coppin et al. [16]	51	T2–T4a	cis-Pt	47		
Shipley et al. [17][a]	190	T2–T4a	cis-Pt	59–74	54	42
Dunst et al. [18]	131	T1–T4	cis-Pt	76	47	75
Housset et al. [19][b]	173	T2–T4	5-FU + cis-Pt	78	66	75
Kachnic et al. [20]	106	T2–T4	cis-Pt	70	52	43
Sauer et al. [21]	79	T1–T4	cis-Pt	76	41	41
Arias et al. [22]	50	T2–T4	cis-Pt	68	48	
Zapatero et al. [23]	33	T2–T4	cis-Pt	ND	65	69

cis-Pt cisplatin, *CPt* carboplatin, *5-FU* 5-fluorouracil, *CR* complete response, *BP* bladder preservation, *ND* not determined
[a]Combination of RTOG trials 8512, 8802, 8903, 9506, 9706, some included neo ± adjuvant chemotherapy
[b]Hypofractionated radiation therapy

quality, and multifocality. Complete histological response following induction chemoradiation is another major prognostic factor of survival and local control in chemoradiation protocols.

When discussing bladder toxicity one can discriminate between "global" injury to the whole bladder and "focal" injury to a part of the bladder. Symptoms of global injury include urinary frequency, urgency, decrease in bladder capacity, and cystitis. Symptoms of focal injury include bleeding, ulceration, stone formation, and fistula. Global injury is most common when the entire bladder is irradiated. Among patients treated with interstitial implants, focal injury dominates and global injury is not a major problem. For both global and focal injury, there appears to be a dose–response relationship. The estimated risk for severe bladder complications is 5–10% after a whole-bladder dose of 50–60 Gy as normalized total dose (NTD) (2 Gy equivalent) and 10–20% after doses of 60–70 Gy. Doses of around 65 Gy delivered to approximately one third to one half of the bladder, or doses of 70–75 Gy to about 20% of the bladder, yield a 5–10% complication rate [26]. For large pelvic treatment fields, the total dose is usually limited to approximately 50 Gy because of small-intestinal toxicity, a reason to consider planning bladder cancer irradiation with empty bladder. In patients treated to small volumes, toxicity occurs only in less than 5% of patients at doses of 70 Gy or more. We should note, however, that, given the possible latency period of several decades between treatment and clinical manifestation of sequelae, reports may have underestimated the late GU toxicity rates. The reported rates of acute side effects might be more accurate [27]. Nevertheless, quality of life has been reported as satisfactory in over two thirds of the patients, 8-years post-chemoradiation [25].

17.4 Bladder-Sparing Radiation Modalities

Selective bladder preservation using trimodality, consisting of external-beam radiation therapy and chemotherapy following transurethral resection of the bladder tumor, is an alternative to radical cystectomy in appropriately selected patients with muscle-invasive bladder cancer [11]. Brachytherapy has been used successfully in association with partial cystectomy for tumors of the dome or vertex (superior portion of the bladder) [28–30]. Brachytherapy dose distributions can yield very abrupt dose gradients allowing for sparing of healthy bladder.

Several new techniques like IGRT or stereotactic body radiation therapy (SBRT) in general can reduce treatment volumes in bladder RT. Using IGRT-based adaptive SBRT, dose distributions similar to those that could only be achieved with brachytherapy, have been demonstrated in prostate [31] and bladder cancers [32]. Notably, these techniques, despite requiring implantation of fiducials, are considerably less invasive than brachytherapy and may yield even better dose distributions particularly at the level of the urethra and the ureters. These improvements may be critical to further reduce the incidence of obstructive urinary symptoms, a non-negligible drawback of brachytherapy due to its high doses to the urethra and ureters. Dose escalation could thus be effected and lead to potential gains in treatment outcomes, provided that the fractionation schedules are calibrated with care. This may be best achieved based on experience gained with brachytherapy.

17.4.1 Brachytherapy

Brachytherapy has been used for select high-risk, superficial, and solitary muscle-infiltrating tumors since the 1980s. Pilot studies have been performed by van der Werf-Messing et al. with preoperative EBRT (10.5 Gy in three fractions) followed the same day by partial cystectomy and intraoperative placement of radium needles [33]. Brachytherapy can be performed for T1–T2 tumors 5 cm or less in diameter. CTV usually includes the macroscopic disease or the tumor bed with a safety margin of 1 cm including the full thickness of the wall. During the placement procedure, the bladder tumor is implanted with plastic tubes spaced at 10- to 15-mm distance and fixed to the skin. Dummy sources are usually loaded to check the position of the plastic tubes under fluoroscopy and record a CT scan performed 3–4 days postoperatively to calculate the dose distribution. The target volume may be delineated using clips placed intraoperatively on the partial cystectomy scar. Iridium-192 wires are inserted 4 to 5 days after the surgical procedure for low-dose-rate (LDR), pulse-dose-rate (PDR), or the high-dose-rate (HDR) techniques. The prescribed dose depends on the previous preoperative EBRT dose and fractionation schedule, and on the dose rate of the brachytherapy technique. When using LDR, the prescribed dose ranges from 25 to 30 Gy – after 40 Gy EBRT at 2 Gy per fraction level – to 60–65 Gy after lower-dose EBRT. When using HDR, optimization of the dose distribution is performed manually according to the modification of the dwell-time position of the HDR iridium source. The total prescription dose is 34 Gy in 10 fractions of 3.4 Gy twice a day with an interfraction interval of 6 h or more.

Local control rates have been reported to be about 70% at 5 years [33–36] (Table 17.2). Disease-free survival was 57% and local progression 25% in selected patients with preoperative EBRT followed by surgical exploration with or without partial cystectomy and insertion of source carrier tubes for afterloading with iridium-192 [30]. De Crevoisier et al. have reported excellent long-term results of periop iridium HDR brachytherapy with an afterloading technique [28]. However, some authors have suggested that LDR yielded better results than HDR. Pos et al. have reported significantly different local control rates at 2 years, which were 72 and 88% for HDR and LDR brachytherapy, respectively [37]. Further studies with sufficient follow-up are therefore warranted to assess the value of LDR and HDR brachytherapy in bladder cancer.

17.4.2 Adaptive Stereotactic Radiotherapy

As mentioned above, brachytherapy in one form or another has been in use for the treatment of muscle-invading tumors, therefore, its role and benefits have

Table 17.2 Brachytherapy for bladder cancer

Author	Number of patients	Clinical stage	Treatment	5-year local control (%)	5-year survival (%)
van der Werf-Messing et al. [33]	328	T2	EBRT, Ra-226	77	56
Nieuwenhuijzen et al. [36]	108	T1–T2	EBRT, Ir-192	73	62
van der Steen-Banasik et al. [35]	76	T1–T2	EBRT, Cs-137, Ir-192	70	57
Blank et al. [34]	122	T1–T2–T3	EBRT, Ir-192	76	73

EBRT External beam radiation therapy, *Ra-226* brachytherapy using radium needles, *Ir-192* brachytherapy with afterloading iridium, *Cs* brachytherapy using Cesium been firmly established for mobile portions of the bladder. It is possible that some of the favorable and promising aspects of brachytherapy treatments can be duplicated and some undesirable characteristics such as its invasive nature may be avoided through the use of IGRT-based adaptive stereotactic body radiotherapy (SBRT) planning and motion-tracking capabilities [31]. As explained above, indications of brachytherapy are limited to mobile portions of the bladder while SBRT may be proposed for posterior wall and lateral wall portions.

Moving tumors that are not dependent on respiration may be difficult or impossible to model. Cardiac movements (though data is scarce and must be further validated) have been modeled [38]. Some tumors are prone to erratic, unpredictable movements. As discussed under the *Image-Guided Physiology and Adaptive Radiation Therapy* heading, bladder filling may be modeled on an individual basis with adequate imaging methods. Bladder filling accounts for the most important inter and intra-fraction variations in terms of shape and volume when fraction duration is quite long, as would be the case in IMRT and SBRT. Other bladder movements like erratic movements due to autonomous nervous system influence on smooth muscles or movements due to the adjacent rectum or prostate are less predictable but also less significant. For instance, prostate can move significantly in only a matter of seconds during treatment delivery. This intrafraction motion is one of the major limiting factors for dose escalation.

In Aluwini's study on prostate cancer [39], it is shown that bladder volume can be reproducible using a prescribed treatment protocol and ultrasound imaging. In that study, all patients followed a low-fiber diet and were given laxatives before and during the radiation course to minimize the daily variations in intestine filling and its effect on prostate movement [39]. Bladder catheters were used to maintain a constant 100 cm^3 in the bladder during CT and MRI imaging and during the radiation course for eight patients. This procedure rendered the two scans compatible for reference. Ultrasound imaging was used to monitor bladder fullness and for corrections as necessary. It was found that catheters were not necessary during the treatment for a steady bladder fullness [39]. Interfraction intraindividual bladder volume variations were 9% in average (range, 3–18%), as measured with US for the first eight consecutive patients with 100 cm^3 saline in the bladder. These US-based estimations were reproducible and precise (data not shown). Conversely, in Aluwini's study, fractions of 45-min duration showed intrapatient bladder volume variations of 35% in average (range, 20–55%) without the catheter use. Due to large increases in bladder volume in a few patients, it was sometimes necessary for them to empty their bladder and to drink 100 cm^3 of fluid 40 min into the fraction before the treatment could resume. The protocol was therefore performed without a catheter in routine practice. Patients were instructed in diet and bowel preparation prior to treatment. Treatments were not interrupted unless absolutely necessary due to excessive filling of the bladder.

Although no such protocol has yet been validated for the treatment of bladder, a similar approach may also be applicable to the SBRT of bladder cancer. Bladder tumor movements to be tracked by the image guidance system can be divided into different types. On the one hand, they are dependent on predictable factors, i.e., bladder filling with a continuous linear rate that has a sigmoid trend after 150 cm^3. These may be estimated on an individual basis using cine-MRI. On the other hand, bladder volume and shape are dependent on interfraction rectal variations that may be best controlled using laxatives and checked on a daily basis with cone beam CT prior to irradiation. In patients that have difficulty emptying their bladder, ultrasound may subsequently indicate a need to catheterize the bladder in some cases [39]. In patients with unstable bladders, urodynamic testing should be carried out prior to simulation, and medication may be necessary. Unless instability is manageable, these troubles may preclude irradiation in such patients. Finally, erratic movements of probably minor significance might occasionally be observed and may be tracked as is the case for prostate.

Due to the nature of the movements and the absence of sufficient contrast between surrounding structures and bladder tumors, image-guided SBRT requires that fiducials or some other localizable marker (e.g., radiofrequency transponders) or contrast material (e.g., lipidiol) be placed to track bladder tumors. The fiducials provide reference positions for the bladder-wall localizations. After surgical resection of the bladder tumor (transurethral resection of the bladder, TURB), pathological examination assesses the quality of the resection. Insertion of at least four gold seeds or titanium clips into the bladder mucosa is then performed under rigid cystoscopy by the urologist as a means to localize the postoperative bed during treatment planning. The implantation of fiducials is performed with local anesthesia using a procedure described earlier [32, 40].

Radiofrequency transponders (Calypso Medical Technologies, Inc., Seattle, WA), real-time tracking software (Acculoc®, Civco Medical Solutions, Kalona, IA; ExacTrac®, BrainLAB AG, Feldkirchen, Germany), and injection of a fatty radio-opaque substance, lipiodol, [41], into the bladder-wall during flexible cystoscopy, are other tracking methods under development. Chai et al. have investigated the usefulness of lipiodol in tracking tumor deformation during partial bladder tumor irradiation. According to the authors, the relative movement of each lipiodol spot pair was correlated with the relative bladder volume to study tumor deformation. Uncertainties in the left–right direction (0.14–0.19 cm) were smaller than those in caudocranial and anteroposterior directions (0.19–0.32 cm). While a lipiodol spot is highly visible on cone beam computed tomography (CBCT), it is unlikely that this procedure (injection under cystoscopy) will gain widespread use due to lipiodol washout during prolonged courses of radiation, and the relatively invasive nature of the procedure when performed daily [41]. Furthermore, the fact that enhancement can be shown far from the original tumor region makes it a cause of error.

In the case of one promising SBRT delivery platform, CyberKnife® (Accuray Incorporated, Sunnyvale, CA), for reliable tracking, fiducials should be inserted, as much as possible, at the periphery of the tumor, with a 15-degree angle and at a distance greater than 2 cm. As shown in prostate cancer, real-time image guidance and automatic correction techniques unique to the CyberKnife system seem adequate to maintain submillimeter targeting accuracy for patients with slow and continuously drifting prostate motion [42]. However, in cases where rapid and erratic prostate motion occurs, more frequent imaging and correction of beam aim are necessary to ensure accuracy. The rate and extent of movement can vary from patient to patient and from fraction to fraction. It is therefore difficult to establish a standard image guidance frequency. For this purpose, Accuray has launched the InTempo™ Adaptive Imaging System, which increases the imaging frequency during periods of rapid and erratic movement. Continual assessment of motion combined with prostate automatic correction for movement in real-time ensures that prescribed doses are delivered to the prostate, and the surrounding sensitive structures are maximally spared.

We have recently reported on a case of bladder cancer of the lateral wall in a heavily pretreated patient [32]. The patient had a contracted bladder with limited capacity, and thus was subject to relatively minimal filling variability. We used a drinking and voiding protocol that entailed no fluids at least 1 h before irradiation and auto-catheterization within the 30 min preceding irradiation, and investigated the individual reproducibility of the bladder shape in this patient, using four implanted fiducials. Individual day-to-day bladder shape changes were investigated for a given fixed bladder volume. In this case study of bladder cancer treated with CyberKnife, bladder volume changes were limited, because the patient had a contracted bladder, due to medical history, with a capacity of 230–250 cm^3 and was catheterized three to five times daily; had no rectal filling due to a previous ileostomy; and was menopausal, therefore had no uterine variations. All these factors worked to limit bladder volume variations.

Due to her surgical and radiation history, and other factors as mentioned above, the patient's bladder deformation pattern was relatively predictable [32]. Shifts in fiducial positions were detected through measuring any changes of distance between fiducial markers. These relative movements of each marker pair (rigid body errors) were correlated with the relative bladder volume to study tumor deformation (Fig. 17.1). The center of gravity of several fiducial markers was used for tumor tracking. A statistically distributed migration was thus assumed to keep the center of the dose distribution fairly constant.

A relatively low-dose hypofractionated reirradiation with CyberKnife was used. Targeting a fraction size below 6 Gy, the linear quadratic formula was used to arrive at an NTD (2 Gy) of 18–20 Gy, which was comparable to the conventional 65-Gy total-dose regimen. As a boost to a chemoradiation protocol, this

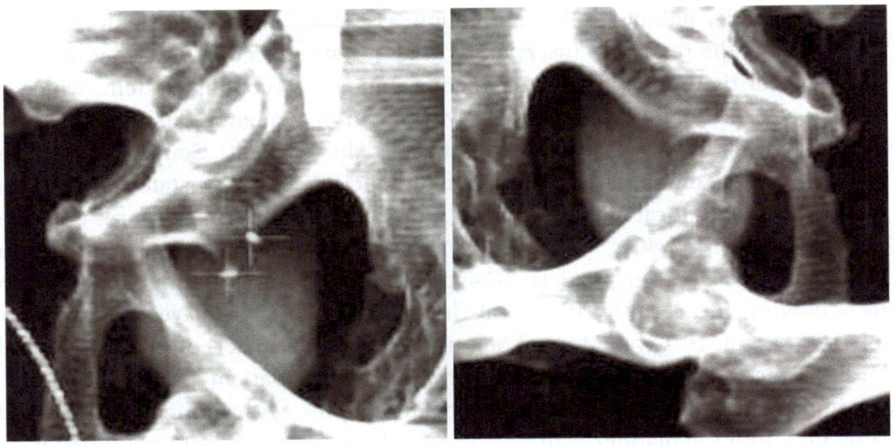

Fig. 17.1 Orthogonal oblique (45°) views obtained from digital reconstructed radiographs to track fiducials (radio-opaque markers shown by crosses) for CyberKnife treatment of bladder cancer. Tumor deformation was studied by correlating the relative bladder volume with any change in distance between fiducial markers

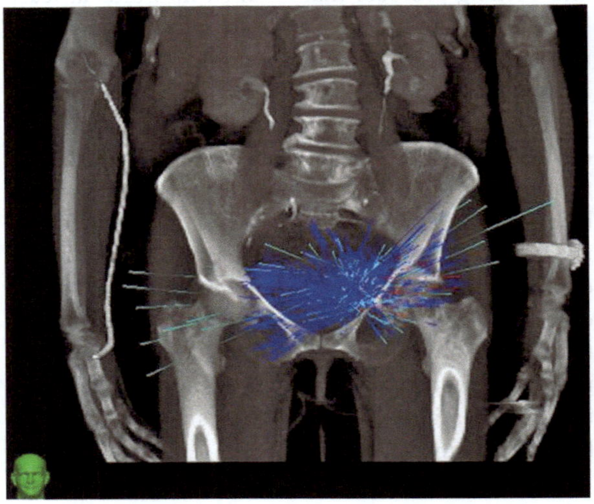

Fig. 17.2 Three-dimensional visualization of beams and isodose distribution for CyberKnife treatment targeting the transurethral bladder resection area. The patient received 24 Gy in four fractions. The dose was prescribed to the 80% isodose line

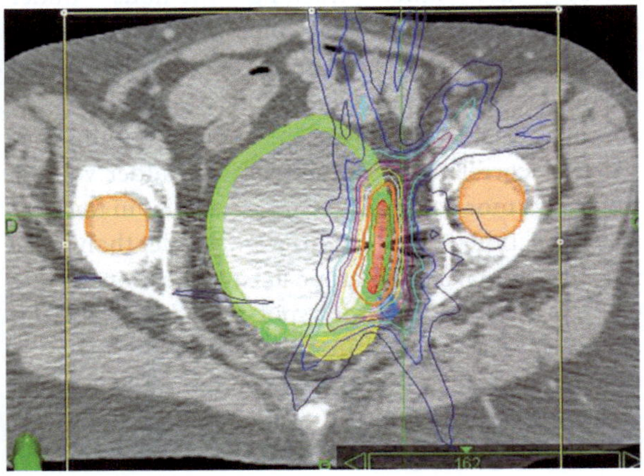

Fig. 17.3 Axial view showing dose distribution around the target transurethral bladder resection area for CyberKnife treatment. The CTV was defined by the four fiducials placed in the periphery of the tumor bed and a 1 cm margin. Constraints were defined for the organs at risk (rectum, bladder minus PTV, anal canal, and femoral heads)

dose was administered in a slightly accelerated fashion, as was radiobiologically attractive for bladder cancer without a significant risk of late detrimental effects. In the end, the patient received 24 Gy in four 6-Gy fractions (Figs. 17.2 and 17.3).

The patient was set-up supine with hands on her sides (Fig. 17.4). Patients with pelvic tumors are currently treated supine with hands on breasts. The patient was asked not to consume any fluids 30 min prior to the CT scan. She was asked to empty her bladder or catheterized 30 min prior to each treatment. A urinary tube or US monitoring was not used, because extensive bladder variations were not expected, and an in-room US device was not available. Axial CT scan images of 1-mm slice thickness were used for delineation and treatment planning. Contouring of the bladder CTV was done by a radiation oncologist, based on a contrast-enhanced diagnostic CT fused with the non-contrast-enhanced planning CT and cystoscopy description. The CTV was defined by the four fiducials placed in the periphery of the tumor bed, and a 1-cm margin. PTV

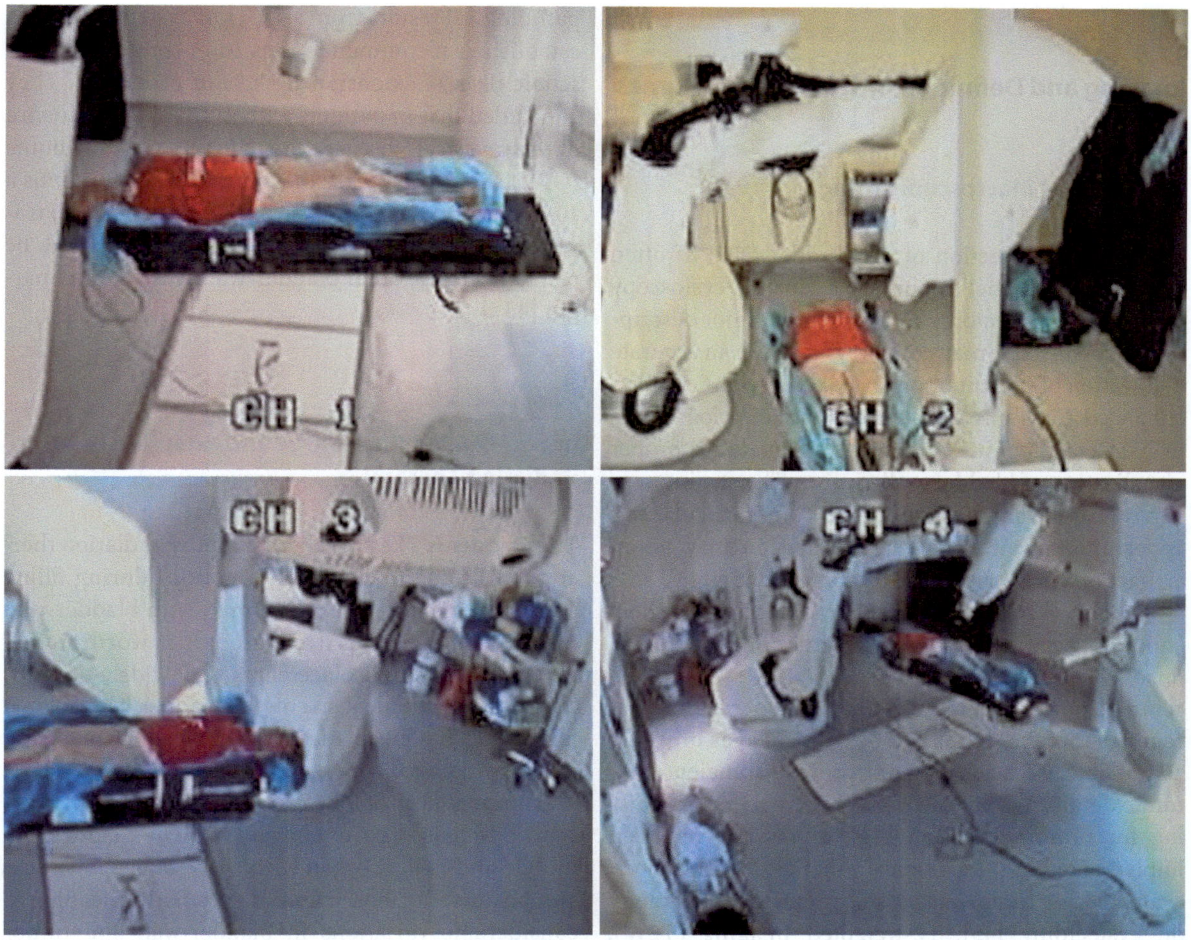

Fig. 17.4 Patient with localized bladder cancer placed in supine position with hands along her body, seen using online video surveillance during CyberKnife stereotactic radiation therapy. A lumbar Xsight® Spine (Accuray) set-up was generated for initial positioning

consisted of the CTV and a 5-mm margin in all directions for targeting uncertainties. Constraints for the organs at risk (rectum, bladder minus PTV, anal canal, and femoral heads) were the usual 2-Gy equivalent constraints assuming an alpha beta ratio of 2, with special care to avoid hot spots. The dose was prescribed to the 80% isodose line that covered 95% of the PTV, with a maximum of 120% of the prescribed dose to the PTV. Cumulative doses from previous treatments were not considered as her last treatment to bladder was in 1994. A lumbar Xsight® Spine (Accuray) set-up was generated for initial positioning. Tracking was performed using the fiducials.

Dose distribution was comparable to HDR brachytherapy treatment, without the use of invasive catheters. It has now been 3 years since her CyberKnife treatment, which proved to be safe and effective [32]. This case study represents the first application of robotic stereotactic radiation therapy for the treatment of a patient with localized bladder cancer who was not eligible for standard treatment due to her medical history of pelvic cancer. The current treatment yielded good immediate tolerance. Further follow-up is warranted to assess long-term outcome of local control and potential complications.

17.5 Imaging and Definition of Treatment Volumes

17.5.1 Definition of Macroscopic Tumor

Transurethral resection of the bladder (TURB) often underestimates the tumor stage during cystoscopy compared to cystectomy. Consequently, tumor description on cystoscopy may not always result in an accurate delineation of the tumor on an axial CT scan. Contrast-enhanced CT scans are used for visualization of the urinary tract, but are not always adequate for proper visualization of bladder-wall tumors. The staging sensitivity based on CT is around 50%. In particular, CT appearance of an extravesical extension may be an artifact of a previous transurethral resection [43].

Indication of a post-TURB irradiation is the most commonly encountered clinical situation in radiation oncology dealing with bladder cancer. Often, the tumor is no longer present. Partial bladder irradiation requires that the tumor bed be delineated as precisely as possible. CT scan may not provide sufficient anatomic details. While MRI cystography seems promising for tumor definition [44], it has not yet been implemented into the clinical practice. MRI has been evaluated for tumor response compared to histology on cystectomy [45]. T2-weighted imaging (T2W), dynamic contrast-enhanced T1-weighted imaging (DCE), and diffusion-weighted magnetic resonance imaging (DWI) were used. DWI was significantly superior to CT with sensitivity/specificity/accuracy of 57%/92%/80%, respectively. Despite the limitations of CT and the advent of new imaging techniques, CT scan remains the reference imaging for treatment planning in radiation therapy. In any case, if several imaging modalities are to be used, image fusion (diagnostic MRI + planning CT) must rely on images of bladder in similar shape and volume.

17.5.2 Definition of Margins: Microscopic Disease in Treatment Planning

The presence and extent of tumor growth beyond the outer bladder-wall may be difficult to measure radiologically. Jenkins et al. correlated CT scans with histopathological results from a series of cystectomies and established recommendations to encompass microscopic disease extension in 90% of cases [43]. They concluded that in patients with radiological evidence of extravesical disease, the clinical target volume (CTV) should comprise the outer bladder-wall plus a 10-mm margin. In patients with no evidence of extravesical disease on CT scans, the CTV should be restricted to the outer bladder-wall plus a 6-mm margin [43].

17.5.3 Image-Guided Physiology and Adaptive Radiation Therapy

The bladder is a key organ for adaptive radiation therapy (ART) due to shape deformations during filling and to the risk of geographic miss with bladder-wall displacements during irradiation. It is worth noting that bladder-wall displacements vary widely depending on the anatomical site on the bladder. The normal filling rate has been measured around 1.5 cm^3/min during prolonged times without drinking.

The pivotal problem in radiotherapy for bladder cancer is caused by organ motion. The bladder is a mobile and hollow organ with changes in shape, size, and position during a course of irradiation, leading to considerable variations in bladder-wall and tumor position. This severely limits the precision of conventional bladder-radiation therapy. Attempts to control bladder volumes during radiotherapy with drinking protocols, restricting fluid intake before treatment, or urinary catheter balloons have so far not been successful in preventing organ motion. In bladder-radiation therapy, the CTV is relatively large as it usually includes the entire bladder into the full dose area. It may consist of the tumor only for partial bladder boost irradiation protocols following completion of mid-dose irradiation of the entire bladder. With the given uncertainty in the target location in the absence of image guidance, CTV to planning target volume (PTV) margins of 2–3 cm are theoretically required to account for organ motion although margins are smaller than that in clinical practice. This implies that, for example, a bladder CTV of 130 cm^3 with a margin of 2 cm will result in a PTV of approximately 600 cm^3. In a study by Cowan et al., the median PTV volume of the whole bladder with a 1.5 cm margin was 815 cm^3, varying between 490 and 1,362 cm^3 [46]. The large PTV volumes imply irradiation of large volumes of healthy tissue, in particular the bladder itself and the small bowel, with consequent and dose-limiting toxicity.

A bladder volume increase of just 50 cm^3 can lead to local bladder-wall displacements of up to 1 cm. This also results in isocenter shifts that can be significant during radiotherapy delivery. Turner et al. have found that the bladder moves more than 1.5 cm at least once in 60% of patients with a maximum displacement of 2.7 cm during conventional irradiation [47]. Individual day-to-day variation in bladder volume can be observed even in volunteers despite specific drinking instructions. While the dominant direction is primarily in the superior, and secondarily in the anterior direction, normal bladder volume changes exhibit more global and more symmetrical expansion patterns compared to diseased ones [48]. Furthermore, diseased bladders do not empty totally after micturition. Diseased bladders also have a tendency to expand away from the involved region, which is roughly reproducible between fractions. Other movements are due to rectal and small-bowel movements. These are generally transient and rapid, not inducing significant bladder displacement, but only momentary deflections of partial bladder-walls [48]. Nevertheless, any diarrhea and stool problems should be reported to the physician. To limit variations in shape and bladder volume, fluid-intake protocols have been proposed; however, they have not proved sufficiently reliable. It is estimated that the use of isotropic margins may not be appropriate in about two thirds of patients due to non-symmetrical bladder expansion [49] with limited variations at the level of the trigone and wide changes at the vertex. Important asymmetrical variations may also be noted in diseased bladders. Individually tailored adequate margins are therefore necessary. This is relevant for whole-bladder irradiation, and even more so for partial-boost irradiation, where the risks of margin breach is critical.

Urodynamic testing may be used to assess individual bladder-filling capacity and voiding perception thresholds. It may therefore be useful to estimate bladder volume changes during a given treatment duration. The need for medications (anticholinergic drugs) may also be assessed by the urologist to reduce unpredictable muscle spasms and movements in cases of unstable bladder, a disorder that might be underestimated in bladder cancer. Such movements may be due to dysautonomic nerve function and irritative syndrome.

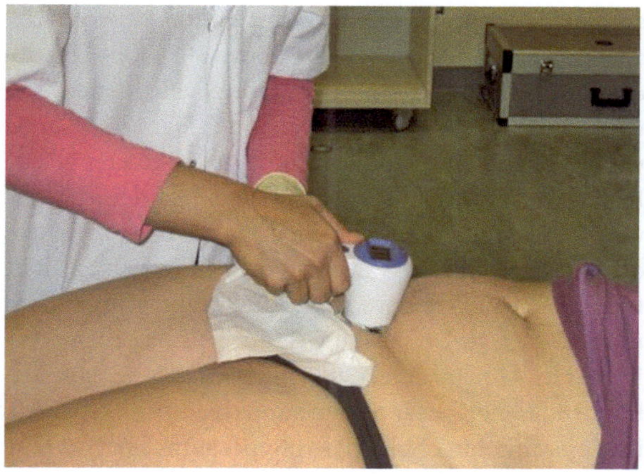

Fig. 17.5 Application of the ultrasound probe on the patient's pelvis prior to and at regular intervals during irradiation. Ultrasound imaging provides a simple and non-invasive method for the measurement of the bladder volume

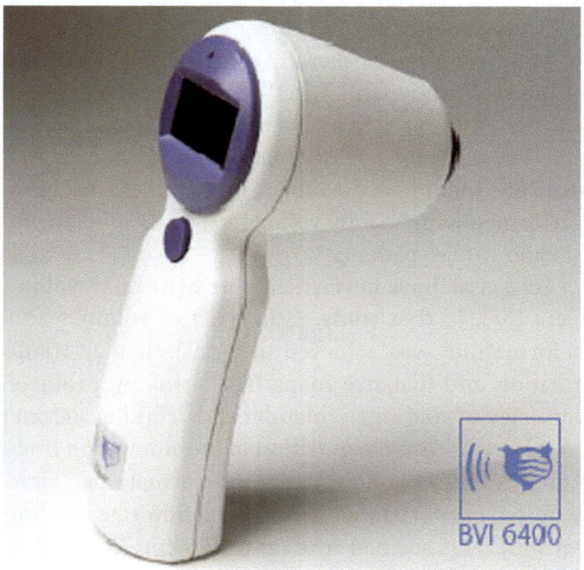

Fig. 17.6 The ultrasound probe (BladderScan®) is a portable, hand-held device utilized for quick and reliable bladder-volume assessment

Ultrasound imaging (US) with a portable, hand-held device (BladderScan® BVI 9000, Verathon Inc., Bothell, WA; Figs. 17.5 and 17.6) provides a simple, non-invasive method of assessing the bladder volume, which is not associated with additional radiation dose. Several studies have shown a strong correlation between US and CT, with an accuracy rate above 90% [50–52]. US can thus be considered a quick and reliable method for the measurement of bladder volume (Fig. 17.7). Large variations in daily bladder volume have been reported. Furthermore, a trend in decreasing bladder volume with increasing number of fractions has been reported during a conventional radiotherapy course [50–52]. It is therefore critical to have some kind of image guidance method such as US for daily setup. This has been confirmed by Aluwini et al. [39]. However, in other studies, important inter-observer variations have been reported in the estimation of bladder volume. Sufficient training and experience is needed. Changes in target position due to rectal and small bowel influences cannot be visualized and no information about isocenter or field position can be inferred. Nevertheless, US provides a relatively low-technology and rapid screening assessment for identifying patients with significant variation in bladder volume.

More recent radiotherapy-oriented investigations of bladder urodynamics [53] have studied cine-MRI and cone-beam CT to assess bladder volume changes and deformations during fractions of 15–20 min and from one fraction to the other. Some studies have been performed with healthy volunteers, while others with bladder cancer patients.

Lotz et al. have performed cine-MRI in 18 volunteers [53]. In that study, estimation of volumes and deformations was achieved using a Delaunay triangulation and distance maps. The drinking protocol consisted of voiding the bladder and drinking 300 cm^3 15 min prior to the acquisition of the simulation fraction. Bladder volumes and deformations were acquired every 10 min for 1 h. The inflow rate was linear [48]. This seemed true up to 150 cm^3 [54] with a sigmoid inflexion after 150 cm^3 [48, 54]. Bladder expansion slightly decreased with time. Bladder-wall displacements of up to 3.5 cm in 10 min were noted for one patient with the high filling rate of 15 cm^3/min. Age influenced the filling rate. Intra-individual intra-fraction variability was low. McBain et al. showed that intrafraction variability in bladder filling between individuals was high, and intraindividual interfraction initial volume variability was high (some had difficulty emptying their bladder) [48], while it was relatively steady according to Mangar et al. [54], potentially due to different subject selection. Initial volume post voiding was 148 ± 88 cm^3 [48] or 113 ± 53 cm^3 [54]. Intraindividual variability in rectal filling was high, ≥40 cm^3 in 33% of individuals, resulting in 0.3–1.2 cm wall displacements and bladder rotation around the left–right axis. A dependency of bladder position was also noted with female menstrual cycle. Larger shape deformations of cranial and posterior portions and smaller variations for smaller retracted bladders were noted. A maximal shift of 2 cm was noted in the first 10 min [53, 55]. In another cine-MRI study by McBain et al. on five volunteers and ten bladder cancer patients, the drinking protocol consisted of drinking abstinence for 1 h before patients emptied their bladder and starting the acquisitions, every 10 min for 28 min [48]. Two such sessions were performed at 3-week intervals for volunteers, or at baseline and after 17 radiotherapy fractions in patients. More symmetrical and global bladder expansions were noted in volunteers. Diseased bladders were less likely to completely empty and expansion occurred away from the cancer-involved region. Maximal wall displacement was reported at or after 28 min with maximal bladder filling. It was maximal superiorly [48, 54]. Although the 1.5 cm CTV–PTV margin was sufficient to account for expansion in the majority of cases in Mangar's study, a breach occurred on the anterior wall consistent with the need of anisotropic margins [48, 54]. Some authors have recommended to perform a tumor boost volume on a full bladder to minimize variations and reduce the margins [46]. A boost volume with 1-cm margins defined on a full bladder treated 40% of the bladder to 60 Gy, compared with 80% of the bladder using an empty bladder protocol with 2-cm margins [46]. Lotz and McBain's studies are contradictory on one major practical issue for radiotherapy planning: the filling rate seemed maximal in the first 10 min in one [53] and after 28 min in the other [48]. Interindividual shape and volume variations can be high but are individually predictable [56].

17.5.3.1 Cone Beam CT Scanner (CBCT)

Image-guided radiotherapy (IGRT) enables correction of positional and deformational errors to the target either by organ deformation or cancer-related shrinkage. In-room soft tissue imaging with kV and MV cone

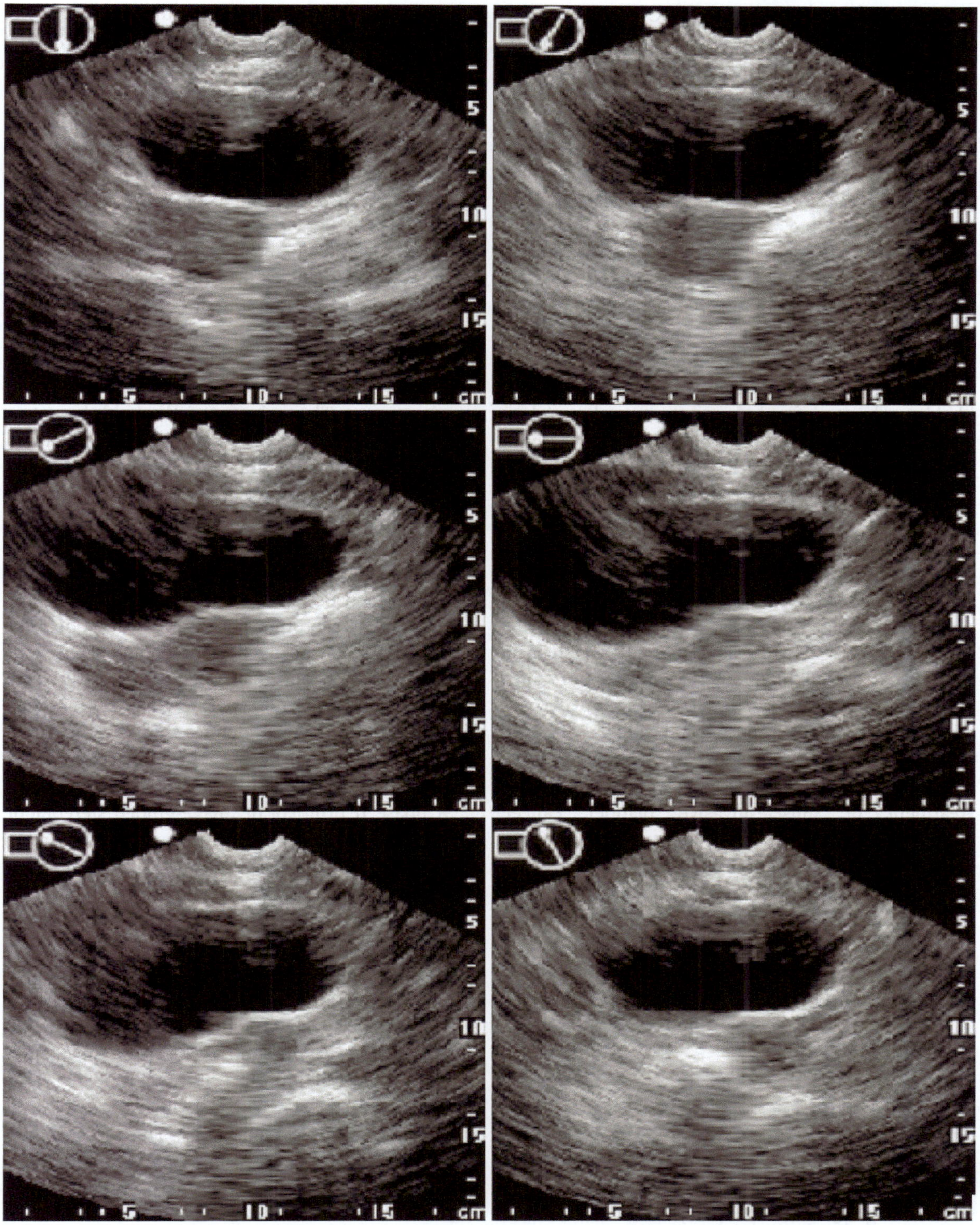

Fig. 17.7 Ultrasound imaging showing visualization of bladder filling during irradiation

beam computed tomography (CBCT) is becoming increasingly prevalent in the radiotherapy planning of bladder cancer. The additional dose received by a kV CBCT to the pelvis is around 0.035 Gy, i.e., approximately 1 Gy for a whole treatment. CBCT can be used on the treatment couch as an offline or online procedure. CBCT prolongs treatment time by several minutes. An offline protocol allows for correction of systematic errors, but cannot correct for random daily movements and volume variations. Prolongation of treatment time by online adaptive radiation delivery may follow a learning curve and may be advantageous to reduce treatment margins, reduce toxicity (reduced irradiated volumes of small bowel), and improve target coverage [57]. Muren et al. correlated the relative bladder volume, defined as repeat scan volume/planning scan volume, and the margins required to account for internal motion from weekly repeat CT scans, with or without fluid intake restrictions in 8 and 20 bladder cancer patients, respectively [58]. Translational movement of the bladder was accounted for by isocenter shifting. Isotropic margins >10 mm were required in 55% of the cases. Drinking restrictions were not sufficient to translate into margin reduction, but the authors planned the treatment on empty bladders in the belief that a full bladder situation was more difficult to standardize and maintain. CT-based IGRT was useful to substantially reduce the margins.

Finally, there remain some uncertainties on the optimal adaptive radiation therapy protocol for the treatment of muscle-invasive bladder cancer. Nevertheless, IGRT has shown a potential for margin reduction and adaptation of treatment delivery on an individual/personalized basis. Based on the almost linear curve of bladder filling, prediction might be relatively easy to model. Prospective IGRT protocols should provide more solid data on the way to predict target position changes and to reduce toxicities.

17.6 Conclusion and Perspectives

It is challenging, if not impossible, to localize the tumor site in a case of bladder cancer using conventional irradiation technologies. Therefore, it is similarly difficult to deliver high-dose, localized radiation to bladder tumors. In order to achieve this goal, brachytherapy has been used successfully over the decades, despite the many inconveniences associated with it, for tumors of the mobile portion and the outcomes have been excellent. The desirable effects of brachytherapy type of radiation delivery appear to be possible to replicate using an advanced treatment planning and delivery system such as the CyberKnife. This type of delivery offers an ideal means of decreasing margins around the tumor, limiting volumes that receive significant doses and optimizing dose-volume histograms (DVHs). Compared with three-dimensional radiotherapy, robotic radiation therapy yields superior DVHs on the healthy bladder and provides excellent coverage for moving targets. These characteristics hold the potential for dose escalation and shortening of overall treatment times to limit tumor repopulation, making robotic radiation therapy convenient for patients. It is of note that, because each fraction duration is quite long (1–1.5 h), bladder surface deformations and volume changes, i.e., the filling rate must be minimized.

The strategy used for this particular patient cannot be extrapolated to other patients. Indeed, individual urodynamics may need to be studied for each patient. Bladder filling owing to its linearity should be estimated or modeled, and strict bowel-related instructions and fluid-intake guidelines should be provided. A urinary catheter is probably necessary for mobile portions of the bladder.

A phase II protocol of image-guided stereotactic tumor bed boost, following transurethral resection and conformal pelvic irradiation with chemotherapy is under evaluation for the treatment of patients with incompletely resected invasive bladder cancer or inoperable patients. The boost dose is 15 Gy in three fractions administered with the CyberKnife system to the TURB bed after conventional irradiation of the pelvis with 45 Gy in 25 fractions (or the NTD equivalent of such in 2 Gy fractions). The NTD equivalent is not increased but more precisely delivers the 2 Gy equivalent of 63–65 Gy with a slightly shortened irradiation course with chemotherapy. The importance of concurrent chemotherapy must also not be underestimated in view of the high rates of distant metastases encountered with muscle-invasive bladder cancer.

Finally, bladder-filling rate is linear up to 150 cm^3; it has a sigmoid trend reproducible and predictable for an individual patient, using a drinking protocol, cine-MRI, and possibly US. Rectal filling is manageable with diet and laxatives, and unpredictable movements may be managed using InTempo-like software. An initial step in our evidence-based approach is the development of an algorithm to model bladder-wall movements during 1-hr fractions and a prediction tool/software for an adaptive CyberKnife treatment of bladder cancer, first for the fixed portion, and, when/if proved reliable, for the mobile portions of the bladder.

References

1. Pos FJ, Hart G, Schneider C et al (2006) Radical radiotherapy for invasive bladder cancer: what dose and fractionation schedule to choose? Int J Radiat Oncol Biol Phys 64: 1168–1173
2. Pos FJ, Koedooder K, Hulshof MC et al (2003) Influence of bladder and rectal volume on spatial variability of a bladder tumor during radical radiotherapy. Int J Radiat Oncol Biol Phys 55:835–841
3. Krengli M, Calvo F et al. (2010) Intraoperative irradiation techniques and results in genitourinary cancer. Springer, Heidelberg
4. Housset M, Durdux C et al (2010) Chemoradiation in bladder cancer. Bull Cancer 97:19–25
5. Pouessel D, Thariat J, Lagrange JL et al (2010) Perioperative strategies in patients with muscle invasive bladder cancer. Bull Cancer 97(Suppl Cancer de la vessie):5–9
6. Thariat J, Caullery M, Ginot A et al (2009) State of the art and advances in radiotherapy for bladder cancer. Prog Urol 19:85–93
7. Marks LB, Carroll PR, Dugan TC et al (1995) The response of the urinary bladder, urethra, and ureter to radiation and chemotherapy. Int J Radiat Oncol Biol Phys 31:1257–1280
8. Maciejewski B, Majewski S (1991) Dose fractionation and tumour repopulation in radiotherapy for bladder cancer. Radiother Oncol 21:163–170
9. Shipley WU (1984) Full-dose irradiation for invasive bladder cancer: prognostic factors and techniques. Urology 23: 95–100
10. Housset M, Maulard C, Chretien Y et al (1993) Combined radiation and chemotherapy for invasive transitional-cell carcinoma of the bladder: a prospective study. J Clin Oncol 11:2150–2157
11. Rodel C, Weiss C, Sauer R (2006) Trimodality treatment and selective organ preservation for bladder cancer. J Clin Oncol 24:5536–5544
12. Poortmans PM, Richaud P, Collette L et al (2008) Results of the phase II EORTC 22971 trial evaluating combined accelerated external radiation and chemotherapy with 5FU and cisplatin in patients with muscle invasive transitional cell carcinoma of the bladder. Acta Oncol 47:937–940
13. Tester W, Porter A, Asbell S et al (1993) Combined modality program with possible organ preservation for invasive bladder carcinoma: results of RTOG protocol 85–12. Int J Radiat Oncol Biol Phys 25:783–790
14. Chauvet B, Felix-Faure C, Davin JL et al (1998) Results of long-term treatment of inoperable cancer of the bladder with cisplatin and concurrent irradiation: prognostic factors of local control and survival. Cancer Radiother 2(Suppl 1):85s–91s
15. Rodel C, Grabenbauer GG, Kuhn R et al (2002) Combined-modality treatment and selective organ preservation in invasive bladder cancer: long-term results. J Clin Oncol 20:3061–3071
16. Coppin CM, Gospodarowicz MK, James K et al (1996) Improved local control of invasive bladder cancer by concurrent cisplatin and preoperative or definitive radiation. The National Cancer Institute of Canada Clinical Trials Group. J Clin Oncol 14:2901–2907
17. Shipley WU, Zietman AL, Kaufman DS et al (2005) Selective bladder preservation by trimodality therapy for patients with muscularis propria-invasive bladder cancer and who are cystectomy candidates–the Massachusetts General Hospital and Radiation Therapy Oncology Group experiences. Semin Radiat Oncol 15:36–41
18. Dunst J, Rodel C, Zietman A et al (2001) Bladder preservation in muscle-invasive bladder cancer by conservative surgery and radiochemotherapy. Semin Surg Oncol 20:24–32
19. Housset MaXB (2002) Intérêt de la radiochimiothérapie concomitante dans le traitement des tumeurs infiltrantes de vessie: à propos de 173 cas. Thèse de Doctorat en médecine, Université René Descartes
20. Kachnic LA, Kaufman DS, Heney NM et al (1997) Bladder preservation by combined modality therapy for invasive bladder cancer. J Clin Oncol 15:1022–1029
21. Sauer R, Dunst J, Altendorf-Hofmann A et al (1990) Radiotherapy with and without cisplatin in bladder cancer. Int J Radiat Oncol Biol Phys 19:687–691
22. Arias F, Dominguez MA, Martinez E et al (2000) Chemoradiotherapy for muscle invading bladder carcinoma. Final report of a single institutional organ-sparing program. Int J Radiat Oncol Biol Phys 47:373–378
23. Zapatero A, MartindeVidales C, Arellano R et al (2009) Updated results of bladder-sparing trimodality approach for invasive bladder cancer. Urol Oncol 28:368–374
24. Efstathiou JA, Bae K, Shipley WU et al (2009) Late pelvic toxicity after bladder-sparing therapy in patients with invasive bladder cancer: RTOG 89–03, 95–06, 97–06, 99–06. J Clin Oncol 27:4055–4061
25. Lagrange JL, Bascoul-Mollevi C, Geoffrois L et al (2010) Quality of life assessment after concurrent chemoradiation for invasive bladder cancer: results of a multicenter prospective study (GETUG 97–015). Int J Radiat Oncol Biol Phys 79:172–178
26. Yan D, Lockman D, Brabbins D et al (2000) An off-line strategy for constructing a patient-specific planning target volume in adaptive treatment process for prostate cancer. Int J Radiat Oncol Biol Phys 48:289–302
27. Viswanathan AN, Yorke ED, Marks LB et al (2010) Radiation dose-volume effects of the urinary bladder. Int J Radiat Oncol Biol Phys 76:S116–S122
28. de Crevoisier R, Ammor A, Court B et al (2004) Bladder-conserving surgery and interstitial brachytherapy for

lymph node negative transitional cell carcinoma of the urinary bladder: results of a 28-year single institution experience. Radiother Oncol 72:147–157
29. Pos F, Moonen L (2005) Brachytherapy in the treatment of invasive bladder cancer. Semin Radiat Oncol 15:49–54
30. Van Poppel H, Lievens Y, Van Limbergen E et al (2000) Brachytherapy with iridium-192 for bladder cancer. Eur Urol 37:605–608
31. Fuller DB, Naitoh J, Lee C et al (2008) Virtual HDR CyberKnife treatment for localized prostatic carcinoma: dosimetry comparison with HDR brachytherapy and preliminary clinical observations. Int J Radiat Oncol Biol Phys 70:1588–1597
32. Thariat J, Trimaud R, Angellier G et al (2010) Innovative image-guided CyberKnife stereotactic radiotherapy for bladder cancer. Br J Radiol 83:e118–e121
33. van der Werf-Messing B, Menon RS, Hop WC (1983) Cancer of the urinary bladder category T2, T3, (NxMo) treated by interstitial radium implant: second report. Int J Radiat Oncol Biol Phys 9:481–485
34. Blank LE, Koedooder K, van Os R et al (2007) Results of bladder-conserving treatment, consisting of brachytherapy combined with limited surgery and external beam radiotherapy, for patients with solitary T1-T3 bladder tumors less than 5 cm in diameter. Int J Radiat Oncol Biol Phys 69:454–458
35. van der Steen-Banasik E, Ploeg M, Witjes JA et al (2009) Brachytherapy versus cystectomy in solitary bladder cancer: a case control, multicentre, East-Netherlands study. Radiother Oncol 93:352–357
36. Nieuwenhuijzen JA, Pos F, Moonen LM et al (2005) Survival after bladder-preservation with brachytherapy versus radical cystectomy; a single institution experience. Eur Urol 48:239–245
37. Pos FJ, Horenblas S, Lebesque J et al (2004) Low-dose-rate brachytherapy is superior to high-dose-rate brachytherapy for bladder cancer. Int J Radiat Oncol Biol Phys 59: 696–705
38. Ernst F, Bruder R, Schlaefer A et al (2011) Forecasting pulsatory motion for non-invasive cardiac radiosurgery: an analysis of algorithms from respiratory motion prediction. Int J Comput Assist Radiol Surg 6:93–101
39. Aluwini S, van Rooij P, Hoogeman M et al (2010) CyberKnife stereotactic radiotherapy as monotherapy for low- to intermediate-stage prostate cancer: early experience, feasibility, and tolerance. J Endourol 24:865–869
40. Hulshof MC, van Andel G, Bel A et al (2007) Intravesical markers for delineation of target volume during external focal irradiation of bladder carcinomas. Radiother Oncol 84:49–51
41. Chai X, van Herk M, van de Kamer JB et al (2010) Behavior of lipiodol markers during image guided radiotherapy of bladder cancer. Int J Radiat Oncol Biol Phys 77:309–314
42. Xie Y, Djajaputra D, King CR et al (2008) Intrafractional motion of the prostate during hypofractionated radiotherapy. Int J Radiat Oncol Biol Phys 72:236–246
43. Jenkins P, Anjarwalla S, Gilbert H et al (2009) Defining the clinical target volume for bladder cancer radiotherapy treatment planning. Int J Radiat Oncol Biol Phys 75: 1379–1384
44. Beer A, Saar B, Zantl N et al (2004) MR cystography for bladder tumor detection. Eur Radiol 14:2311–2319
45. Yoshida S, Koga F, Kawakami S et al (2010) Initial experience of diffusion-weighted magnetic resonance imaging to assess therapeutic response to induction chemoradiotherapy against muscle-invasive bladder cancer. Urology 75:387–391
46. Cowan RA, McBain CA, Ryder WD et al (2004) Radiotherapy for muscle-invasive carcinoma of the bladder: results of a randomized trial comparing conventional whole bladder with dose-escalated partial bladder radiotherapy. Int J Radiat Oncol Biol Phys 59:197–207
47. Turner SL, Swindell R, Bowl N et al (1997) Bladder movement during radiation therapy for bladder cancer: implications for treatment planning. Int J Radiat Oncol Biol Phys 39:355–360
48. McBain CA, Khoo VS, Buckley DL et al (2009) Assessment of bladder motion for clinical radiotherapy practice using cine-magnetic resonance imaging. Int J Radiat Oncol Biol Phys 75:664–671
49. Wright P, Redpath AT, Hoyer M et al (2008) The normal tissue sparing potential of adaptive strategies in radiotherapy of bladder cancer. Acta Oncol 47:1382–1389
50. Fiorino C, Foppiano F, Franzone P et al (2005) Rectal and bladder motion during conformal radiotherapy after radical prostatectomy. Radiother Oncol 74:187–195
51. Stam MR, van Lin EN, van der Vight LP et al (2006) Bladder filling variation during radiation treatment of prostate cancer: can the use of a bladder ultrasound scanner and biofeedback optimize bladder filling? Int J Radiat Oncol Biol Phys 65:371–377
52. Ahmad R, Hoogeman MS, Quint S et al (2008) Inter-fraction bladder filling variations and time trends for cervical cancer patients assessed with a portable 3-dimensional ultrasound bladder scanner. Radiother Oncol 89:172–179
53. Lotz HT, van Herk M, Betgen A et al (2005) Reproducibility of the bladder shape and bladder shape changes during filling. Med Phys 32:2590–2597
54. Mangar SA, Miller NA et al (2007) Evaluating the impact of volume limitation as a method of reducing the internal margin of the PTV in bladder radiotherapy. Clin Oncol (R Coll Radiol) 19:S38–S39
55. Lotz HT, Pos FJ, Hulshof MC et al (2006) Tumor motion and deformation during external radiotherapy of bladder cancer. Int J Radiat Oncol Biol Phys 64:1551–1558
56. Krywonos J, Fenwick J, Elkut F et al (2010) MRI image-based FE modelling of the pelvis system and bladder filling. Comput Methods Biomech Biomed Engin 13: 669–676
57. Burridge N, Amer A, Marchant T et al (2006) Online adaptive radiotherapy of the bladder: small bowel irradiated-volume reduction. Int J Radiat Oncol Biol Phys 66: 892–897
58. Muren LP, Redpath AT, Lord H et al (2007) Image-guided radiotherapy of bladder cancer: bladder volume variation and its relation to margins. Radiother Oncol 84:307–313

Stereotactic Body Radiotherapy for Gynecologic Malignancies

18

Daniel S. Higginson, Mahesh A. Varia, and David E. Morris

CONTENTS

18.1 Abstract

This chapter provides a review of the applications of stereotactic body radiotherapy (SBRT) as a treatment modality for gynecological malignancies.

SBRT may be an alternative for patients with difficult anatomy or disease extension to challenging sites not suitable for boost with brachytherapy or conventional radiation. SBRT is a safely tolerated means of boosting gross residual or recurrent disease in the periaortic nodal chain, leading to effective salvage therapy in carefully selected patients. SBRT may also have an important role in the treatment of oligometastatic disease.

18.2 Introduction

Radiotherapy is an indispensible treatment modality for malignancies of the female gynecologic tract. Yet there remain common clinical scenarios, both in the primary and recurrent setting, in which normal tissue tolerances to radiotherapy limit its clinical effectiveness. While small volumes of the uterine corpus, cervix, and upper vaginal mucosa can tolerate very high doses of radiation (>100 Gy) [1], the tissue tolerances of surrounding whole organs, such as small bowel (45 Gy), bladder (65 Gy), and rectum (60 Gy) limit the capacity to safely deliver a curative dose (70–85 Gy) to a tumor with conventional techniques [2].

L.E. Ponsky et al. (eds.), *Treating Prostate Cancer and Related Genitourinary Applications*, Robotic Radiosurgery,
DOI 10.1007/978-3-642-11495-3_18,

Robotic stereotactic body radiotherapy (SBRT) is a new technical innovation that allows for highly conformal targeting of radiation to tumors using multiple beams and stereotactic tracking to account for internal organ motion secondary to respiration, peristalsis, and fluctuations in bladder and rectum filling. In several important ways, SBRT has great potential for use in gynecologic malignancies. First, the vagina, uterus, and the cervix can tolerate very high doses of radiation based upon analogous toxicity and outcome data with the use of high-dose-rate (HDR) brachytherapy (BT) and intraoperative radiotherapy (IORT). Second, the uterus, cervix, and the vaginal cuff are subject to large inter- and intrafractional displacements during a radiation treatment course and thus fiducial tracking is highly advantageous. Third, fiducials can be directly placed in the vaginal cuff/cervix by experienced radiation oncologists. Fourth, there are a number of situations in which SBRT may be an alternative or supplement to BT boost when BT is medically, anatomically, or dosimetrically constrained. In addition, SBRT can offer novel noninvasive avenues for dose escalation in clinical sites not previously possible.

Two sites of disease have generated much interest in SBRT: (1) pelvic and periaortic lymph nodes and (2) extensive parametrial disease. These sites are uniquely challenging to boost with BT or conventional radiation and remain sites for tumor recurrence. Lymph node metastases are not readily accessible for BT and are typically in close proximity to loops of small bowel, limiting conventional external-beam dose. Locally advanced cervical cancer, in particular, frequently spreads laterally into the parametrial tissues, outside of the area treated to a high dose with BT.

This chapter provides a review of the technological innovations and clinical experience with SBRT and discusses the potential of SBRT for improving local tumor control in clinical situations not amenable to current treatment methods.

18.3 Cervical Carcinoma

18.3.1 Background

A curative course of radiation for cervical carcinoma consists conventionally of two parts: (1) external-beam radiation therapy (EBRT) to treat the primary cervical site, regional spread, and the pelvis and periaortic lymph node chain as indicated, and (2) a boost to gross disease. An intracavitary brachytherapy (IC-BT) boost, as opposed to 3D conformal RT or intensity-modulated radiotherapy (IMRT) or SBRT, remains the standard of care for almost all patients as it affords two inherent advantages relative to all varieties of teletherapy: (1) extremely high doses are applied near the source with rapid dose fall off and (2) the fixation of the source adjacent to tumor, greatly reducing geo-

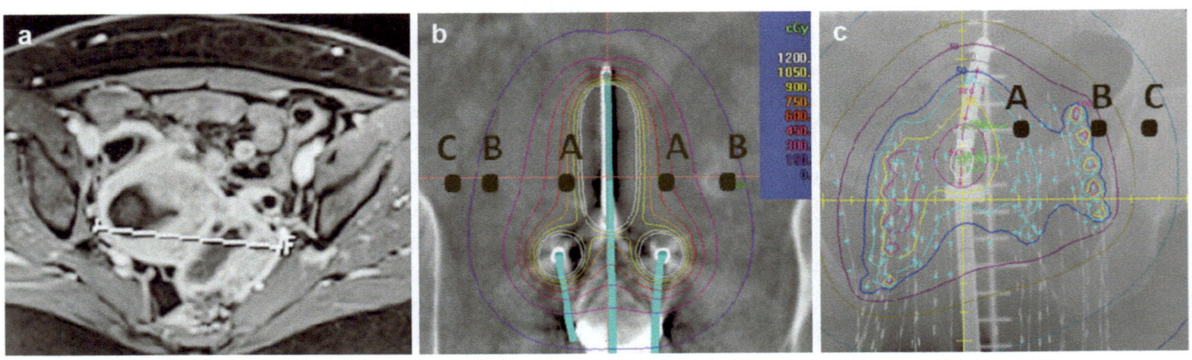

Fig. 18.1 The difficulty surrounding pelvic side wall disease and brachytherapy. (**a**) is an axial MRI image of a patient with stage IIIB cervical squamous cell carcinoma, with nearly complete sidewall to sidewall disease. (**b**) displays a coronal image of an HDR IC-BT implant with the isodose lines labeled. *Points A, B, and C* are displayed. Point A is located 2 cm superior to the external cervical os and 2 cm lateral, corresponding approximately to the position that the uterine artery crosses the ureter. Point B is 3 cm lateral to point A and represents parametrial tissue. Point C is 1 cm lateral to the point B and represents the pelvic sidewall. (**c**) exhibits the isodose distribution of an LDR IS-BT implant for a stage IIIB cervical squamous cell carcinoma, demonstrating improved pelvic sidewall coverage. In this image 30 Gy was prescribed to the royal blue isodose line

metric uncertainty. Still, there are a number of clinical situations in which SBRT can be considered, either as a supplement to BT or as an alternative.

SBRT, with the typical dose rates of 3–10 Gy/min per beam, is most analogous to HDR BT (>12 Gy/h) [3]. With HDR intracavitary applications (see Fig. 18.1a, b), BT delivers very high doses (>13 Gy) to tissues immediately adjacent to the source while point A (Fig. 18.1b), 2 cm away, typically receives 6 Gy. Points B and C, which correspond anatomically to the parametria and pelvic sidewall, receive only 1/3 and 1/5 of this dose and thus underdosing of large tumors with gross parametrial disease approaching the sidewall is a long recognized problem with IC-BT [4]. Interstitial LDR brachytherapy, as seen in panel C, can provide better coverage of disease extending to the sidewall.

18.3.2 SBRT as a Substitute for Brachytherapy

SBRT can be considered a substitute for BT for patients exhibiting difficult anatomy, such as patients with narrow, stenotic vaginas, noncanalizable cervical ossa, or obliterated vaginal fornices. Situations arise where patients refuse IC-BT or may be medically at high risk for such procedures. Finally, some patients' primary tumors are too extensive, even after receiving the initial course of EBRT, to be adequately covered with IC-BT, and may not be ideal candidates for an interstitial implant.

Both IMRT and interstitial brachytherapy (IS-BT) are also considered alternatives to IC-BT for large tumors. IS-BT, in experienced hands, is arguably associated with improved local control for stage IIIB tumors [5–8]; however, not all investigators agree and the modality itself is technically challenging and highly invasive [6]. The technique has not disseminated into routine use in the United States as evidenced by one patterns-of-care analysis, which found only 1% utilization in community practices versus 9% in academic centers [9].

IMRT has also been proposed as an alternative to BT, but multiple dosimetric studies have concluded that although IMRT achieves superior dose homogeneity and superior coverage of tumor in some cases, it cannot spare normal tissues as well as BT [10–13]. One study found up to a twofold increase in the volume of normal tissue receiving 60 Gy when IMRT plans are developed with the same dosimetric constraints as BT [10, 14].

There are not yet enough data to comment on the clinical efficacy of SBRT boosts relative to BT. The available series report its use in patients with tumors too advanced for BT (thus making direct comparisons difficult) or involve too few cervical cancer patients [15]. As compared to IMRT boosts, robotic SBRT adds the benefit of stereotactic tracking, which reduces setup error and accounts for internal target motion (discussed in Sect. 18.8). With smaller, more highly conformal CTV-PTV margins and a greatly increased number of radiation beams and angles of beam entry, there is an improved shaping of dose around a smaller target compared to IMRT. Additionally, the multiplicity of beams can more adeptly mimic the dose escalation effect of BT.

Molla and colleagues have used stereotactic guidance with SBRT as a final boost to treat seven cervical cancer patients after surgery [15]. Each patient received conventional, four-field pelvic irradiation to 45–50.4 Gy prior the SBRT boost of 14 Gy in two fractions with 4–7 days between fractions. The target consisted of the vaginal vault with a 6- to 10-mm expansion to create a PTV. Only one patient recurred at a median 12.6-month follow-up and one late grade 3 rectal bleeding toxicity was observed. Although these results were encouraging, the patients under study typically had no gross residual disease, making direct comparisons to BT in cervix cancer difficult.

Guckenberger et al. has treated 12 cervical cancer patients with SBRT at the time of recurrence after surgery and therefore, each had gross disease [16]. Patients received conventional pelvic EBRT to 50 Gy with concurrent weekly cisplatin chemotherapy. SBRT was chosen as a final boost instead of vaginal BT in these patients because of the size or peripheral location of the recurrence. The typical dose was 15 Gy in three fractions delivered every other day within 1 week and prescribed to the 65% isodose line with a 5-mm PTV margin on the GTV. The local control rate was 81%, but only 34% survival was demonstrated at 3 years for all patients, including some endometrial cancer patients [16].

Deodata et al. has treated two patients with SBRT for gross disease after prior surgery or prior chemoradiation. The group employed 25 Gy in five fractions or 30 Gy in six fractions on consecutive days and none of the patients had evidence of disease at 19 and 28 months [17].

In a comparison between teletherapy of any variety and BT boost, one must recognize that BT inherently delivers an inhomogeneous escalation of dose next to the source (>13 Gy in HDR BT), an effect that is difficult to mimic with EBRT. This heterogeneity may be of clinical benefit, as reported in prostate cancer ^{125}I brachytherapy [18]. CyberKnife® (Accuray Incorporated, Sunnyvale, CA) SBRT has been the most likely platform to mimic the heterogeneity of brachytherapy [19].

18.3.3 SBRT in Addition to Brachytherapy

Several investigators have suggested combining BT and IMRT boosts, thereby taking advantage of the best properties of BT (less geometric uncertainty, central dose escalation) and the advantages of IMRT (ability to treat the distant parametrial disease near the sidewall) [10, 11, 20]. In our view, further study is warranted to determine whether SBRT as well can supplement IC-BT and thereby offer an alternative to IS-BT for patients with advanced parametrial disease.

This approach is supported by one dosimetric study in which six patients with advanced cervical tumors that were deemed unfavorable for IC-BT. They were planned with EBRT to the whole pelvis (45 Gy/25 fractions) and a boost of 28 Gy in four fractions. The boost was planned using IC-BT, IMRT, IS-BT, or IC-BT and IMRT together. In the combined scenario, IMRT was optimized to cover areas undertreated by IC-BT while the IC-BT applicator was in situ. As expected, the analysis found that target coverage (volume receiving greater than 85 Gy) was significantly higher with the use of IMRT or IS-BT versus IC-BT alone (95–98% vs. 74%). IMRT alone, however, increased the volume receiving over 60 Gy (V60) by 83% relative to IC-BT, increasing dose to normal tissue. However, IC-BT combined with IMRT improved coverage to 95%, while increasing V60 by only 33% relative to IC-BT [11].

Combined BT and SBRT or IMRT boosts would need to proceed with caution as increasing doses to pelvic structures carry the risk of increased severe late toxicity. Barillot and colleagues analyzed 642 patients over three decades of radiation therapy as doses and practices of EBRT and BT varied and found that the volume in the pelvis receiving more than 60 Gy (termed HWT in the paper) through EBRT and/or BT combined correlated with increased grade 3 rectal and soft tissue toxicity [14].

Logsdon and Eifel reviewed 1,096 patients who received definitive treatment for IIIB cervical cancer at MD Anderson [21]. Over the years, the dose delivered to the pelvis via EBRT declined as dose delivered through BT increased. They found that those patients who received more than 52 Gy of EBRT to the central pelvis experienced higher rates of grade 3–5 toxicity (57–68%) versus patients receiving less than 52 Gy (20–33%). Between 1960 and 1981, when patients commonly received >52 Gy, the risk of fatal complications was 8–15%, compared to 0% after 1981 when few patients received >52 Gy via EBRT. Thus, any effort to add additional dose to the pelvis, whether targeted with SBRT or IMRT, would need to be carefully considered.

18.3.4 Periaortic and Pelvic Node Boosts

18.3.4.1 Primary Setting

In addition to parametrial disease, the second area that is difficult to boost to a high dose consists of macroscopically positive pelvic and periaortic lymph nodes. Although not a part of International Federation of Gynecology and Obstetrics (FIGO) staging for cervical cancer, node positivity signifies a worse prognosis across each clinical stage [22]. Periaortic node metastases portend a particularly poor prognosis with one study finding a hazard ratio of 5.88 for disease recurrence compared to those without PA nodes metastases [22].

There are several reports suggesting a deficiency of dose to positive periaortic nodes attenuates survival (see Table 18.1). In the Gynecologic Oncology Group (GOG) 125 study of cervical cancer patients with biopsy confirmed periaortic node metastases treated with 45 Gy and concurrent 5-FU/cisplatin chemotherapy, Varia et al. observed 50% 3-year overall survival in patients with normal size nodes on CT, but 27% 3-year survival for enlarged nodes on CT imaging. In Radiation Therapy Oncology Group (RTOG) 01-16, 26 patients with positive PA nodes, confirmed by surgery or by imaging, were administered 45 Gy with 3D conformal boosts to 54–59.6 Gy. Despite the boost dose above 45 Gy, periaortic node persistence or recurrence was thought to be the pri-

Table 18.1 Extended-field radiation to positive periaortic nodes from cervical carcinoma primary tumors

First author	Assessment of PANs	*N*	Final dose to PAN	RT prescription and technique	LRF (5 years)	OS (5 years)	Grade 3–5 toxicity
Kim et al. [23]	PET-CT, MRI, or L	33	59.4 Gy	45 Gy to T12-L1 superior border. Boost to 59.4 Gy.	30%[a]	47%	SBO requiring surgery(2 pts), rectovaginal fistula (2 pts), ureteral stricture(3 pts).
Grigsby et al. [24] RTOG 92-10	B	30	54–58	48 Gy to T12-L1 superior border. Boost to 54–58 Gy.	50% (2y)	29% (4 y)	50% overall grade 4 toxicity. 34% grade 3–4 GI late toxicity.
Eifel et al. [25] RTOG 90-01	B or L	195	45	45 Gy to L1-L2 superior border. No boosts.	34%	52%	14% late grade 3–5 GI, GU toxicity. 3 treatment related deaths.
Small et al. [26] RTOG 01-16	B, CT, or MRI	26	54–59.6	45 Gy to T11-12 superior border. Boost to 54–59.6 Gy.	46%[b]	60% (1.5y)	40% late grade 3,4 toxicity, primarily bowel toxicity. 8 pts underwent surgery.
Varia et al. [27] GOG 125	B	86	45	45 Gy to L1–2 superior border. No boosts.	27%	39% (3 y)	14% late GI toxicity, primarily involving rectum. No SBO.
Kidd et al. [28]	PET-CT	23	50.4	50.4 Gy via IMRT to superior level of the renal vessels.	–	–	6% in all 135 patients in the series.

PAN periaortic nodes or periaortic node region, *RT* radiotherapy, *LRF* locoregional failure, *OS* overall survival, *3D CRT* three dimensional conformal radiotherapy, *SBO* small bowel obstruction, *B* biopsy, *L* lymphangiogram, *CT* computed tomography, *PET* positron emission tomography, *MRI* magnetic resonance imaging

[a]Obtained from Table 5 in the paper

[b]Eleven of 26 patients had persistent or recurrent regional lymph nodes

mary pattern of failure [26]. Eleven of 16 treatment failures at 4 months involved either isolated nodes (ten patients) or local and regional failures (one patient). In a retrospective review of 198 patients with regional failures after definitive radiation for cervix cancer, 58% experienced in-field nodal failures. Of all the 1,894 patients treated from 1980 to 2000, 452 experienced locoregional failure (LRF) and 43% of the LRF were regional only and 72% contained some element of regional failure [29].

The dose-limiting structures for boosting positive lymph nodes are bowel, kidneys, and spinal cord. For patients with positive periaortic or high pelvic lymph nodes, the periaortic lymph node chain is conventionally irradiated to 45 Gy with AP and PA fields with or without two lateral fields. This technique results in at least 14% late grade 3–5 toxicity [25, 27] and efforts to boost the PA nodes to a higher dose (54–59.6 Gy) with 3D conformal radiotherapy were met with 40–50% grade 3–5 toxicity (see Table 18.2) [24, 26]. In RTOG 01-16, 40% late GI toxicity was observed, with eight patients requiring subsequent surgery [26].

SBRT constitutes another means of boosting grossly enlarged nodes in the primary setting while minimizing additional dose to small bowel and adjacent normal organs. The available literature regarding SBRT, however, describes its use only in the recurrent PA node setting [34–36]. A reasonable extrapolation from this data can be made in terms of local control and toxicity (see Sect. 18.3.4.2) because these patients did not receive prior periaortic chain irradiation as a part of their primary treatment.

We have treated one patient in the primary setting who had stage IB2 poorly differentiated squamous-cell carcinoma with three closely approximated positive left pelvic nodes on PET-CT imaging. The patient received EBRT consisting of 45 Gy to the pelvis with a sidewall boost to 54 Gy with concurrent cisplatin weekly chemotherapy. She underwent HDR IC-BT, 30 Gy to point A in five applications, and then SBRT was used to boost the positive pelvic nodes. Tracking fiducials were placed and then the gross nodal disease was irradiated to 12 Gy in three fractions on nonconsecutive days, prescribed to the 79% isodose line, using the CyberKnife SBRT system (see Fig. 18.2). With

Table 18.2 Salvage radiotherapy for isolated periaortic node recurrences from cervical carcinoma primaries

First author	Assessment of PAN	N	Final dose to PAN	RT prescription and technique	Concurrent chemotherapy	LRF (5 years)	OS (5 years)	Grade 3–5 toxicity
EBRT								
Chou et al. [30]	CT or B	14	45 Gy	4 field box EBRT.	Weekly cisplatin	–	51%	–
Singh et al. [31]	CT	7	45–50.4 Gy	Conventional EBRT.	Navelbine, irinotecan, or cisplatin	–	100%	Grade 3 enteritis (1 pt)
Kim et al. [32]	CT or MRI	12	60 Gy	Conventional AP/PA EBRT. 1.2 Gy BID.	Paclitaxel or cisplatin	67%	19% (3y)	Grade 3–4 hematologic toxicity (2pts)
Grigsby et al. [33]	CT	20	46.4 Gy[a]	Conventional EBRT.	None	–	0	–
SBRT								
Choi et al. [34]	CT or PET-CT	28	33–45 Gy/3 fractions	SBRT alone (25pts). 27–45 Gy of EBRT and SBRT (3pts).	Mixed usage of cisplatin based chemotherapy[b]	33%	50%	Grade 3+ hematologic toxicity (5 pts); ureteral stricture (1 pt)

PAN periaortic nodes, *CT* computed tomography, *B* biopsy, *MRI* magnetic resonance imaging, *PET* positron emission tomography, *AP/PA* anterior-posterior and posterior-anterior, *BID* twice a day, *RT* radiotherapy, *LRF* locoregional failure, *OS* overall survival
[a]Median dose
[b]Two patients received chemotherapy before SBRT, 9 patients received concurrent SBRT, and 14 received chemotherapy after SBRT

2-year follow-up, the patient had no evidence of disease and no toxicity.

18.3.4.2 Recurrent Setting

Isolated periaortic node recurrence is a well-characterized outcome affecting 1.7–12% of patients following definitive radiation or surgery for cervical carcinoma initially localized to the pelvis [30, 31, 37]. The success of salvage radiotherapy is traditionally thought to be very low, with Grigsby and colleagues reporting no survivors and 50% LRF in 20 patients [33]. Three series reporting the use of periaortic node irradiation and concurrent chemotherapy found improved long-term survival (see Table 18.2).

Choi and colleagues treated 30 patients with isolated periaortic node recurrences after prior definitive treatment for cervical (28 patients) and endometrial (2 patients) carcinoma [34]. Four of the 30 patients received 27–45 Gy of EBRT to the periaortic LN chain in addition to SBRT. One of the four patients received one fraction of 13 Gy after 45 Gy of EBRT and the three other patients received three fractions of 10–11 Gy after 27–45 Gy of EBRT. All four patients were alive without recorded grade 3 or 4 toxicity [34]. The remaining 26 patients received SBRT alone using the CyberKnife SBRT system. Gold fiducials were placed percutaneously, two each to three successive vertebrae near the target. The PTV was defined as GTV + 2 mm. Doses of 33–45 Gy in three fractions were prescribed to the 73–87% isodose lines. The overall local control at 4 years was 67% and overall survival was 50%. Larger PTVs corresponded to worse disease-free survival: 26% vs. 65% for PTVs more or less than 17 cc, respectively. Symptomatic patients, i.e., those with leg edema or lower back pain, exhibited less favorable 4-year overall survival (19% vs. 64%), a finding also seen in other series [30, 33]. Toxicity was limited to grade 3 hematologic toxicity in five patients who received concurrent or adjuvant chemotherapy and one patient who had a urethral stricture [34].

We have treated seven patients with CyberKnife stereotactic SBRT with isolated periaortic node recurrences (cervix, two patients; endometrial, three patients; ovarian, two patients). Four of the seven patients received 45 Gy of conventional EBRT in addition to SBRT. Doses have ranged between 30 Gy in five fractions to 20 Gy in four fractions, prescribed to the 58–80% isodose lines and delivered on nonconsecutive days. The volume of small bowel receiv-

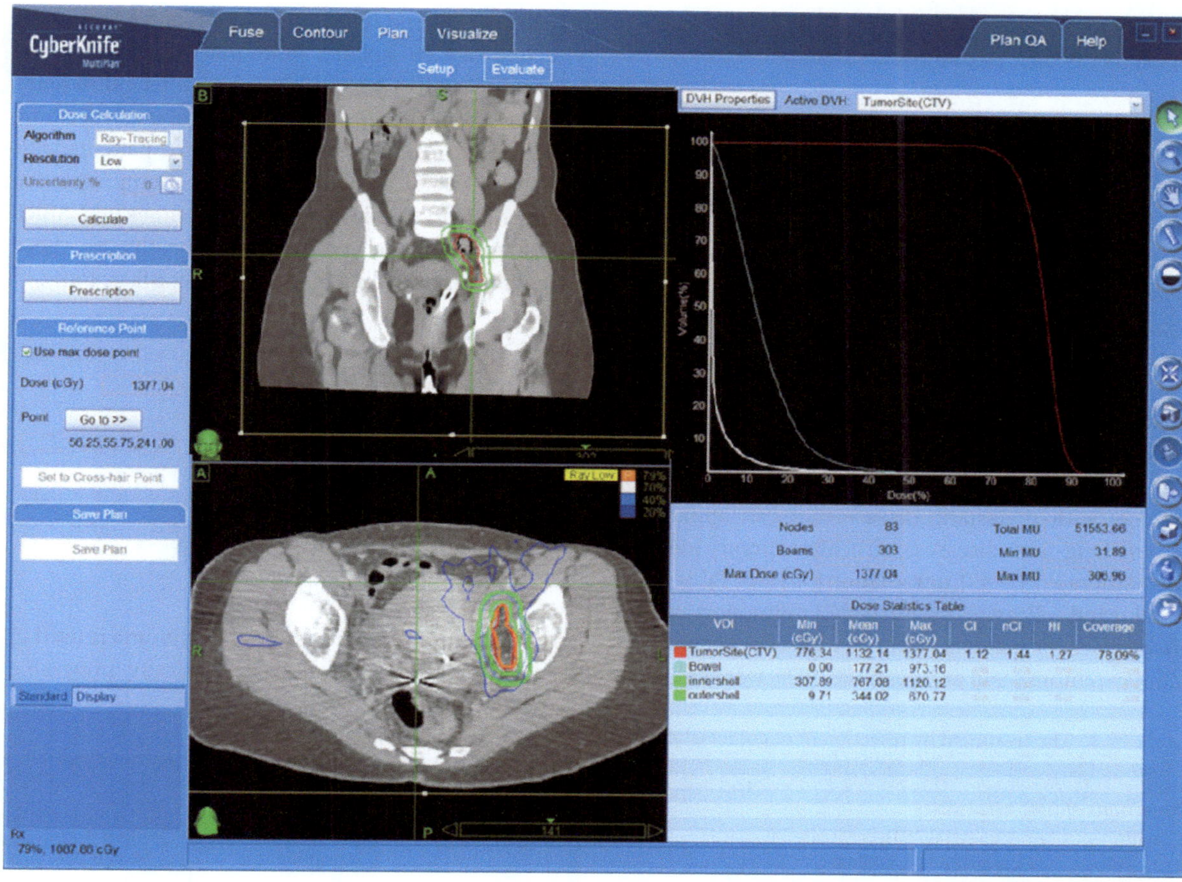

Fig. 18.2 CyberKnife SBRT treatment plan for a patient with IB2 squamous cell carcinoma of the cervix with three PET positive pelvic lymph nodes. Tracking fiducials were used and the gross nodal disease was irradiated to 1,200 12 Gy in 3 fractions, prescribed to the 79% isodose line

ing 25 Gy was evaluated and a limit of 3 cc to this dose was deemed acceptable. Three patients had no evidence of disease at 7, 14, and 30 months. One patient developed a local failure, one failed distantly, one had simultaneous local and distant failure, and one deceased with an unknown pattern of failure. No grade 3–5 toxicity was noted.

18.3.5 Central Recurrences

A central recurrence following definitive radiotherapy is a much more difficult clinical scenario than following definitive surgery. Repeat EBRT for pelvic recurrences is associated with a high incidence of acute and late toxicity [38, 39], typically the only other option available being pelvic exenteration, an intervention limited to a highly selected group of patients, with prior early-stage disease and long disease-free interval, who are young and have good performance status. One group has used SBRT in the recurrent setting (cervix: one patient, endometrial: one patient, and ovarian: three patients) for palliative purposes, using fiducial markers and the CyberKnife SBRT system [40]. Three patients had previous EBRT alone and two had prior EBRT and BT. Doses of 15–24 Gy in three fractions to the 70–80% isodose line were employed, and at a median of 9 months, four of five patients had controlled pelvic disease. One patient had no evidence of disease at 10 months. One patient developed a bowel obstruction requiring surgery due to progressive disease and one patient developed bladder failure.

18.3.6 Oligometastatic Disease

The treatment of oligometastatic disease, i.e., the use of SBRT to treat a limited number of metastatic sites, has some theoretical justification in cervical cancer. First, a small but significant percentage (10–16%) of cervical cancer patients with distant supraclavicular nodes can apparently still be cured with radiotherapy [22, 41]. Second, systemic chemotherapy is limited to a survival benefit of a few months [42, 43] and thus the local control potential of SBRT in patients with limited or isolated metastatic disease with or without addition of chemotherapy may provide longer disease-free survival and potential for cure. Third, there are a few reports of patients with metastatic disease that can apparently achieve long-term disease control after surgery [44–46], chemotherapy [47–49], or radiation [50] (see Table 18.3). Anraku and colleagues performed 71 pulmonary metastasectomies for patients with cervical squamous-cell or adenocarcinoma and at 5 years, 40–47% were still alive [51]. Yamamoto and colleagues found that for 23 patients with one or two isolated pulmonary metastases, the 5-year disease-free survival was 42% after pulmonary metastasectomy [45]. Consideration of metastasectomy is itemized as one of several options for patients with limited metastatic disease in the National Comprehensive Cancer Network Clinical Practice Guidelines [55]. SBRT can be an attractive noninvasive alternative for those not eligible or unwilling to undergo metastasectomy.

18.4 Endometrial Carcinoma

18.4.1 Background

Radiation therapy in endometrial carcinoma is used in the adjuvant setting or for use in medically inoperable

Table 18.3 The treatment by resection of oligometastatic disease in gynecologic malignancies

Author	Patients	N	F/U (years)	5y OS (%)	10y OS (%)	Toxicity	Comments
Resections of lung metastases							
Clavero et al. [44]	Endometrial (60), cervical (7), ovarian (2), vaginal (1)	70	3	47	34	1 death, 26% complication rate	Median DFS 8 months; 8 pts disease free
Yamamoto et al. [45]	Cervical	29	4.3	33	–	NS	42% 5y DFS in 23 pts with 1–2 mets.
Lim et al. [46]	Cervical	23	1.5	88[a]	–	No deaths, 26% complication rate	16 pts disease free at 18 m. median f/u
Anraku et al. [51]	All	133	3.3	55	45	1% morbidity, 1% mortality	25 pts alive with >8 years f/u
	Cervical SCC	58		47			
	Cervical AD	13		40			
	Endometrial	23		76			
	Choriocarcinoma	16		87			
	Leiomyosarcoma	11		38			
Logmans et al. [52]	Cervical (4), endometrial (1), ovarian (1)	6	3.7	100[b]	–	NS	5/6 patients have no evidence of disease with 3.1–4.5y f/u
Resections of liver metastases							
Lim et al. [53]	Ovarian	14	2	51	–	No deaths, 11 complications	23% 5y PFS
Chi et al. [54]	Cervical (2), endometrial (2), ovarian (7), fallopian tube (1)	12	2.1	50[c]	–	No deaths, 8% complications	3 patients NED at 8, 17, 38 months.

NS not stated, *DFS* disease free survival, *PFS* progression free survival, *NED* no evidence of disease, *SCC* squamous cell carcinoma, *AD* adenocarcinoma, *Mets* metastases, *f/u* follow-up

[a] At 18 month median follow-up

[b] At 3.7 year median follow-up

[c] Estimated from Fig. 19.1 at 24 months

patients. For early, stage I endometrial carcinoma, vaginal cylinder BT is used only when clinical and pathologic factors predict for a clinically significant rate of recurrence [56–58]. SBRT is an attractive modality for use as a substitute for BT in the medically inoperable patient when anatomical limitations or procedural risks preclude tandem and ovoid IC-BT. Finally, SBRT may also be an effective way of boosting periaortic and pelvic lymph nodes, along with pelvic and vaginal cuff recurrences.

18.4.2 SBRT as a Substitute for Brachytherapy

18.4.2.1 Endometrial Boosts

For medically inoperable patients with disease confined to the uterus with a minor degree of myometrial invasion on MRI, we administer eight applications of tandem HDR BT: five with both tandem and ovoid applications and three with a tandem application only. A dose of 8–10 Gy with each application prescribed to 1 cm lateral to the tandem taking into account the uterine anatomy on imaging. For patients with advanced features, a course of pelvic EBRT to 45 Gy would then be followed with five applications of tandem and ovoid IC-BT.

There have been situations in our practice in which IC-BT has been anatomically difficult or when the depth of myometrial invasion led us to choose a radiosurgical boost to the endometrium. One such patient presented with grade 3 clear cell adenocarcinoma of the endometrium with clinical extension into the cervix. The patient received 48.8 Gy of EBRT to the pelvis and a subsequent SBRT boost to the gross disease of 20 Gy in five fractions, prescribed to the 59% isodose line and delivered on nonconsecutive days (see Fig. 18.3). She developed grade 3 rectal bleeding 8 months following treatment that was controlled with Argon laser photocoagulation. She died a month later at age 91 of unclear reasons.

18.4.2.2 Vaginal Cuff Recurrences

The typical paradigm to treat vaginal cuff recurrences after surgery is EBRT to the pelvis (45 Gy) followed by vaginal cylinder BT. The BT consists of 5 Gy prescribed to 5-mm depth into the vaginal mucosa when the lesion is superficial. For some patients, the depth of the recurrent disease away from the vaginal mucosa may be on the order of several centimeters and thus these tumors would not be adequately treated with vaginal cylinder BT.

Guckenberg treated seven patients of similar description with a combination of EBRT and SBRT boost. The boost consisted of 15 Gy in three fractions prescribed to the 65% isodose line and delivered every other day within 1 week. The PTV was a 5-mm expansion of CTV, which in turn was a 2- to 3-mm expansion of GTV [16]. At 22 months median follow-up, only one local endometrial recurrence was noted. Kunos et al. treated one patient with a 6-cm vaginal cuff recurrence, who had had a prior vaginal cylinder therapy. The group gave 45 Gy of pelvic EBRT followed by a CyberKnife SBRT boost, consisting of 15 Gy in three fractions prescribed to the 70% isodose line. The patient suffered grade 3 fatigue and failed distantly in the lungs and mediastinum, but 19 months following therapy she had no evidence of disease in the pelvis [40]. They also treated four other patients with analogous vaginal cuff recurrences from ovarian and cervix malignancies with up to 24 Gy in three fractions.

Our group has used SBRT for three such patients with vaginal cuff disease, albeit from vaginal, bladder, and cervical primaries (see Fig. 18.4). Our rationale for using SBRT instead of BT was (1) thickness of the lesions and (2) proximity of adjacent small bowel. Each of our patients underwent a course of pelvic radiation (reirradiation in the case of a patient with vaginal carcinoma) followed by 20 or 25 Gy in five fractions prescribed to the 55–77% isodose lines delivered by CyberKnife SBRT on nonconsecutive days. One patient has no evidence of disease at 10 months. One patient recurred locally and was deceased at 7 months. A third patient achieved local control but failed distantly and was alive at 15 months.

18.4.2.3 Adjuvant Vaginal Cuff Irradiation

Vaginal cuff BT results in excellent control following surgery, is relatively easy to perform, exhibits few side effects, and can be performed in most patients. Nevertheless, two clinical papers indicate that either

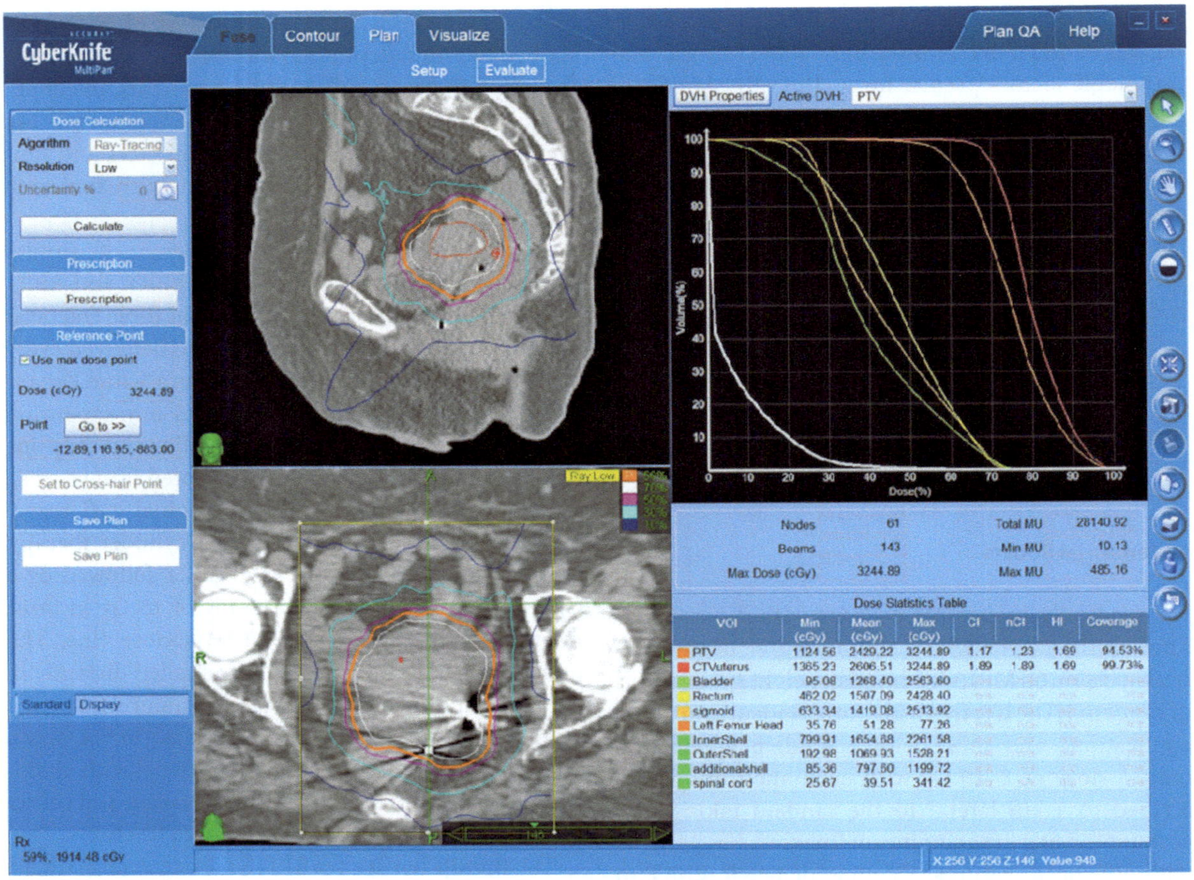

Fig. 18.3 CyberKnife SBRT treatment plan for a patient medically inoperable due to old age, obesity and heart disease. She was diagnosed with grade 3 clear cell adenocarcinoma of the endometrium with clinical extension into the cervix and deep penetration into the myometrium on imaging. She received 48.8 Gy of EBRT to the pelvis and a subsequent boost to the gross disease of 20 Gy in 5 fractions, prescribed to the 59% isodose line. She developed grade 3 rectal bleeding 8 months following treatment and was managed with argon laser coagulation

IMRT or SBRT may substitute for vaginal cuff BT in the adjuvant setting. This effort is motivated by dosimetric analyses suggesting IMRT is capable of decreased rectal dose, comparable coverage, and reduced inhomogeneity compared to HDR BT [13]. In addition, the Molla group has suggested that IMRT can improve CTV coverage near the apex of the vagina [15]. In our view, vaginal cylinder BT should still be considered the standard of care, because the treatment is well tolerated and the Post-Operative Radiation Therapy in Endometrial Carcinoma (PORTEC) randomized study showed a less than 3% vaginal recurrence rate, suggesting the dose inhomogeneity generated by BT may not be harmful.

Molla et al. treated nine patients with endometrial carcinoma following surgery. Each received 45–50.4 Gy of pelvic EBRT followed by a stereotactic radiotherapy boost of 14 Gy in two fractions delivered to the vaginal cuff with 4–7 days between fractions. No recurrences were seen, but one patient developed grade 3 rectal bleeding [15]. Macchia and colleagues enrolled 12 patients with IB or IC endometrial carcinoma into a prospective trial [59]. Following surgery, each patient received five fractions of IMRT in 1 week to the upper two-thirds of the vagina. A radio-opaque applicator was inserted into the vagina and a 5-mm PTV margin was employed. Six patients received 25 Gy in five fractions and six patients received 30 Gy in five fractions. No recurrences were observed in a 15-month follow-up period. No grade 3 toxicity was observed.

The interpretation of these two series must take into consideration that early endometrial cases recur,

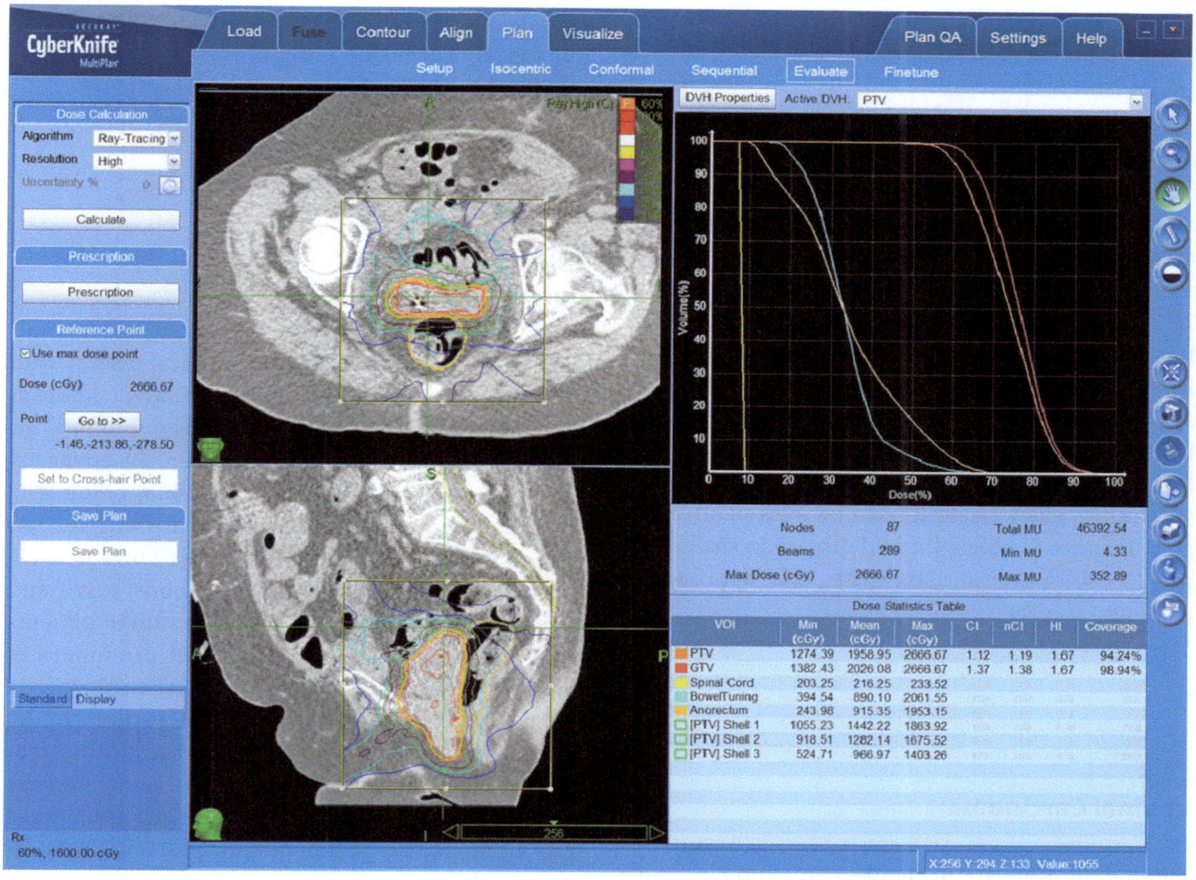

Fig. 18.4 CyberKnife SBRT treatment plan for a 77-year-old patient who underwent cystectomy for T2N0 muscle-invasive bladder cancer, but 10 months following surgery, a 3 cm mass was found within the anterior portion of the remaining vaginal cuff. Further surgery was not deemed appropriate and therefore she received 45 Gy in 1.8 Gy fractions to the pelvis followed by CyberKnife SBRT, 16 Gy in 4 fractions prescribed to the 60% isodose line. There is no evidence of disease at 10 months follow-up

at most, 26% of the time without radiation and 6% after whole pelvic radiation [57]. Therefore a very low recurrence rate is the expected outcome.

18.4.3 Periaortic and Pelvic Lymph Node Boosts

In our practice, patients with node-positive endometrial carcinoma receive three cycles of chemotherapy followed by adjuvant radiation to the pelvis and possibly periaortic lymph node chain. The course of radiation is followed again by three cycles of chemotherapy. There have been situations in which we have boosted periaortic nodes in the recurrent setting, sometimes detected after periaortic lymph node dissections and the initial course of chemotherapy. If the periaortic nodal chain has not been previously irradiated, we will deliver 45 Gy to the periaortic nodes followed by a course of SBRT. We have treated one patient with 30 Gy in five fractions, one patient with 25 Gy in five fractions, and one patient with 20 Gy in four fractions. Two of three patients were alive with no evidence of disease and no late toxicity.

Likewise, Choi and colleagues treated two patients with recurrent endometrial carcinoma in PA nodes, one of whom had prior EBRT to 36 Gy. The patients received 39 and 33 Gy in three fractions, respectively. Both had a partial response and were alive at 26- and 15-month follow-up with no grade 3 or 4 toxicity.

18.4.4 Oligometastatic Disease

The use of metastasectomy of limited sites of disease in endometrial carcinoma can result in surprising 5- and 10-year survival (see Table 18.3). Anraku and colleagues resected 133 uterine pulmonary metastases (23 were endometrial) with 1% mortality and morbidity with the 5-year survival reaching 75.7% [51]. Clavero et al. also resected 60 endometrial pulmonary metastases with 1.4% mortality and 25.7% perioperative complications. Five- and 10-year survival was 46.8% and 34.2%, respectively [44], indicating that a plurality of patients could achieve long-term control with resection of limited metastatic sites. Likewise, SBRT can be used in an analogous manner to ablate limited disease in the lung or liver, but long-term data with this approach is lacking.

18.5 Vaginal Carcinoma

The standard of care in vaginal carcinoma is similar to cervix cancer in that an initial course of EBRT to the pelvis with concurrent chemotherapy is followed by a BT boost. The choice of BT technique depends upon the depth of invasion into the vaginal mucosa and the traditional teaching is that lesions greater than 5-mm depth at the end of EBRT are not suitable for vaginal cylinder BT and require IS-BT. There are two areas in which even IS-BT is difficult. First, the posterior vaginal wall may not be suitable for an interstitial implant due to the limited thickness of the rectovaginal septum and the high risk for rectovaginal fistula. Second, the vaginal cuff region carries a risk of injury to the bladder or the bowel that may be adherent to the cuff.

We treated one patient with a periurethral vaginal adenocarcinoma with SBRT following 45 Gy to the pelvis delivered traditionally through EBRT, using 25 Gy in five fractions. Eighteen months following radiotherapy, she had no evidence of disease in the pelvis but developed a lung metastasis. Treatment was complicated by grade 2 radiation cystitis and she already had a vesicovaginal fistula due to tumor invasion into the bladder before treatment began.

18.6 Vulvar Carcinoma

Vulvar carcinoma is primarily a surgical disease with radiotherapy reserved for postoperative adjuvant therapy based on surgical pathology findings for recurrent disease and for locoregionally advanced tumors. Vulvar carcinoma is a malignancy of the skin, which raises concern about late toxicity with the use of high doses per fraction. The use of SBRT is likely limited to the recurrent setting or to boost pelvic and periaortic nodes. Kunos et al. treated three patients with recurrent vulvar squamous-cell carcinoma in the labia who had received prior EBRT to the pelvis and genitalia. Each received 8 Gy × 3 fractions to the 70–80% isodose line with the CyberKnife SBRT system. All three patients recurred locoregionally near or just outside of the treated area. The treatments were accompanied by skin desquamation in the treatment field, focal necrosis where tumor resolved, and pain [60].

18.7 Ovarian Carcinoma

18.7.1 Oligometastatic Disease

The modus operandi in ovarian cancer is maximally debulking surgery followed by adjuvant chemotherapy. The use of an extensive local treatment, i.e., surgery, in the setting of intra-abdominal metastatic disease in some ways supports the use of SBRT for limited sites of disease in some cases (see Table 18.3). In our experience, we use SBRT for situations in which a patient has had prior surgery and after adjuvant chemotherapy is left with limited periaortic nodes, isolated lung metastases, or a lesion at the vaginal cuff. We have used similar techniques and dose prescriptions as described in other sections.

18.8 Technical Considerations

18.8.1 Setup Error and Intra- and Interfractional Organ Movement

In gynecologic malignancies, internal target motion is likely the dominant source of error with manual setups (see Table 18.4) [66, 69]. Kaatee and colleagues found that standard deviations of typical setup errors measure only 1–3 mm, compared to 3–5 mm for movement of internally placed radiopaque markers on the cervix [66].

With robotic SBRT, setup errors are reduced significantly through the use of internal fiducial markers that are recognized on continuous orthogonal kV imaging that localizes an image center to submillimeter accuracy. The linear accelerator is mounted on a robotic arm, allowing rapid adjustments in the radiation beam to track and match the image center as it moves during treatment. Yamamoto and colleagues found that the use of fiducial markers and orthogonal imaging reduces the standard deviations of systematic setup error from 3.8–4.9 to 2.3–2.7 mm [70]. With real-time tracking, a small degree of systematic setup error is still possible, because the fiducial markers can move internally relative to each other or even fall out as tumor regresses. Yamamoto found that, of the 12 patients enrolled, two had dropped a marker before treatment had begun and the median change in distances between markers was 0.8 mm (range 0–2.8 mm) [70].

Both the cervix and the uterus are subject to large interfractional shifts secondary to tumor regression and bladder and rectum filling, potentially on the order of centimeters of movement over the initial course of the EBRT (see Table 18.4). Multiple studies have suggested that tumor volume regresses by a median of 46–62% after an initial course of pelvic EBRT [61, 67, 71]. Huh et al. found that the uterus shifts more than 30° in 18% of patients and that the cervical canal shortens by a median of 1.4 cm. Of the 44 patients with an anteroflexed uterus, five converted into a retroflexed uterus after treatment. Consistently, these studies indicate that the clinical target volume can change in unpredictable ways between fractions.

Intrafractional motion may be significantly less important than interfractional movement. Using cinematic MRI and a protocol that obtains images of 1-min duration at 4-min intervals, Chan and colleagues found that points of interest at the cervical os, canal, and uterine fundus move only 1–3 mm over 30 min [63]. Yamamoto also found intrafractional movement of fiducial markers to be within 1–4 mm over 10 min. Put together, these imaging studies suggest that fiducial markers can reduce setup error and are needed in SBRT to account for sizable interfractional changes, whereas real-time tracking needs only to adapt to a few millimeters of intrafractional movement.

18.8.2 Patient Setup and Treatment Planning

Fiducial markers are inserted through the vagina into cervix, paracervical tissues, vaginal cuff, or visible tumor if possible. For pelvic or periaortic nodes, markers are placed within an enlarged node or in nearby tissues with CT guidance by an interventional radiologist. When this is technically impossible, we have used the Xsight® Spine Tacking System (Accuray) if the node of interest is within 6 cm of a vertebral body. We wait 7–10 days after fiducial placement before CT simulation to allow the fiducials to settle into a consistent position.

For central pelvic lesions, we perform the CT simulation while the patient is immobilized with a vacuum mattress with the patient's arms at their sides (Vac-Lok cushion, Civco Medical Solutions, Orange City, IA, USA). We place a foley catheter, drain the bladder, and perform an initial CT simulation without bladder or bowel contrast. In our experience, placement of immobilization devices into the vagina displaces the fiducials in unpredictable directions, making image guidance and tracking difficult and thus we do not use them. The CT needs to obtain adequate imaging of the target with wide margins in the superior and inferior directions to visualize and plan for nonaxial radiation beams. We use a maxi-

Table 18.4 Inter- and intrafractional internal target/organ movement. A variety of statistical approaches are employed in each paper. Some papers analyze movement of the 'center of mass' of the target; others analyze movement of each of the six borders individually

Author	Method	*N*		Displacements S-I (mm) Mean	S-I (mm) Range	A-P (mm) Mean	A-P (mm) Range	R-L (mm) Mean	R-L (mm) Range
Intrafractional displacements									
Beadle et al. [61]	Bladder full/empty CTs	16	Cervix	5	(0.1–9)[a]	5	(0.1–11)	2	(0.3–6)
Buchali et al. [62]	Bladder, rectum full/empty CTs	29	Cervix	4	(1–6)[b]	N.S.	–	N.S.	–
Chan et al. [63]	Intrascan cine-MRI	20	Cervix	−0.5	(−4 to 4)[c]	−0.1	(−4 to 4)	–	–
Collen et al. [64]	Daily post-treament MVCT	10	Cervix	2	(+/−8) S.[d]	0.4	(+/−10) A.	0.2	(+/−5) R.
				0.5	(+/−5) I.	3	(+/−12) P.	4	(+/−5) L.
Buchali et al. [62]	Bladder, rectum full/empty CTs	14	Uterus	7	(3–15)[b]	4	(1–9)	N.S.	–
Chan et al. [63]	Intrascan cine-MRI	20	Uterine fundus	−3	(−9 to 7)[c]	1	(−6 to 4)	–	–
Chan et al. [63]	Intrascan cine-MRI	20	Uterine canal	−2	(−5 to 4)[c]	0.3	(−5 to 4)	–	–
Collen et al. [64]	Daily post-treatment MVCT	10	Uterus	6	(+/−12) S.[d]	3	(+/−12) A.	0.6	(+/−8) R.
				5	(+/−11) I.	0.3	(+/−12) P.	0.7	(+/−8) L.
Interfractional displacements									
Beadle et al. [61]	Weekly CTs	16	Cervix	21	(12–33)[a]	16	(5–25)	8	(4–14)
Huh et al. [65]	MRI before and after RT	66	Cervix	9	(+/−8)[d]	–	–	–	–
Kaatee et al. [66]	Radio-opaque markers, daily fluoroscopy	10	Cervix	3[e]	(+/−5)	2	(+/−5)	1	(+/−3)
Lee et al. [67]	Radio-opaque marker	17	Cervix	8	(36)[f]	16	(23)	10	(24)
Lee et al. [68]	Weekly CTs	13	Uterus	8	(+/−2) S.[g]	2	(+/−11) A.	3	(+/−10) R.
						6	(+/−12) P.	3	(+/−13) L.
Huh et al. [65]	MRI before and after RT	66	Uterus	6	(+/−9)[d]	2	(+/−7)	–	–

S-I superior-inferior dimension, *A-P* anterior-posterior dimension, *R-L* right-left dimension, *CT* computed tomography, *Cine-MRI* cinetographic magnetic resonance imaging, *MVCT* megavoltage CT, *S* superior, *I* inferior, *A* anterior, *P* posterior, *R* right, *L* left, *N.S.* not stated

[a]Mean (range). Center of mass technique

[b]Median (range). Center of mass technique

[c]Mean (90th percentile prediction interval). Single points analyzed and intervals reflect movement in a 3D coordinate system

[d]Mean (± SD)

[e]Mean (±SD)

[f]Median (maximum displacement)

[g]Mean (±SD). Each border analyzed separately

mum of 3-mm CT slice thickness. Caution is exercised to ensure that the full circumference of obese women is captured on the CT images. A second scan is often performed with IV, bladder, or bowel contrast for more accurate target delineation. If a pelvic MRI is obtained to better visualize primary tumors, we leave the foley catheter in place after the CT simulation and direct our radiology center to obtain the images in the treatment position. The additional scans are registered to the noncontrast CT for treatment planning.

Once the desired dose and fractionation have been selected, our goal is to create a plan that delivers 100% coverage to the GTV and at least 95% coverage to the PTV with prescriptions to the 50–80% isodose lines and conformality indices less than 1.5. We verify that plans do not contain excessive islands of dose in the skin or soft tissues (point dose <6–10 Gy per fraction). We limit the maximum point dose to the spinal cord, small bowel, rectum, colon, and stomach to less than 30 Gy total in three to five fractions and less than 10 Gy in a single fraction [72]. We allow only 3 cc or less of small bowel to receive >25 Gy. The dose to kidney is limited to 1/3 the volume receiving greater than 15 Gy and we minimize the volume receiving >20 Gy [73]. For patients who have also received EBRT, we mimic the BT dose constraints in the International Commission of Radiation Units Report 38 [74] or the recommendations of the working group for gynecologic brachytherapy of the Group European de Curitherapie/European Society for Therapeutic Radiology and Oncology (GYN GEC ESTRO) [75]. According to the GYN GEC ESTRO data, the minimum dose to the most exposed 2 cc of the bladder can be no more than 100 Gy via EBRT and BT combined ($D_{2cc} < 100$ Gy) and the minimum dose to the most exposed 2 cc of the rectum can be no more than 75 Gy ($D_{2cc} < 75$ Gy) [75].

During a CK treatment, which can take over 1 h to perform, the foley catheter is left to drain continuously. This improves patient comfort during the entire treatment and yields greater reproducibility of the internal organ positions. We frequently prescribe a low-dose anxiolytic 20 min prior to treatment. Using the analogy of our experiences with HDR BT, we do not deliver treatments on consecutive days.

18.9 Conclusions

SBRT is a promising, noninvasive, emerging technology for use in gynecologic malignancies. With short term follow-up, it appears that SBRT techniques can provide a new option for local tumor control in selected patients with recurrent cervical and endometrial carcinoma in the periaortic nodal chain and can provide curative therapy with additional radiation in those who do not have other metastatic disease. SBRT is a sophisticated tool to complement conventional EBRT with its ability to deliver highly conformal dose, minimize the risk of late toxicity, and potentially dose-escalate. SBRT may also be useful as a supplement to BT or a substitute for BT for patients with large tumors or difficult anatomy. Like IMRT, SBRT should be considered a second-line option rather than a replacement of BT. As more experience is gained with this technique, more mature results will provide information on treatment outcomes with its use. SBRT techniques are providing treatment options for situations that could not be readily addressed by conventional techniques.

References

1. Gunderson LJ, Tepper JE (2007) Clinical radiation oncology. Elsevier, Philadelphia, pp 1323–1357
2. Emami B, Lyman J, Brown A et al (1991) Tolerance of normal tissue to therapeutic irradiation. Int J Radiat Oncol Biol Phys 21:109–122
3. Gunderson LJ, Tepper JE (2007) Clinical radiation oncology. Churchhill Livingstone, an imprint of Elsevier Inc, Philadelphia, pp 255–282
4. Chao KS, Williamson JF, Grigsby PW et al (1998) Uterosacral space involvement in locally advanced carcinoma of the uterine cervix. Int J Radiat Oncol Biol Phys 40:397–403
5. Hughes-Davies L, Silver B, Kapp DS (1995) Parametrial interstitial brachytherapy for advanced or recurrent pelvic malignancy: the Harvard/Stanford experience. Gynecol Oncol 58:24–27
6. Monk BJ, Tewari K, Burger RA et al (1997) A comparison of intracavitary versus interstitial irradiation in the treatment of cervical cancer. Gynecol Oncol 67:241–247
7. Gaddis O Jr, Morrow CP, Klement V et al (1983) Treatment of cervical carcinoma employing a template for transperineal interstitial Ir192 brachytherapy. Int J Radiat Oncol Biol Phys 9:819–827

8. Syed AM, Puthawala AA, Abdelaziz NN et al (2002) Long-term results of low-dose-rate interstitial-intracavitary brachytherapy in the treatment of carcinoma of the cervix. Int J Radiat Oncol Biol Phys 54:67–78
9. Erickson B, Eifel P, Moughan J et al (2005) Patterns of brachytherapy practice for patients with carcinoma of the cervix (1996–1999): a patterns of care study. Int J Radiat Oncol Biol Phys 63:1083–1092
10. Georg D, Kirisits C, Hillbrand M et al (2008) Image-guided radiotherapy for cervix cancer: high-tech external beam therapy versus high-tech brachytherapy. Int J Radiat Oncol Biol Phys 71:1272–1278
11. Assenholt MS, Petersen JB, Nielsen SK et al (2008) A dose planning study on applicator guided stereotactic IMRT boost in combination with 3D MRI based brachytherapy in locally advanced cervical cancer. Acta Oncol 47:1337–1343
12. Malhotra HK, Avadhani JS, de Boer SF et al (2007) Duplicating a tandem and ovoids distribution with intensity-modulated radiotherapy: a feasibility study. J Appl Clin Med Phys 8:2450
13. Aydogan B, Mundt AJ, Smith BD et al (2006) A dosimetric analysis of intensity-modulated radiation therapy (IMRT) as an alternative to adjuvant high-dose-rate (HDR) brachytherapy in early endometrial cancer patients. Int J Radiat Oncol Biol Phys 65:266–273
14. Barillot I, Horiot JC, Maingon P et al (2000) Impact on treatment outcome and late effects of customized treatment planning in cervix carcinomas: baseline results to compare new strategies. Int J Radiat Oncol Biol Phys 48:189–200
15. Molla M, Escude L, Nouet P et al (2005) Fractionated stereotactic radiotherapy boost for gynecologic tumors: an alternative to brachytherapy? Int J Radiat Oncol Biol Phys 62:118–124
16. Guckenberger M, Bachmann J, Wulf J et al (2010) Stereotactic body radiotherapy for local boost irradiation in unfavourable locally recurrent gynaecological cancer. Radiother Oncol 94:53–59
17. Deodato F, Macchia G, Grimaldi L et al (2009) Stereotactic radiotherapy in recurrent gynecological cancer: a case series. Oncol Rep 22:415–419
18. Ling CC, Roy J, Sahoo N et al (1994) Quantifying the effect of dose inhomogeneity in brachytherapy: application to permanent prostatic implant with 125I seeds. Int J Radiat Oncol Biol Phys 28:971–978
19. Fuller DB, Naitoh J, Lee C et al (2008) Virtual HDR CyberKnife treatment for localized prostatic carcinoma: dosimetry comparison with HDR brachytherapy and preliminary clinical observations. Int J Radiat Oncol Biol Phys 70:1588–1597
20. Macdonald DM, Lin LL, Biehl K et al (2008) Combined intensity-modulated radiation therapy and brachytherapy in the treatment of cervical cancer. Int J Radiat Oncol Biol Phys 71:618–624
21. Logsdon MD, Eifel PJ (1999) Figo IIIB squamous cell carcinoma of the cervix: an analysis of prognostic factors emphasizing the balance between external beam and intracavitary radiation therapy. Int J Radiat Oncol Biol Phys 43:763–775
22. Kidd EA, Siegel BA, Dehdashti F et al (2010) Lymph node staging by positron emission tomography in cervical cancer: relationship to prognosis. J Clin Oncol 28:2108–2113
23. Kim YS, Kim JH, Ahn SD et al (2009) High-dose extended-field irradiation and high-dose-rate brachytherapy with concurrent chemotherapy for cervical cancer with positive para-aortic lymph nodes. Int J Radiat Oncol Biol Phys 74:1522–1528
24. Grigsby PW, Heydon K, Mutch DG et al (2001) Long-term follow-up of RTOG 92-10: cervical cancer with positive para-aortic lymph nodes. Int J Radiat Oncol Biol Phys 51:982–987
25. Eifel PJ, Winter K, Morris M et al (2004) Pelvic irradiation with concurrent chemotherapy versus pelvic and para-aortic irradiation for high-risk cervical cancer: an update of radiation therapy oncology group trial (RTOG) 90-01. J Clin Oncol 22:872–880
26. Small W Jr, Winter K, Levenback C et al (2007) Extended-field irradiation and intracavitary brachytherapy combined with cisplatin chemotherapy for cervical cancer with positive para-aortic or high common iliac lymph nodes: results of ARM 1 of RTOG 0116. Int J Radiat Oncol Biol Phys 68:1081–1087
27. Varia MA, Bundy BN, Deppe G et al (1998) Cervical carcinoma metastatic to para-aortic nodes: extended field radiation therapy with concomitant 5-fluorouracil and cisplatin chemotherapy: a Gynecologic Oncology Group study. Int J Radiat Oncol Biol Phys 42:1015–1023
28. Kidd EA, Siegel BA, Dehdashti F et al (2010) Clinical outcomes of definitive intensity-modulated radiation therapy with fluorodeoxyglucose-positron emission tomography simulation in patients wtih locally advanced cervical cancer. Int J Radiat Oncol Biol Phys 77:1085–1091
29. Beadle BM, Jhingran A, Yom SS et al (2010) Patterns of regional recurrence after definitive radiotherapy for cervical cancer. Int J Radiat Oncol Biol Phys 76:1396–1403
30. Chou HH, Wang CC, Lai CH et al (2001) Isolated paraaortic lymph node recurrence after definitive irradiation for cervical carcinoma. Int J Radiat Oncol Biol Phys 51:442–448
31. Singh AK, Grigsby PW, Rader JS et al (2005) Cervix carcinoma, concurrent chemoradiotherapy, and salvage of isolated paraaortic lymph node recurrence. Int J Radiat Oncol Biol Phys 61:450–455
32. Kim JS, Kim SY, Kim KH et al (2003) Hyperfractionated radiotherapy with concurrent chemotherapy for para-aortic lymph node recurrence in carcinoma of the cervix. Int J Radiat Oncol Biol Phys 55:1247–1253
33. Grigsby PW, Vest ML, Perez CA (1994) Recurrent carcinoma of the cervix exclusively in the paraaortic nodes following radiation therapy. Int J Radiat Oncol Biol Phys 28:451–455
34. Choi CW, Cho CK, Yoo SY et al (2009) Image-guided stereotactic body radiation therapy in patients with isolated para-aortic lymph node metastases from uterine cervical and corpus cancer. Int J Radiat Oncol Biol Phys 74:147–153
35. Kim MS, Yoo SY, Cho CK et al (2009) Stereotactic body radiotherapy for isolated para-aortic lymph node recurrence after curative resection in gastric cancer. J Korean Med Sci 24:488–492
36. Kim MS, Yoo SY, Cho CK et al (2009) Stereotactic body radiation therapy using three fractions for isolated lung recurrence from colorectal cancer. Oncology 76:212–219
37. Carl UM, Bahnsen J, Rapp W (1992) Radiation therapy of para-aortic lymph nodes in gynaecologic cancers:

techniques, results and complications. Strahlenther Onkol 168:383–389
38. Randall ME, Evans L, Greven KM et al (1993) Interstitial reirradiation for recurrent gynecologic malignancies: results and analysis of prognostic factors. Gynecol Oncol 48:23–31
39. Russell AH, Koh WJ, Markette K et al (1987) Radical reirradiation for recurrent or second primary carcinoma of the female reproductive tract. Gynecol Oncol 27:226–232
40. Kunos C, Chen W, DeBernardo R et al (2009) Stereotactic body radiosurgery for pelvic relapse of gynecologic malignancies. Technol Cancer Res Treat 8:393–400
41. Qiu JT, Ho KC, Lai CH et al (2007) Supraclavicular lymph node metastases in cervical cancer. Eur J Gynaecol Oncol 28:33–38
42. Moore DH, Blessing JA, McQuellon RP et al (2004) Phase III study of cisplatin with or without paclitaxel in stage IVB, recurrent, or persistent squamous cell carcinoma of the cervix: a gynecologic oncology group study. J Clin Oncol 22:3113–3119
43. Long HJ 3rd, Bundy BN, Grendys EC Jr et al (2005) Randomized phase III trial of cisplatin with or without topotecan in carcinoma of the uterine cervix: a Gynecologic Oncology Group Study. J Clin Oncol 23:4626–4633
44. Clavero JM, Deschamps C, Cassivi SD et al (2006) Gynecologic cancers: factors affecting survival after pulmonary metastasectomy. Ann Thorac Surg 81:2004–2007
45. Yamamoto K, Yoshikawa H, Shiromizu K et al (2004) Pulmonary metastasectomy for uterine cervical cancer: a multivariate analysis. Ann Thorac Surg 77:1179–1182
46. Lim MC, Lee HS, Seo SS et al (2010) Pathologic diagnosis and resection of suspicious thoracic metastases in patients with cervical cancer through thoracotomy or video-assisted thoracic surgery. Gynecol Oncol 116:478–482
47. Khoury-Collado F, Bowes RJ, Jhamb N et al (2007) Unexpected long-term survival without evidence of disease after salvage chemotherapy for recurrent metastatic cervical cancer: a case series. Gynecol Oncol 105:823–825
48. Ota S, Sugiyama T, Ushijima K et al (2001) Remission of metastatic cervical adenocarcinoma with weekly paclitaxel. Int J Gynecol Cancer 11:167–168
49. Hindenburg AA, Matthews L (2003) Complete and sustained remission of refractory cervical cancer following a single cycle of capecitabine. A case report. Int J Gynecol Cancer 13(6):898-900
50. Vrdoljak E, Hamm W, Omrcen T et al (2004) Long-lasting complete remission of a patient with cervical cancer FIGO IVB treated by concomitant chemobrachyradiotherapy with ifosfamide and cisplatin and consolidation chemotherapy–a case report. Eur J Gynaecol Oncol 25:247–249
51. Anraku M, Yokoi K, Nakagawa K et al (2004) Pulmonary metastases from uterine malignancies: results of surgical resection in 133 patients. J Thorac Cardiovasc Surg 127:1107–1112
52. Logmans A, ten Kate M, van Lent M (2000) Metastasectomy, a feasible treatment in selected cases with gynecologic malignancy. Eur J Obstet Gynecol Reprod Biol 91:165–167
53. Lim MC, Kang S, Lee KS et al (2009) The clinical significance of hepatic parenchymal metastasis in patients with primary epithelial ovarian cancer. Gynecol Oncol 112:28–34
54. Chi DS, Fong Y, Venkatraman ES et al (1997) Hepatic resection for metastatic gynecologic carcinomas. Gynecol Oncol 66:45–51
55. National Comprehensive Cancer Network Clinical Practice Guidelines in Oncology (2010) Cervical Cancer. V.1.2010 ed
56. Creutzberg CL, van Putten WL, Koper PC et al (2000) Surgery and postoperative radiotherapy versus surgery alone for patients with stage-1 endometrial carcinoma: multicentre randomised trial. PORTEC Study Group. Post Operative Radiation Therapy in Endometrial Carcinoma. Lancet 355:1404–1411
57. Keys HM, Roberts JA, Brunetto VL et al (2004) A phase III trial of surgery with or without adjunctive external pelvic radiation therapy in intermediate risk endometrial adenocarcinoma: a Gynecologic Oncology Group study. Gynecol Oncol 92:744–751
58. Nout RA, Smit VT, Putter H et al (2010) Vaginal brachytherapy versus pelvic external beam radiotherapy for patients with endometrial cancer of high-intermediate risk (PORTEC-2): an open-label, non-inferiority, randomised trial. Lancet 375:816–823
59. Macchia G, Cilla S, Ferrandina G et al (2010) Postoperative intensity-modulated radiotherapy in low-risk endometrial cancers: final results of a Phase I study. Int J Radiat Oncol Biol Phys 76:1390–1395
60. Kunos C, von Gruenigen V, Waggoner S et al (2008) Cyberknife radiosurgery for squamous cell carcinoma of vulva after prior pelvic radiation therapy. Technol Cancer Res Treat 7:375–380
61. Beadle BM, Jhingran A, Salehpour M et al (2009) Cervix regression and motion during the course of external beam chemoradiation for cervical cancer. Int J Radiat Oncol Biol Phys 73:235–241
62. Buchali A, Koswig S, Dinges S et al (1999) Impact of the filling status of the bladder and rectum on their integral dose distribution and the movement of the uterus in the treatment planning of gynaecological cancer. Radiother Oncol 52:29–34
63. Chan P, Dinniwell R, Haider MA et al (2008) Inter- and intrafractional tumor and organ movement in patients with cervical cancer undergoing radiotherapy: a cinematic-MRI point-of-interest study. Int J Radiat Oncol Biol Phys 70:1507–1515
64. Collen C, Engels B, Duchateau M et al (2010) Volumetric imaging by megavoltage computed tomography for assessment of internal organ motion during radiotherapy for cervical cancer. Int J Radiat Oncol Biol Phys 77(5):1590–1595, Epub 2010 Apr 6
65. Huh SJ, Park W, Han Y (2004) Interfractional variation in position of the uterus during radical radiotherapy for cervical cancer. Radiother Oncol 71(1):73–79
66. Kaatee RS, Olofsen MJ, Verstraate MB et al (2002) Detection of organ movement in cervix cancer patients using a fluoroscopic electronic portal imaging device and radiopaque markers. Int J Radiat Oncol Biol Phys 54:576–583
67. Lee CM, Shrieve DC, Gaffney DK (2004) Rapid involution and mobility of carcinoma of the cervix. Int J Radiat Oncol Biol Phys 58:625–630
68. Lee JE, Han Y, Huh SJ et al (2007) Interfractional variation of uterine position during radical RT: weekly CT evaluation. Gynecol Oncol 104:145–151

69. Santanam L, Esthappan J, Mutic S et al (2008) Estimation of setup uncertainty using planar and MVCT imaging for gynecologic malignancies. Int J Radiat Oncol Biol Phys 71:1511–1517
70. Yamamoto R, Yonesaka A, Nishioka S et al (2004) High dose three-dimensional conformal boost (3DCB) using an orthogonal diagnostic X-ray set-up for patients with gynecological malignancy: a new application of real-time tumor-tracking system. Radiother Oncol 73:219–222
71. van de Bunt L, van der Heide UA, Ketelaars M et al (2006) Conventional, conformal, and intensity-modulated radiation therapy treatment planning of external beam radiotherapy for cervical cancer: the impact of tumor regression. Int J Radiat Oncol Biol Phys 64:189–196
72. Kavanagh BD, Pan CC, Dawson LA et al (2010) Radiation dose-volume effects in the stomach and small bowel. Int J Radiat Oncol Biol Phys 76:S101–S107
73. Milano MT, Constine LS, Okunieff P (2008) Normal tissue toxicity after small field hypofractionated stereotactic body radiation. Radiat Oncol 3:36
74. ICoRUa (1985) M. ICRU report 38: Dose and volume specification for reporting intracavitary therapy in gynecology. International Commission on Radiation Units and Measurements, Bethesda
75. Georg P, Lang S, Dimopoulos JC et al (2011) Dose-volume histogram parameters and late side effects in magnetic resonance image-guided adaptive cervical cancer brachytherapy. Int J Radiat Oncol Biol Phys 79(2):356–362, Epub 2010 Apr 10

Advances in Prostate Imaging: Implications for Prostate Cancer Diagnosis and Treatment

19

Russell N. Low

CONTENTS

19.1 Abstract

Prostate imaging can be accomplished with numerous techniques including computed tomography (CT), ultrasound, and magnetic resonance (MR) imaging. Each of these imaging tools relies on different physical properties of the tissue being evaluated to create an anatomic image. Ultimately, the goal of the numerous imaging strategies is to increase the conspicuity of the tumor, leading to improved diagnosis and staging. For the radiologist, the prostate gland presents challenges due to the simultaneous presence of normal tissue, and benign and malignant diseases that can produce very similar changes in the tissue characteristics on the CT scan, sonogram, and MR image. Distinguishing normal from diseased tissue or benign from malignant processes within the prostate gland is challenging when based solely upon anatomic images. Newer imaging techniques that focus on functional or metabolic imaging rather than simple anatomic changes may provide insight into prostate cancers by allowing us to investigate changes that occur in the prostate gland on a cellular level. A synthesis of high-resolution anatomic imaging with functional and metabolic imaging may provide new tools for understanding prostate cancer.

19.2 Introduction: Goals of Prostate Imaging

Imaging has gained importance in prostate cancer detection, staging, treatment planning and delivery, and follow-up. Initially, the information imaging provides may guide treatment selection and treatment planning. There are several goals when imaging the

L.E. Ponsky et al. (eds.), *Treating Prostate Cancer and Related Genitourinary Applications*, Robotic Radiosurgery,
DOI 10.1007/978-3-642-11495-3_19,

prostate gland. For primary prostate cancer, accurate depiction of the tumor location, volume, and extent is essential for pretreatment staging. This assessment includes determination of the presence or absence of transcapsular tumor extension or involvement of the neurovascular bundle and adjacent structures, findings that are critical for prostate cancer staging. Similarly, detecting nodal and osseous metastases or distant metastases affects tumor staging and prognosis. All of these factors may affect selection of treatment options.

For patients undergoing radiation therapy, imaging studies for treatment planning should determine the location, volume, and borders of the prostate gland and separate the gland from adjacent structures such as the seminal vesicles, rectum, urethra, and bladder. Imaging with high spatial resolution and accurate registration of the images with the treatment planning CT scan are essential elements for this pre-radiation therapy planning. It should be noted that various imaging modalities are also employed in the setup of patients prior to treatment and in the actual delivery of radiation therapy, including cone-beam CT, in-room CT imaging, the MV CT imaging capability of the helical tomotherapy device, and orthogonal kV X-ray imaging.

For the patient who has undergone radiation treatment for prostate cancer, imaging studies can be utilized in conjunction with serial serum prostate-specific antigen (PSA) values to assess the tumors response to therapy. In this evaluation of therapy response, newer functional and metabolic types of imaging may play an important role. For the patient with treated prostate cancer, imaging studies, including MRI and CT, are utilized to determine the presence of local residual or recurrent tumor, or distant metastases.

19.3 Transrectal Ultrasound

Transrectal ultrasound is the most widely used imaging study for prostate cancer and is the study of choice for image guidance of prostate biopsies. Systematic needle biopsy obtaining 18-gauge cutting needle biopsy cores from six or more areas or sextants, as well as from any suspicious areas, is performed with transrectal ultrasound guidance. The reported sensitivity from a single biopsy session is 70–80% for the detection of cancer [1].

Potential underdiagnosis of prostate cancer can be reduced by obtaining more cores to sample larger areas of the prostate gland. While most cancers appear as hypoechoic regions in the prostate gland, the sensitivity and specificity of this finding without biopsy is of limited value. Local staging of prostate cancer with transrectal ultrasound detecting extracapsular extension or seminal vesicle involvement has been described [2, 3], but is not its typical role.

19.4 Computed Tomography

CT measures the attenuation of X-rays by different tissues. CT has excellent spatial resolution and speed of data acquisition. However, its range of contrast within soft tissues is much more limited, which, at times, limits the ability of CT to distinguish normal tissues from tumors. For prostate imaging, CT shows poor definition of intraprostatic anatomy and limited separation of the prostate from adjacent structures, including the levator ani muscles. For this reason, CT plays essentially no role in prostate cancer detection or local staging. CT is usually reserved for advanced cases of prostate cancer with gross extraprostatic tumor extension and nodal or distant metastases [4, 5]. These are patients with PSA level greater than 20 ng/mL, Gleason score >7, or clinical tumor stage T3 or higher [6]. As more patients are currently diagnosed with earlier-stage disease, the incidence of metastases from prostate cancer at presentation has diminished as has the role of CT in their imaging evaluation [7]. For the patient undergoing radiation treatment, CT plays an additional important role in treatment planning. Treatment planning CT scans are used to determine the contours of the prostate gland and its relationship to adjacent vital structures.

19.5 Magnetic Resonance Imaging

19.5.1 The High-Field MR Scanner

High-field-strength MR imaging (MRI) systems consist of a superconducting magnet, a source for radiofrequency (RF) waves, and coils. An MR scan is essentially a map of the hydrogen protons in the organ being imaged. Hydrogen is the most abundant atom in the body and is capable of being magnetized when placed into a magnetic field. When an object is placed into the bore of the MR scanner, its hydrogen protons align with the magnetic field. Pulses of specific radiofrequency waves are then briefly applied to create an electromagnetic field that tilts the hydrogen protons off the axis of the magnetic field. When the RF pulse is turned off, the hydrogen protons relax and realign with the magnetic field of the scanner. During this process of relaxation, the hydrogen atoms emit a signal that is detectable by the coils which serve as antennas. The hydrogen atoms thus, alternately absorb and emit radio wave energy as they resonate between their resting magnetized state and the excited RF state. By detecting the strength and location of the emitted radio waves, the MR scanner reconstructs an anatomic image of the tissue being imaged.

Anatomic localization of the hydrogen atoms producing the radio wave signal is accomplished by applying additional magnetic field gradients during the scan. When these magnetic gradients are turned on, the magnetic field will vary depending on the position within the patient. A slice selection gradient is used to select the anatomic volume of interest to be scanned. Within that volume of tissue, the position of each point is encoded vertically and horizontally by applying phase gradients in one direction and frequency-encoding gradients in the opposite direction. This series of magnetic gradients allow the RF pulse to selectively excite specific slices of tissue and to determine the location within each slice that the signal originates.

Since the relaxation properties of hydrogen within normal and diseased tissues are different, MR images can more clearly delineate tumors from normal tissues. Compared to CT scanning, which relies solely upon differential attenuation of X-rays by tissues, MR imaging provides a much clearer depiction of soft tissue tumors as well as other diseases, including inflammation, infection, and ischemia.

19.5.2 General Clinical Principles of MRI

MRI is characterized by its excellent soft tissue contrast allowing one to depict many types of tumors and to accurately determine the location and spread of malignancy. The ability to distinguish normal tissue from tumors with high contrast and spatial resolution is a unique feature of MRI, that is to this point unmatched by other imaging techniques. MRI is used clinically to evaluate all forms of malignancy in the head, neck, spine, chest, abdomen, pelvis, and extremities. This widespread adoption of MRI for cancer imaging has occurred over a relatively short time period and reflects the flexibility and robustness of the technique.

MRI is also characterized by its ability to evaluate numerous features of a tumor by manipulating imaging parameters or by using exogenous contrast materials. When one performs an MR scan, imaging parameters that alter the appearance of the tissues being imaged are selected. The classic T1-weighted and T2-weighted MR images are created by altering imaging parameters to accentuate T1 or T2 relaxation of tissues. These images accentuate different features of a tumor and often alter the appearance of the tumor relative to the adjacent normal soft tissues. Newer contrast mechanisms utilized by MRI include diffusion-weighting, which looks at the microscopic motion of water protons in tissues. Tumors often show restriction of water mobility, making them distinct from normal tissues on diffusion-weighted imaging (DWI). Exogenous contrast materials such as gadolinium chelates can be administered intravenously to assess the differential enhancement of tumors and normal tissues. Dynamic contrast-enhanced (DCE) imaging of the prostate gland provides functional information reflecting angiogenesis of prostate cancers. Finally, the metabolic assessment provided by magnetic resonance spectroscopy (MRS) provides insight into prostate cancer metabolism on a cellular level.

19.5.3 Technical Advances in MR Imaging of the Prostate

Recent advances in MR imaging hardware and software have resulted in improvements in image quality, signal, resolution, and speed of data acquisition. Prostate MR imaging can be performed with many different scanners, coils, and pulse sequences. Results may be influenced by these technical differences in the manner in which prostate MR examinations are performed.

Hardware advances include higher-field-strength scanners, systems with larger, high-performance-gradient systems combined with more receiver channels, and endorectal receiving coils designed for prostate imaging. MR scanner field strength is measured in Tesla (T) and is a primary factor in determining the signal-to-noise ratio (SNR) of an MR system. The signal obtained from the MR scanner increases linearly with the magnetic field strength. Currently available commercial high-field MR scanners have field strengths of 1.5 and 3.0 T. MR scanners operating at 3.0 T have approximately double the SNR, which can be used to produce higher-resolution images or faster dynamic imaging during DCE of the prostate.

MR scanners with larger, high-performance gradient systems are now available that can produce higher-resolution images with improved image quality. Currently available commercial MR scanners have gradient amplitudes of 50 mT/m and slew rate (the rate of change of the gradient amplitude) of 200 T/m/s. Improvements in spatial and temporal resolution are a direct result of these high-performance gradient systems. DWI particularly benefits from these MR system hardware advances. These high-performance gradient systems are ideally suited for prostate MR imaging, which focuses on small FOV imaging with high spatial and temporal resolution.

Increasing numbers of receiver channels on new MR scanners, when combined with new phased-array surface coils with more coil elements, also improve image quality and SNR. New MR scanners with 32 independent channels are now available from all major manufacturers.

For prostate MR imaging, coil selection includes phased-array surface coils and endorectal coils. Endorectal coils are inserted into the patient's rectum, placing the receiving coil near the prostate gland and producing images with high SNR, although with a smaller imaging area. The endorectal coils are attached to a balloon that is inflated in the rectum to provide stability of the coil. The inflated balloon often deforms the contours of the adjacent prostate gland, which may affect fusion of the MR images with the treatment planning CT scan. Alternatively, surface phased-array coils are placed on the anterior pelvic wall and produce less SNR but are better tolerated by patients, do not deform the contours of the prostate gland, and provide a larger area of coverage.

Software advances for MR imaging include the development of 3D volumetric acquisitions, which acquire an entire volume of data at one time rather than in a slice-by-slice acquisition. Volumetric imaging can be more efficient, providing high-resolution imaging in a shorter scan time. For prostate imaging, 3D T2-weighted FSE images of the prostate gland can be utilized with excellent results. 3D T1-weighted imaging can also be performed before and after contrast administration for DCE MRI. DWI sequences have also been further optimized for more robust prostate imaging. Finally, sequences with more robust fat and water separation using Dixon-based techniques are now available to achieve more homogeneous fat suppression on pre- and postcontrast imaging of the prostate gland and pelvis.

19.5.4 Detection and Local Staging of Primary Prostate Cancer

The excellent soft tissue contrast of MR imaging makes it an ideal exam for evaluation of prostate cancer [8, 9]. The reported accuracy for anatomic MR imaging in staging prostate cancer varies widely from 54% to 96% [10–18].

Initial reports focused on the use of unenhanced T2-weighted images to depict prostate cancers as low-signal-intensity lesions within the normally

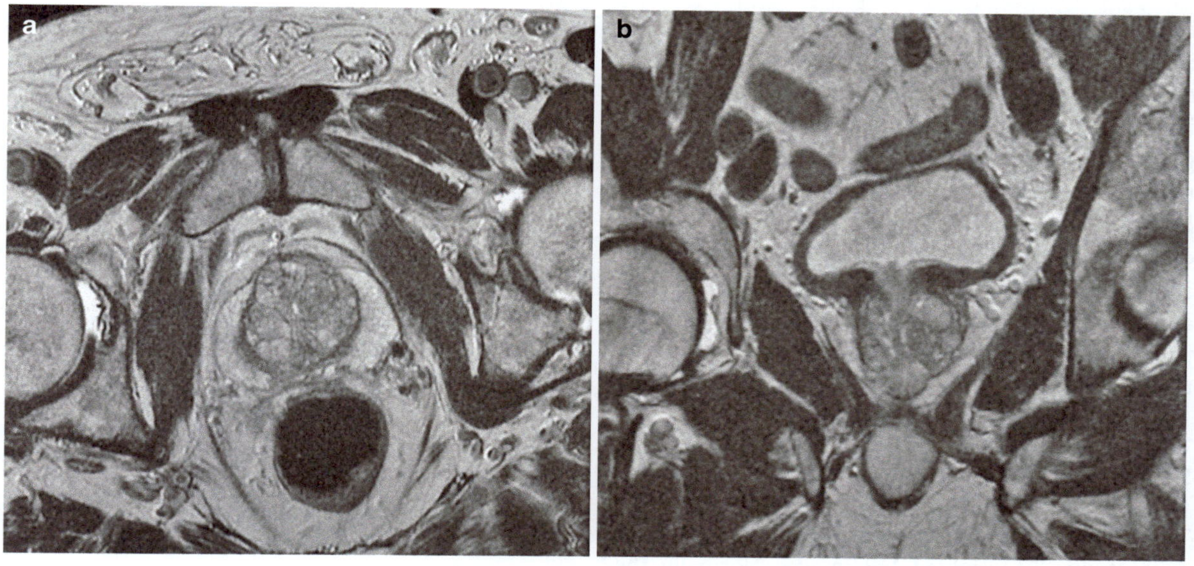

Fig. 19.1 T2-weighted images of the prostate gland in the axial (a) and coronal (b) planes demonstrate the zonal anatomy of the prostate gland. The normal peripheral zone is high signal intensity. Tumors in the peripheral zone are depicted as areas of low signal intensity. This patient shows characteristic changes of benign prostatic hypertrophy in the transitional zone

hyperintense peripheral zone [19] (Fig. 19.1). Detection of prostate cancer has been most effective for tumors located in the peripheral zone, which accounts for 75–85% of prostate cancers [20–24]. Nonperipheral-zone tumors, which may account for the remaining 15–25% of prostate cancers, are more challenging to detect on MR imaging, as they can look identical to the adenomatous nodules of benign prostatic hypertrophy. Features on anatomic MR images that favor the presence of a transitional and central zone prostate cancer include homogeneous low T2 signal intensity, ill-defined margins, lack of a capsule, lenticular shape, and invasion of the anterior fibromuscular stroma [25].

Reports about the sensitivity of T2-weighted MRI for detecting prostate cancer vary widely. A meta-analysis of 146 studies of prostate MRI at 1.5 T showed widely varying performance with a maximum combined sensitivity and specificity of 71% [26]. The improved SNR of prostate imaging using 3 T MR scanners should result in improved accuracy in prostate cancer detection and staging. This comparison will depend on selection of surface phased-array coils versus endorectal coils. It has been noted that the improved SNR at 3 T can compensate for the reduced signal when using a surface coil, providing images similar to 1.5 T prostate imaging with an endorectal coil. In a comparison of prostate cancer imaging at 1.5 T using a combined endorectal coil and phased-array surface coil and 3.0 T using a phased-array surface coil alone, Beyersdorf et al. noted an identical local staging accuracy of 73% [27]. Use of an endorectal coil combined with a 3 T scanner can provide further improvement in prostate cancer detection. In an ROC analysis or prostate MRI performed at 3 T, Heijmink et al. observed that endorectal coil imaging resulted in a significant improvement in prostate cancer detection and staging compared to surface coil imaging. With endorectal coil imaging, the area under the curve (AUC) for localization of prostate cancer was significantly increased, from 0.62 to 0.68 ($P<0.001$). Endorectal coil imaging significantly increased the AUC for staging, and sensitivity of detection of locally advanced disease by experienced readers from 7% to a range of 73–80% [28].

19.5.4.1 Extracapsular Tumor Spread and Neurovascular Bundle Involvement

Criteria for detecting extracapsular extension of prostate cancer includes asymmetry of the neurovascular bundle, gross tumor surrounding the neurovascular bundle, angulation of the prostate gland contour and irregular or spiculated margin, obliteration of the rectoprostatic angle, capsular retraction, a tumor-capsule interface of >1 cm, and a breach of the capsule with gross tumor extension [9, 16, 29–31]. MR imaging has reported 13–95% sensitivity and 49–97% specificity for depicting extracapsular extension of prostate cancer [18, 32–38]. Endorectal coil MR imaging using a 3 T scanner yielded a local staging accuracy of 94% and sensitivity of 88% for experienced readers compared to 81% and 50% for a less experienced reader, respectively [18].

19.5.4.2 Seminal Vesicle Involvement

Tumor extension into the seminal vesicles is depicted on anatomic T2-weighted MR images. Normally, the seminal vesicles are composed of clusters of rounded fluid intensity structures, which are hyperintense on T2-weighted images. A tumor involving the seminal vesicles is depicted as focal low signal intensity or a low-signal-intensity mass within the seminal vesicles. Additional findings include a diffusely enlarged low-signal-intensity seminal vesicle, obliteration of the angle between the prostate and the seminal vesicles, and direct tumor extension from the base of the prostate into the seminal vesicles. MR imaging has a 23–80% sensitivity and 81–90% specificity for depicting seminal vesicle involvement of prostate cancer [39].

19.5.5 Functional MR Imaging of Prostate Cancer

19.5.5.1 Diffusion-Weighted MR Imaging

Diffusion is a physical property that describes the microscopic random movement of molecules in response to thermal energy. Also known as Brownian motion, diffusion may be affected by the biophysical properties of tissues such as cell organization and density, microstructure, and microcirculation. In water, molecules undergo free thermally driven diffusion without restriction. However, in tissues, the movement of molecules is modified by their interactions with cell membranes and macromolecules. In highly cellular tissues, such as most solid tumors, movement of water molecules in the extracellular space is restricted by the higher density of the hydrophobic cellular membranes [40]. Conversely, in necrotic or cystic areas, the migration of water molecules is unimpeded. DWI thus provides unique information that reflects cellular density, the tortuosity of the extracellular space, and the integrity of cellular membranes [40]. It is an important point that restriction of diffusion can occur in benign and malignant processes.

DWI utilizes pulse sequences and techniques that are sensitive to very small-scale motion of water protons at the microscopic level. For example, single-shot echo planar imaging (EPI), DW imaging is utilized to provide very rapid imaging sensitive to subtle small-scale alternations in diffusion.

In the DW pulse sequence paired diffusion-sensitizing gradients are centered on either side of the 180° refocusing pulse. In the absence of motion, water molecules will acquire phase information from the first diffusion gradient that will be refocused by the second diffusion gradient with no net change in signal. However, with moving water molecules, the situation is different. The water molecules will accumulate phase information from the first gradient that will not be completely refocused by the second diffusion gradient due to movement of the water molecules producing a loss of signal. The paired diffusion gradients will thus detect water motion as areas of signal loss. Tumors with a higher cellular density possess more cell membranes per unit volume which restricts mobility of water molecules and diffusion. These tumors will exhibit restricted diffusion and corresponding high signal on DW imaging.

The sensitivity of the DWI sequence to water motion can be varied by changing the b-value, which changes the amplitude of the paired bipolar diffusion-sensitizing gradients. For prostate imaging, one typically acquires at least two b-values, a 0 s/mm^2 one combined with a second, high b-value of 1,000–1,500 s/mm^2. Acquiring additional b-values will improve the accuracy of the quantitative data obtained from DW imaging. Higher b-values result in more diffusion weighting with better background suppression, at the expense of reduced signal and increasing artifacts. At our institution, we typically use three b-values of 0, 500, and 1,500 s/mm^2.

DW images can be evaluated qualitatively by observing changes in signal intensity from areas of the image with minimal restriction of water, such as the normal prostate parenchyma, to those with high restriction of water diffusion, such as tumors. Areas of restricted water diffusion are displayed as areas of high signal intensity. Simple visual inspection of magnitude DW images can lead to a potential pitfall and image misinterpretation since the observed signal represents the combination of effects from water diffusion and T2 relaxation. Tissues with prolonged T2 relaxation may appear bright on a DW image representing "T2 shine through." Elimination of high signal from T2 prolongation can be achieved using ADC maps that depict changes in signal intensity that are solely due to water diffusion. On the ADC map, a tumor with restricted diffusion is displayed as an area with low signal intensity as opposed to the DW image in which the tumor is of high signal intensity (Fig. 19.2).

Quantitative analysis of DW images can be performed if at least two *b*-values are obtained. Obtaining additional *b*-values will increase the accuracy of measurements. This quantitative analysis can be performed easily on the MR scanner or workstation, generating ADC parametric maps that are independent of field strength and T2 shine through. By drawing regions of interest on the ADC map over tissues of interest, a numerical value known as the apparent diffusion coefficient (ADC) is generated. The ADC value can help to characterize tumors as benign or malignant and can assess interval change in a tumor in response to therapy. Areas of highly cellular tumor with restricted diffusion demonstrate low ADC values, while tissues with free water diffusion demonstrate high ADC values. It has also been observed quantitatively that following therapy tumors show a significant increase in ADC values with a corresponding loss of signal on visual inspection of the DW image.

In an ROC analysis comparing whole mount prostatectomy sections to MRI, Haider et al. [41] found that combined T2 and DWI MRI ($A_z = 0.89$) was better than T2 imaging alone ($A_z = 0.81$) in detecting prostate cancer within the peripheral zone. For tumors within the transitional zone, both T2 imaging and DWI performed less well with no added value from the DWI MRI. In a similar study, Lim et al. [15] found that the addition of the DWI ADC map to T2-weighted images improved the sensitivity (78–88% vs. 67–74%) and specificity (88–89% vs. 77–79%) for detecting prostate cancer using multiple observers. Measurements of the volume of tumor in the peripheral zone on MRI compared to prostatectomy specimens was significantly more accurate when combining DWI ADC values and T2 images compared to T2 images alone [42].

The distinction between transitional zone prostate cancer and areas of benign adenomatous hyperplasia is challenging. Conventional T1-weighted and T2-weighted MR imaging are relatively poor in detecting the 15–25% of prostate cancers that occur in the transitional zone. Similarly on DWI tumors and BPH often show similar restriction of water movement and thus identical signal changes on DWI. Another type of DWI is diffusion tensor imaging or fiber tracking that measures the directionality as well as the magnitude of water diffusion. In the prostate, the anatomic direction of the fiber bundles is oriented in a superior to inferior direction in the peripheral zone and transitional zone. BPH maintains the directionality in the superior to inferior direction, whereas prostate cancer disrupts these superior to inferior fiber bundles. The fractional anisotropy (FA) is a quantitative value derived from diffusion tensor imaging that gives information about the shape of the *diffusion* tensor at each *voxel*. The fractional anisotropy reflects differences between an isotropic diffusion and a linear diffusion. The FA range is between 0 and 1 (0 = isotropic diffusion, 1 = highly directional).

In a study on diffusion tensor MRI of prostate cancer, Manenti et al. [43] found that the mean FA values in the neoplastic lesion (0.27 ± 0.05) were significantly lower ($P < 0.05$) than in the normal peripheral area and in the normal central and adenomyomatous area.

DWI provides a new contrast mechanism for evaluation of prostate cancers. By imaging microscopic motion of water molecules, DWI yields new qualitative and quantitative information about tumors that can be used to improve tumor detection, characterize some tumors, and monitor and predict response to treatment.

19.5.5.2 Dynamic Contrast-Enhanced MR Imaging

DCE MR imaging is another form of functional imaging that noninvasively provides information about tissue vascularity [44, 45] Following injection of an exogenous contrast material such a small-molecular-weight gadolinium chelate, the contrast material distributes between the plasma space and the extravascular extracellular space (EES). Tumor neoangiogenesis results in a greater number of abnormal leaky capillaries that allows the contrast to more easily diffuse rapidly from the plasma space into the EES during the first pass and to subsequently rediffuse back into the plasma space. During the DCE experiment, tumors demonstrate more rapid

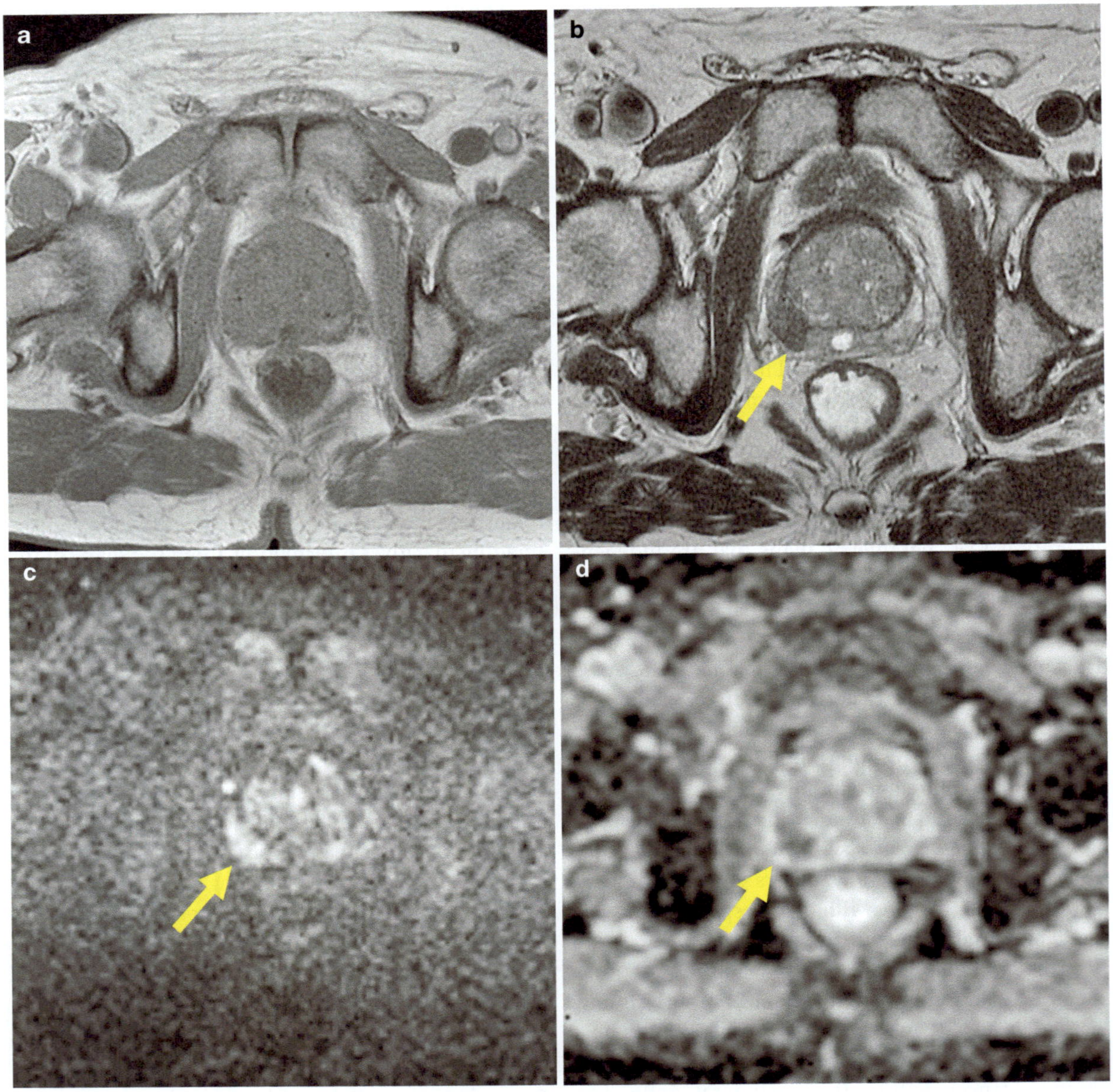

Fig. 19.2 Patient with prostate cancer. (**a, b**) T1-weighted MR image (**a**) is useful to depict postbiopsy hemorrhage but does not typically show prostate cancers. T2-weighted image (**b**) depicts the right posterolateral tumor (*arrow*). (**c, d**) Diffusion-weighted (b-value 1,500 s/m^2) MRI magnitude image (**c**) shows a faint hyperintense tumor in the right posterolateral peripheral zone. The diffusion-weighted MRI ADC map (**d**) demonstrates the low signal intensity tumor to much better advantage. ADC maps removed the T2 contribution from the image and are essential for prostate cancer imaging. (**e, f**) The DCE colorized parametric maps demonstrate the areas of increased permeability within the prostate gland. The RGB map (**e**) and the permeability map (**f**) show the right posterolateral tumor (*arrows*). These hypervascular areas correspond with angiogenesis. Notice that benign prostatic hypertrophy in the transitional zone is also characterized by angiogenesis. The assessment of prostate cancer on DCE images is confined to the peripheral zone where areas of colorization are suspicious for prostate cancer

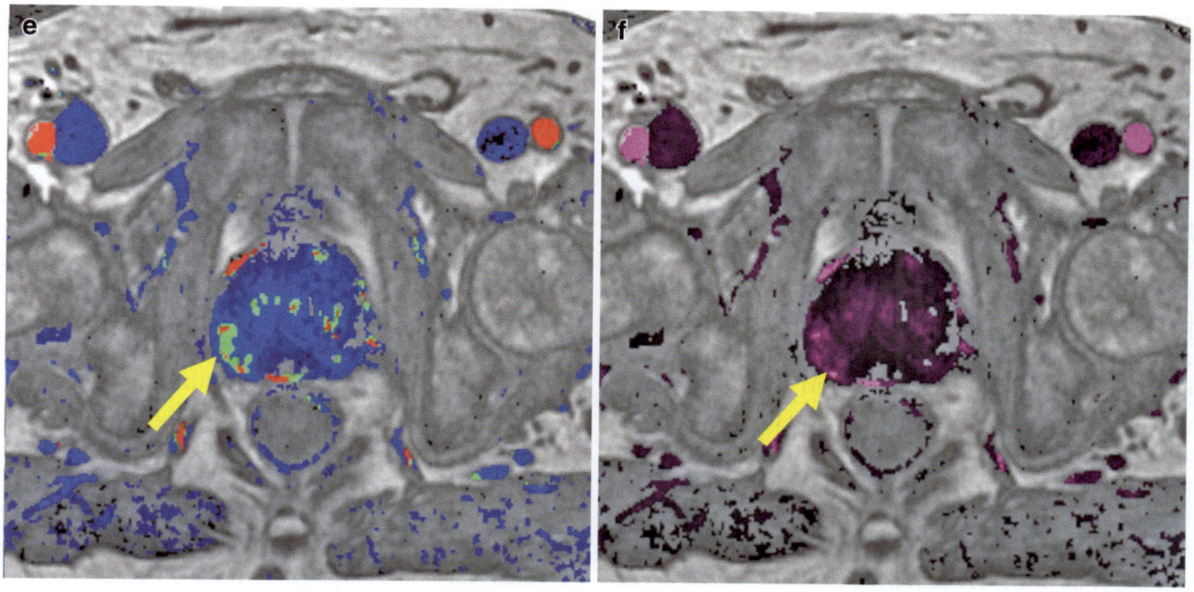

Fig. 19.2 (continued)

enhancement and washout of the contrast material compared to normal tissues. DCE provides insight into the pharmacokinetic properties of tumors that are occurring at a cellular level [44, 45].

In a DCE MRI experiment, intravenous gadolinium is injected and the tissue of interest is repeatedly imaged while the contrast material distributes between the capillaries of the plasma space into the EES. As imaging continues, the material will washout from the EES back into the plasma space. A typical DCE experiment might include rapid imaging over the tumor every 10 s for 6 min. The DCE experiment thus generates hundreds of images acquired during 30–40 passes through the tumor during the period of imaging.

The injected gadolinium chelate causes T1 shortening and an increased signal on a T1-weighted MR image. Measuring changes in signal intensity of the tissue over time after injection of the gadolinium reflects gadolinium concentration and indirectly the vascularity of tumors and normal tissues. The Toft's two-compartment model predicts the distribution of contrast material between the plasma space and the EES [46–48] and has been applied to prostate DCE imaging. Pharmacokinetic parameters are used to describe the movement of contrast material between these two spaces. K^{trans} is the forward transfer constant and reflects the capillary permeability multiplied by the capillary surface area. *K*-ep is the washout of contrast material from the EES back into the plasma space. EVF is the volume of the extracellular extravascular space. Tumors are characterized by abnormal leaky capillaries and demonstrate higher values for K^{trans} and K_{ep} compared to normal tissues. Tumors are also characterized by increased cellular density and thus also show a lower EVF.

The analysis of the hundreds of images in the DCE dataset is performed by perfusion software programs providing quantitative and qualitative information. For enhancing voxels, the transfer constant K^{trans} (permeability surface area product per unit volume of tissue, min^{-1}) and the rate constant k_{ep} (efflux rate from EES back to plasma, min^{-1}) are calculated fitting the gadolinium concentration curves to the Toft's model. The EVF per unit volume of tissue v_e is calculated as $K^{trans}/k_{ep.}$ The analysis also produces colorized parametric maps of the tumor and surrounding tissues in which the parametric values K^{trans}, K_{ep}, and EVF are color-encoded and superimposed upon gray-scale anatomic images. These colorized parametric maps are thus based on signal changes, which are defined by the physiology of normal tissues and tumors.

This type of DCE analysis allows the radiologist to assess areas on the colorized parametric maps with higher vascularity. In some cases, this DCE analysis may allow one to distinguish malignant from benign tissues. Following therapy, there are predictable changes in tumor vascularity that are reflected in the DCE experiment by a reduction in K^{trans} and K_{ep}, and an increase in EFV.

DCE has been utilized for detection and staging of primary prostate cancer [10, 18, 44, 49–51]. Prostate cancers show increased vascularity with elevated K^{trans}, K_{ep}, and lower EVF than normal peripheral zone parenchyma [11, 52–54]. On the colorized parametric maps, peripheral zone tumors are depicted as regions of increased vascularity compared to the adjacent peripheral zone [55]. However, within the transitional zone, nodules of benign adenomatous hyperplasia are also characterized by neoangiogenesis [56]. Prostate cancer and BPH often demonstrate an identical appearance on DCE imaging. We currently limit our analysis of the DCE images to changes that occur within the peripheral zone of the prostate.

The addition of the DCE-colorized parametric maps to T2-weighted images improves sensitivity and staging accuracy, detecting tumors not evident on T2-weighted images alone [12, 57]. Kim et al. noted that the sensitivity and accuracy for depicting prostate cancer in the peripheral zone was 96% and 97% on the DCE parametric maps compared to 75% and 53% on T2-weighted images [57]. Cornud et al. have compared DCE and T2-weighted MRI to prostatectomy specimens and noted that quantitative DCE MRI is more accurate than T2W imaging for tumor localization of nonpalpable cancer greater than 0.2 cm^3 [58]. For prostate cancer staging, DCE images combined with T2-weighted anatomic images can improve the detection of extracapsular tumor spread [12, 13] and involvement of the neurovascular bundle [59].

19.5.5.3 MR Spectroscopy

MR spectroscopy (MRS) provides metabolic information by analyzing the spectra reflecting the relative concentrations of metabolites in the cell cytoplasm and extracellular space [31, 60, 61]. On MRS, prostate cancer is characterized by lower levels of citrate and higher levels of choline and creatinine than are present in normal prostatic tissue and BPH. Normal prostate tissue is characterized by high citrate levels. In prostate cancer, the citrate levels decline as citrate production is converted to citrate oxidation. High turnover of phospholipid in the cell membranes of proliferating and growing cancer cells leads to an increase in choline levels in cancer cells [9, 62].

The spectral peaks of creatinine and choline are very near one another and may be inseparable. On MRS, prostate cancer is thus characterized by an increase in the ratio of choline and creatinine to citrate [31, 62, 63]. Within the peripheral zone, voxels in which the ratio of choline and creatinine to citrate is at least two standard deviations (SD) above the mean represent possible cancer [64]. Voxels with a choline to citrate level of three SD or more above the mean are highly suggestive of prostate cancer [65].

The combination of MRS and MRI can improve prostate cancer detection in the peripheral zone [66–69]. Scheidler and colleagues noted that the combination of MRS and MRI demonstrated a 91% sensitivity and 95% specificity for prostate cancer detection compared to 77% and 81% for MRI alone, and 63% and 75% for MRS alone. Tumor detection on MRS may be related to tumor aggressiveness. In one study, tumor depiction on MRS was 44% for Gleason grade 6 tumors and 90% for Gleason grade 8 and 9 tumors [70].

The use of MRS for detecting transitional zone prostate cancer has also been described. However the choline:citrate ratio in the transitional zone varies more widely in the normal transitional zone and may overlap with that of prostate cancer [71].

19.6 Imaging in Treatment Planning for Radiation Therapy

Image-based computer treatment planning has evolved to the current 3D conformal radiation therapy approach that allows for precise definition of target and nontarget tissues. The ability to deliver higher doses to the targeted tissues with enhanced precision and sparing of adjacent tissues demands more accurate image-guidance techniques. Image guidance with CT has been incorporated into treatment planning rooms for more accurate depiction of the prostate and adjacent anatomic structures.

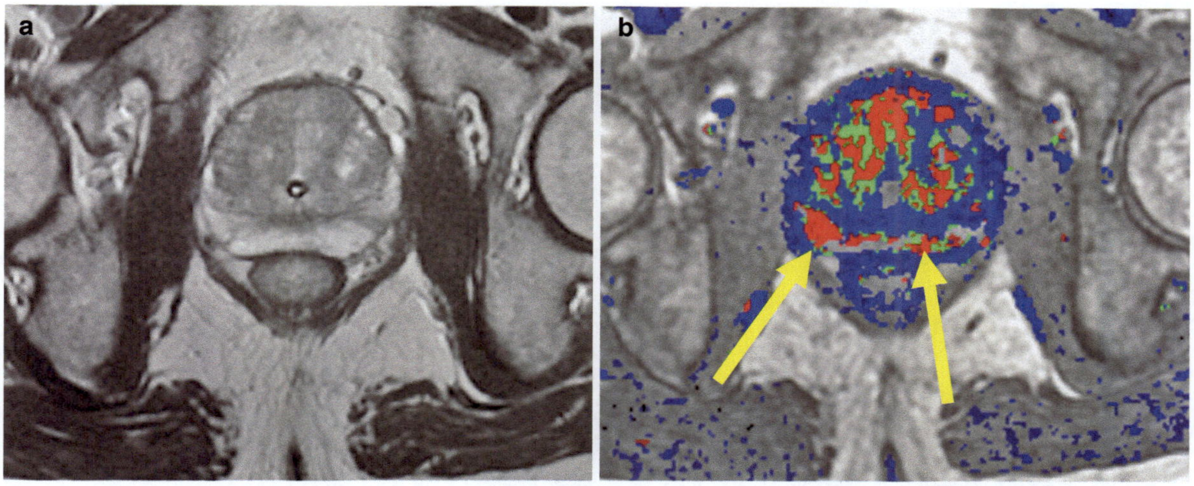

Fig. 19.3 Patient with prostate cancer being evaluated for CyberKnife SBRT. T2-weighted image (**a**) shows small volume faint low signal areas in the peripheral zone. The DCE colorized parametric map (**b**) shows much more extensive bilateral peripheral zone tumor (*arrows*). The more extensive tumor on the DCE map correlated with findings of sextant biopsy. In many cases the DCE-colorized parametric maps are superior for depicting prostate cancer compared to conventional T2-weighted images

The ability with modern radiation therapy to apply different doses to anatomic subregions of the prostate and tumor requires even more precise anatomic definition. This concept of "dose painting" allows for targeting the peripheral zone and defined prostate cancers with higher doses and for sparing of the normal rectum and urethra. The ability to fuse MR images with treatment planning CT scans takes advantage of the superior soft tissue resolution of MRI compared to CT. MR imaging can much more precisely define the zonal anatomy of the prostate and the borders of the prostate with the bladder, rectum, and seminal vesicles. MR imaging also better defines the apex of the prostate, the length and position of the membranous urethra, and the position of the penile bulb.

The evolving concepts of focal treatment of prostate cancers with directed precision radiation therapy may be possible with new techniques such as CyberKnife® SBRT (Accuray Incorporated, Sunnyvale, CA). MR imaging can provide accurate depiction of the location and volume of the prostate cancer and will be a key element in these more directed therapies. The ability to coregister and fuse the DCE-colorized parametric maps that accurately define the prostate cancer with the treatment planning CT scan may provide a valuable tool for precise targeting of the prostate cancer (Fig. 19.3).

19.6.1 Assessing Response to Therapy of Prostate Cancer

Imaging studies have been used to evaluate response of prostate cancer to radiation therapy and androgen deprivation [72–74]. Serial PSA measurements remain the gold standard for evaluating therapeutic response. However, PSA assessment can be challenging with a slow response to treatment that may only reach a nadir after 2 or 3 years. In addition, temporary false-positive elevations of PSA in the absence of residual or recurrent tumor occur in all forms of radiation therapy. This "PSA bounce" was noted to occur in 32% of 295 patients following brachytherapy who were followed for 3 years [75]. An accurate imaging study would be useful as an adjunct to serial PSA values and clinical assessment to follow treatment response.

The challenge in assessing patients following treatment for prostate cancer is to reliably distinguish treated normal tissues and BPH from residual or recurrent prostate cancer. Superimposed prostatitis can also confound interpretation. Radiation therapy itself produces changes in the prostate gland which must be distinguished from tumor. These radiation-induced changes may be related to postradiation edema and or fibrosis. T2-weighted MR images

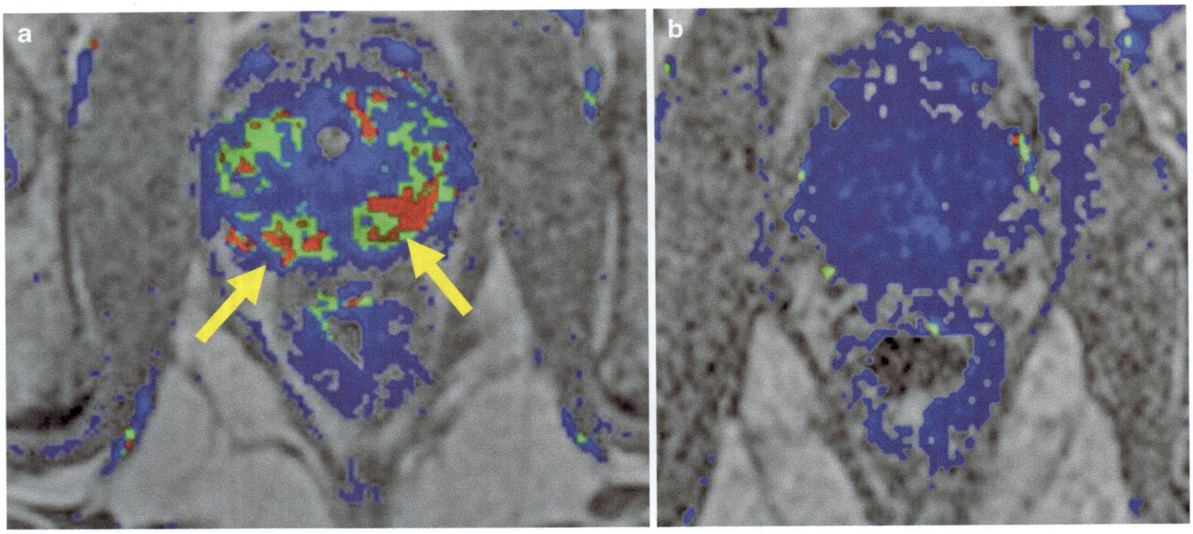

Fig. 19.4 Patient with prostate cancer. Pre-CyberKnife SBRT DCE MRI (**a**) shows large bilateral peripheral zone tumors (*arrows*) and benign prostatic hypertrophy. Follow-up DCE MRI (**b**) obtained 24 months after CyberKnife SBRT shows complete resolution of tumor. The homogeneous blue colorization of the prostate gland is normal following treatment. The quantitative analysis of tumor permeability showed a decrease in the tumor Ktrans from 1.31 min pre CyberKnife to 0.14 min following radiation treatment

typically show diffuse abnormal signal following radiation treatment, which can degrade image quality and preclude accurate assessment for residual tumor. Other types of MR imaging, such as DCE or MRS, may provide a more reliable assessment of the prostate gland following radiation therapy.

Following external-beam radiation therapy, MRS shows a time-dependent loss of the prostatic metabolites choline, creatinine, and citrate. In one study, the mean time to disease resolution assessed by MRS and MRI was 40.3 months [76]. With brachytherapy alone or combined with external-beam radiation therapy or androgen deprivation, metabolic atrophy on MRS preceded PSA nadir in most patients except those treated with all three methods. In these patients, metabolite and PSA nadirs occurred simultaneously [76]. Similar changes were noted on MRS, following androgen deprivation therapy, resulting in total metabolic atrophy on MRS in 25% of patients on long term therapy [77].

DCE has been used to assess patients following external-beam radiation therapy [73]. In six patients, prostate cancer showed a significant decrease in perfusion and increase in extraction coefficient following IMRT. In our experience, patients treated with CyberKnife radiation therapy can be effectively monitored with DCE MRI (Fig. 19.4). Following CyberKnife treatment, prostate cancer shows a consistent decline in the parametric values K^{trans} and K_{ep} and an increase in EVF. On the colorized parametric maps, the enhancing colorized tumors resolve by 6–12 months after CyberKnife radiation therapy with the gland then assuming a homogenous appearance [78]. Other changes that occur with radiation treatment on DCE include a decline in perfusion of the entire prostate gland. In some cases, focal nonenhancing areas develop, which are thought to represent areas of necrosis. Quantitatively, the decline in the prostate cancer's parametric values correlates with the decline in serial PSA values following treatment. Potential false-positive results on DCE MRI may be related to prostatitis, which can also produce areas of increased vascularity. Anecdotally, we have observed similar changes in prostate cancer on DCE MRI following androgen deprivation therapy.

19.7 Imaging of Recurrent Prostate Cancer

Tumor recurrence following prostatectomy or radiation therapy is indicated by a rising PSA value and/or a palpable nodule or induration on DRE (Fig. 19.5). An elevated serum PSA following treatment for prostate

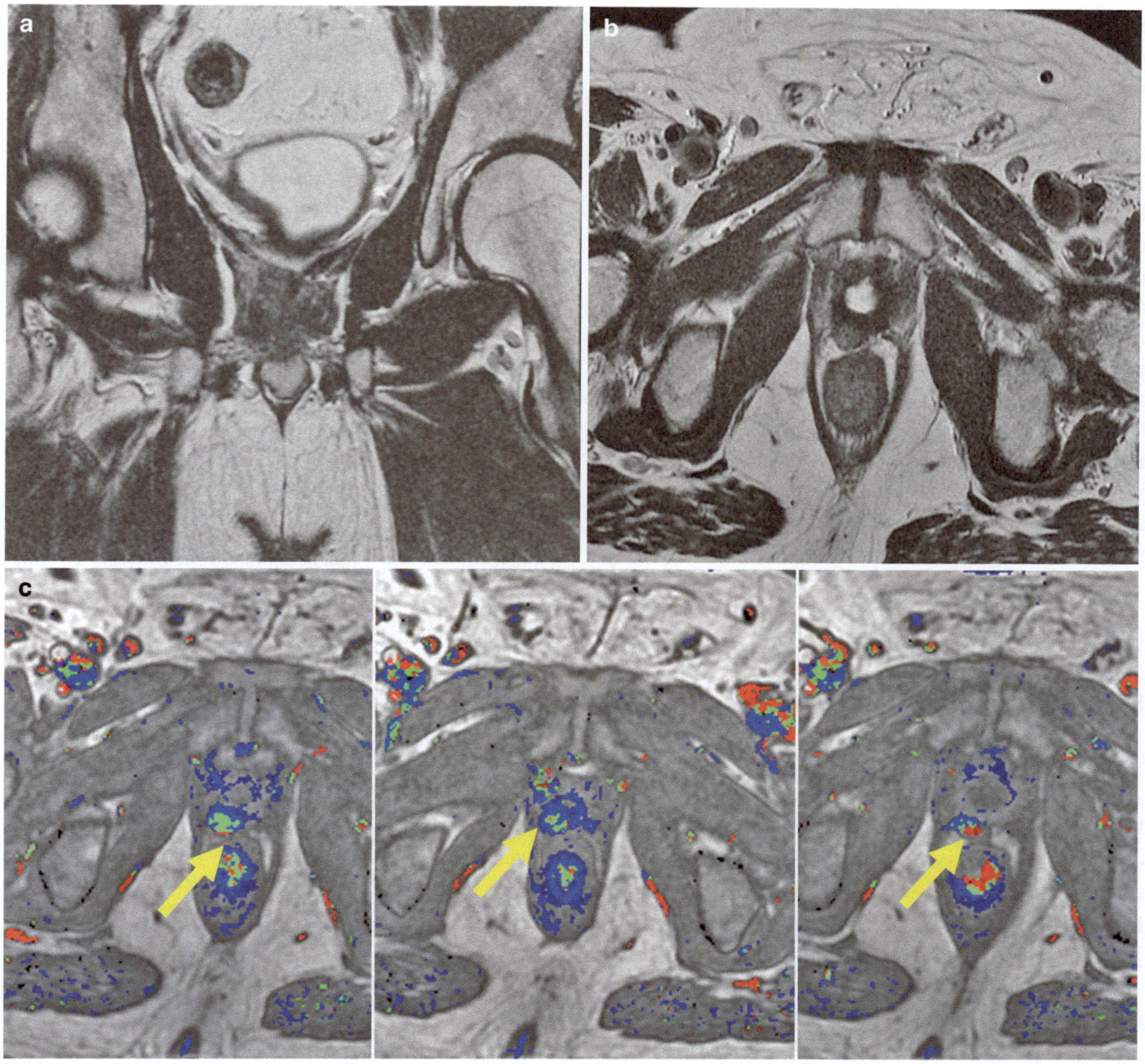

Fig. 19.5 Patient with a rising serum PSA value following prostatectomy. Coronal (**a**) and axial (**b**) T2-weighted images do not clearly show recurrent tumor (**c**) Patient with a rising serum PSA value following prostatectomy. Three sections from the DCE MRI shows enhancing tumor in the prostate bed. Findings were confirmed by biopsy and the patient was treated with salvage CyberKnife radiotherapy

cancer may indicate a PSA relapse, local recurrence in the prostate or post-prostatectomy bed, or distant metastases usually to lymph nodes or osseous structures. The rate of biochemical relapse following radical prostatectomy ranges from 10% to 53% [79–86]. Following external-beam radiation therapy for prostate cancer, the reported 5-year PSA relapse rate ranges from 15% for low-risk patients to 67% for high-risk patients [87, 88].

Imaging evaluation in the setting of suspected local recurrence includes transrectal ultrasound, CT, and MR imaging. CT is relatively insensitive for depicting local recurrence. In one study, CT detected only 36% of recurrent tumors [89]. Endorectal MR imaging has been shown to be more accurate for detecting local tumor recurrence in patients with prostate cancer with 95% sensitivity and 100% specificity [90, 91]. The role of MRS in the setting of local tumor recurrence has also been described [92, 93] and may further improve the accuracy of detecting recurrent prostate cancer.

DCE prostate MRI can be used to detect tumor recurrence following therapy. Haider et al. found that DCE MRI performs better than T2-weighted imaging in the detection and localization of recurrent prostate cancer in the peripheral zone after EBRT [94]. Casciani et al. found that the 91% of recurrent prostate cancers after prostatectomy showed rapid and early enhancement on DCE, resulting in a sensitivity of 88% compared to 48% for MRI alone [95]. DCE MRI is also useful for localization of prostate cancer before repeat biopsy. In 93 patients with abnormal PSA levels and negative prostate biopsy who underwent MRI to guide repeat biopsy, Cheikh et al. observed a per-patient sensitivity of 47.8% for T2-weighted imaging compared to 82.6% for DCE [96].

19.8 Future Directions for Prostate Imaging

Functional MR imaging provides insight into phenomena occurring within prostate tumors at a cellular level [62, 97]. Individual measurements of K^{trans} and K_{ep} on DCE, ADC values on DWI, and metabolite concentrations on MRS may correlate with histopathologic features of prostate cancers and normal prostate tissue [97]. MR imaging with a multiparametric analysis will allow one to effectively combine the information from multiple image contrasts into one comprehensive evaluation of prostate cancer. A multiparametric analysis would combine the information from conventional T2-weighted MR imaging, DWI, MRS, and DCE MRI to predict the presence of prostate cancer in an individual region of the prostate [98]. Comparing DWI, MRS, and DCE, Riches et al. found that the combination of two functional parameters resulted in significant improvements in prostate cancer detection over the use of any single parameter, but that the addition of a third parameter did not further increase tumor detection [99]. Employing a multiparametric MRI at 3T Tukbey et al. found that the combination of T2-weighted MRI, MRS and DCE MRI had a higher sensitivity for peripheral zone tumors than each of the sequences alone [100]. Software programs might allow the user to weight the different contrast mechanisms and could generate a single colorized map that shows the likelihood of prostate cancer in different parts of the gland based upon this multiparametric analysis. This type of approach to imaging prostate cancer would simplify image analysis and improve the accuracy of prostate cancer detection.

References

1. Roehl KA, Antenor JA, Catalona WJ (2002) Serial biopsy results in prostate cancer screening study. J Urol 167: 2435–2439
2. Ukimura O, Troncoso P, Ramirez EI et al (1998) Prostate cancer staging: correlation between ultrasound determined tumor contact length and pathologically confirmed extraprostatic extension. J Urol 159:1251–1259
3. Ohori M, Shinohara K, Wheeler TM et al (1993) Ultrasonic detection of non-palpable seminal vesicle invasion: a clinicopathological study. Br J Urol 72:799–808
4. Rorvik J, Halvorsen OJ, Albrektsen G et al (1998) Lymphangiography combined with biopsy and computer tomography to detect lymph node metastases in localized prostate cancer. Scand J Urol Nephrol 32:116–119
5. Oyen RH, Van Poppel HP, Ameye FE et al (1994) Lymph node staging of localized prostatic carcinoma with CT and CT-guided fine-needle aspiration biopsy: prospective study of 285 patients. Radiology 190:315–322
6. O'Dowd GJ, Veltri RW, Orozco R et al (1997) Update on the appropriate staging evaluation for newly diagnosed prostate cancer. J Urol 158:687–698
7. Wolf JS Jr, Cher M, Dall'era M et al (1995) The use and accuracy of cross-sectional imaging and fine needle aspiration cytology for detection of pelvic lymph node metastases before radical prostatectomy. J Urol 153:993–999
8. Futterer JJ (2007) MR imaging in local staging of prostate cancer. Eur J Radiol 63:328–334
9. Hricak H, Choyke PL, Eberhardt SC et al (2007) Imaging prostate cancer: a multidisciplinary perspective. Radiology 243:28–53
10. Zhu Y, Williams S, Zwiggelaar R (2006) Computer technology in detection and staging of prostate carcinoma: a review. Med Image Anal 10:178–199
11. Buckley DL, Roberts C, Parker GJ et al (2004) Prostate cancer: evaluation of vascular characteristics with dynamic contrast-enhanced T1-weighted MR imaging–initial experience. Radiology 233:709–715
12. Bloch BN, Furman-Haran E, Helbich TH et al (2007) Prostate cancer: accurate determination of extracapsular extension with high-spatial-resolution dynamic contrast-enhanced and T2-weighted MR imaging–initial results. Radiology 245:176–185
13. Sauvain JL, Palascak P, Gomez W et al (2010) MRI and prostatic cancer: measurements of kinetic perfusion parameters of gadolinium with a computerized-aided diagnostic tool (CAD). Prog Urol 20:121–129

14. Low RN, Diffusion-Weighted MR (2009) Imaging for whole body metastatic disease and lymphadenopathy. Magn Reson Imaging Clin N Am 17:245–261
15. Lim HK, Kim JK, Kim KA et al (2009) Prostate cancer: apparent diffusion coefficient map with T2-weighted images for detection–a multireader study. Radiology 250:145–151
16. Outwater EK, Petersen RO, Siegelman ES et al (1994) Prostate carcinoma: assessment of diagnostic criteria for capsular penetration on endorectal coil MR images. Radiology 193:333–339
17. Cornud F, Flam T, Chauveinc L et al (2002) Extraprostatic spread of clinically localized prostate cancer: factors predictive of pT3 tumor and of positive endorectal MR imaging examination results. Radiology 224:203–210
18. Futterer JJ, Engelbrecht MR, Huisman HJ et al (2005) Staging prostate cancer with dynamic contrast-enhanced endorectal MR imaging prior to radical prostatectomy: experienced versus less experienced readers. Radiology 237:541–549
19. Hricak H, White S, Vigneron D et al (1994) Carcinoma of the prostate gland: MR imaging with pelvic phased-array coils versus integrated endorectal–pelvic phased-array coils. Radiology 193:703–709
20. McNeal JE, Redwine EA, Freiha FS et al (1988) Zonal distribution of prostatic adenocarcinoma. Correlation with histologic pattern and direction of spread. Am J Surg Pathol 12:897–906
21. Noguchi M, Stamey TA, Neal JE et al (2000) An analysis of 148 consecutive transition zone cancers: clinical and histological characteristics. J Urol 163:1751–1755
22. Stamey TA, Donaldson AN, Yemoto CE et al (1998) Histological and clinical findings in 896 consecutive prostates treated only with radical retropubic prostatectomy: epidemiologic significance of annual changes. J Urol 160:2412–2417
23. Reissigl A, Pointner J, Strasser H et al (1997) Frequency and clinical significance of transition zone cancer in prostate cancer screening. Prostate 30:130–135
24. Augustin H, Erbersdobler A, Graefen M et al (2003) Biochemical recurrence following radical prostatectomy: a comparison between prostate cancers located in different anatomical zones. Prostate 55:48–54
25. Akin O, Sala E, Moskowitz CS et al (2006) Transition zone prostate cancers: features, detection, localization, and staging at endorectal MR imaging. Radiology 239:784–792
26. Engelbrecht MR, Jager GJ, Laheij RJ et al (2002) Local staging of prostate cancer using magnetic resonance imaging: a meta-analysis. Eur Radiol 12:2294–2302
27. Beyersdorff D, Taymoorian K, Knosel T et al (2005) MRI of prostate cancer at 1.5 and 3.0T: comparison of image quality in tumor detection and staging. AJR Am J Roentgenol 185:1214–1220
28. Heijmink SW, Futterer JJ, Hambrock T et al (2007) Prostate cancer: body-array versus endorectal coil MR imaging at 3T–comparison of image quality, localization, and staging performance. Radiology 244:184–195
29. Yu KK, Hricak H, Alagappan R et al (1997) Detection of extracapsular extension of prostate carcinoma with endorectal and phased-array coil MR imaging: multivariate feature analysis. Radiology 202:697–702
30. Yu KK, Scheidler J, Hricak H et al (1999) Prostate cancer: prediction of extracapsular extension with endorectal MR imaging and three-dimensional proton MR spectroscopic imaging. Radiology 213:481–488
31. Claus FG, Hricak H, Hattery RR (2004) Pretreatment evaluation of prostate cancer: role of MR imaging and 1H MR spectroscopy. Radiographics 24(Suppl 1):S167–S180
32. Bartolozzi C, Menchi I, Lencioni R et al (1996) Local staging of prostate carcinoma with endorectal coil MRI: correlation with whole-mount radical prostatectomy specimens. Eur Radiol 6:339–345
33. Comud F, Belin X, Flam T et al (2003) Local staging of prostate cancer by endorectal MRI using fast spin-echo sequences: prospective correlation with pathological findings after radical prostatectomy. Br J Urol 77:843–850
34. Ikonen S, Karkkainen P, Kivisaari L et al (1998) Magnetic resonance imaging of clinically localized prostatic cancer. J Urol 159:915–919
35. Ikonen S, Karkkainen P, Kivisaari L et al (2001) Endorectal magnetic resonance imaging of prostatic cancer: comparison between fat-suppressed T2-weighted fast spin echo and three-dimensional dual-echo, steady-state sequences. Eur Radiol 11:236–241
36. Perrotti M, Kaufman RP Jr, Jennings TA et al (1996) Endorectal coil magnetic resonance imaging in clinically localized prostate cancer: is it accurate? J Urol 156:106–109
37. Presti JC Jr, Hricak H, Narayan PA et al (1996) Local staging of prostatic carcinoma: comparison of transrectal sonography and endorectal MR imaging. AJR Am J Roentgenol 166:103–108
38. Rorvik J, Halvorsen OJ, Albrektsen G et al (1999) MRI with an endorectal coil for staging of clinically localised prostate cancer prior to radical prostatectomy. Eur Radiol 9:29–34
39. Sala E, Akin O, Moskowitz CS et al (2006) Endorectal MR imaging in the evaluation of seminal vesicle invasion: diagnostic accuracy and multivariate feature analysis. Radiology 238:929–937
40. Koh DM, Collins DJ (2007) Diffusion-weighted MRI in the body: applications and chal-lenges in oncology. AJR Am J Roentgenol 188:1622–1635
41. Haider MA, van der Kwast TH, Tanguay J et al (2007) Combined T2-weighted and diffusion-weighted MRI for localization of prostate cancer. AJR Am J Roentgenol 189:323–328
42. Mazaheri Y, Hricak H, Fine SW et al (2009) Prostate tumor volume measurement with combined T2-weighted imaging and diffusion-weighted MR: correlation with pathologic tumor volume. Radiology 252:449–457
43. Manenti G, Carlani M, Mancino S et al (2007) Diffusion tensor magnetic resonance imaging of prostate cancer. Invest Radiol 42:412–419
44. Padhani AR, Gapinski CJ, Macvicar DA et al (2000) Dynamic contrast enhanced MRI of prostate cancer: correlation with morphology and tumour stage, histological grade and PSA. Clin Radiol 55:99–109
45. Padhani AR, Husband JE (2000) Dynamic contrast-enhanced MRI studies in oncology with an emphasis on quantification, validation and human studies. Clin Radiol 56:607–620

46. Tofts PS, Kermode AG (1991) Measurement of the blood-brain barrier permeability and leakage space using dynamic MR imaging. 1. Fundamental concepts. Magn Reson Med 17:357–367
47. Tofts PS (1997) Modeling tracer kinetics in dynamic Gd-DTPA MR imaging. J Magn Reson Imaging 7:91–101
48. Tofts PS, Brix G, Buckley DL et al (1999) Estimating kinetic parameters from dynamic contrast-enhanced T(1)-weighted MRI of a diffusable tracer: standardized quantities and symbols. J Magn Reson Imaging 10:223–232
49. Alonzi R, Padhani AR, Allen C (2007) Dynamic contrast enhanced MRI in prostate cancer. Eur J Radiol 63:335–350
50. Jackson AS, Reinsberg SA, Sohaib SA et al (2009) Dynamic contrast-enhanced MRI for prostate cancer localization. Br J Radiol 82:148–156
51. Hara N, Okuizumi M, Koike H et al (2005) Dynamic contrast-enhanced magnetic resonance imaging (DCE-MRI) is a useful modality for the precise detection and staging of early prostate cancer. Prostate 62:140–147
52. Ocak I, Bernardo M, Metzger G et al (2007) Dynamic contrast-enhanced MRI of prostate cancer at 3T: a study of pharmacokinetic parameters. AJR Am J Roentgenol 189:849
53. Macura KJ (2008) Multiparametric magnetic resonance imaging of the prostate: current status in prostate cancer detection, localization, and staging. Semin Roentgenol 43:303–313
54. Franiel T, Ludemann L, Rudolph B et al (2009) Prostate MR imaging: tissue characterization with pharmacokinetic volume and blood flow parameters and correlation with histologic parameters. Radiology 252:101–108
55. Engelbrecht MR, Huisman HJ, Laheij RJ et al (2003) Discrimination of prostate cancer from normal peripheral zone and central gland tissue by using dynamic contrast-enhanced MR imaging. Radiology 229:248–254
56. Ren J, Huan Y, Wang H et al (2008) Dynamic contrast-enhanced MRI of benign prostatic hyperplasia and prostatic carcinoma: correlation with angiogenesis. Clin Radiol 63:153–159
57. Kim JK, Hong SS, Choi YJ et al (2005) Wash-in rate on the basis of dynamic contrast-enhanced MRI: usefulness for prostate cancer detection and localization. J Mang Reson Imaging 22:639–646
58. Cornud F, Beuvon F, Thevenin F et al (2009) Quantitative dynamic MRI and localisation of non-palpable prostate cancer. Prog Urol 19:401–413
59. Ogura K, Maekawa S, Okubo K et al (2001) Dynamic endorectal magnetic resonance imaging for local staging and detection of neurovascular bundle involvement of prostate cancer: correlation with histopathologic results. Urology 57:721–726
60. Coakley FV, Qayyum A, Kurhanewicz J (2003) Magnetic resonance imaging and spectros-copic imaging of prostate cancer. J Urol 70:S69–S76
61. Katz S, Rosen M (2006) MR imaging and MR spectroscopy in prostate cancer management. Radiol Clin North Am 44:723–734, viii
62. Choi YJ, Kim JK, Kim N et al (2007) Functional MR imaging of prostate cancer. Radiographics 27:63–77
63. Carroll PR, Coakley FV, Kurhanewicz J (2006) Magnetic resonance imaging and spectroscopy of prostate cancer. Rev Urol 8(Suppl 1):S4–S10
64. Kurhanewicz J, Vigneron DB, Hricak H et al (1996) Three-dimensional H-1 MR spectroscopic imaging of the in situ human prostate with high (0.24–0.7-cm^3) spatial resolution. Radiology 198:795–805
65. Males RG, Vigneron DB, Star-Lack J et al (2000) Clinical application of BASING and spectral/spatial water and lipid suppression pulses for prostate cancer staging and localization by in vivo 3D 1H magnetic resonance spectroscopic imaging. Magn Reson Med 43:17–22
66. Scheidler J, Hricak H, Vigneron DB et al (1999) Prostate cancer: localization with three-dimensional proton MR spectroscopic imaging–clinicopathologic study. Radiology 213:473–480
67. Vilanova JC, Barceló J (2007) Prostate cancer detection: magnetic resonance (MR) spectros-copic imaging. Abdom Imaging 32:253–261
68. Kurhanewicz J, Swanson MG, Nelson SJ et al (2002) Combined magnetic resonance imaging and spectroscopic imaging approach to molecular imaging of prostate cancer. J Magn Reson Imaging 16:451–463
69. Reinsberg SA, Payne GS, Riches SF et al (2007) Combined use of diffusion-weighted MRI and 1H MR spectroscopy to increase accuracy in prostate cancer detection. AJR Am J Roentgenol 188:91–98
70. Zakian KL, Sircar K, Hricak H et al (2005) Correlation of proton MR spectroscopic imaging with gleason score based on step-section pathologic analysis after radical prostatectomy. Radiology 234:804–814
71. Zakian KL, Eberhardt S, Hricak H et al (2003) Transition zone prostate cancer: metabolic characteristics at 1H MR spectroscopic imaging–initial results. Radiology 229:241–247
72. Pickett B, Kurhanewicz J, Coakley F et al (2004) Use of MRI and spectroscopy in evaluation of external beam radiotherapy for prostate cancer. Int J Radiat Oncol Biol Phys 60:1047–1055
73. Franiel T, Ludemann L, Taupitz M et al (2009) MRI before and after external beam intensity-modulated radiotherapy of patients with prostate cancer: the feasibility of monitoring of radiation-induced tissue changes using a dynamic contrast-enhanced inversion-prepared dual-contrast gradient echo sequence. Radiother Oncol 93:241–245
74. Mueller-Lisse UG, Swanson MG, Vigneron DB et al (2001) Time-dependent effects of hormone-deprivation therapy on prostate metabolism as detected by combined magnetic resonance imaging and 3D magnetic resonance spectroscopic imaging. Magn Reson Med 46:49–57
75. Toledano A, Chauveinc L, Flam T et al (2006) PSA bounce after permanent implant prostate brachytherapy may mimic a biochemical failure: a study of 295 patients with a minimum 3-year followup. Brachytherapy 5:122–126
76. Pickett B, Ten Haken RK, Kurhanewicz J et al (2004) Time to metabolic atrophy after permanent prostate seed implantation based on magnetic resonance spectroscopic imaging. Int J Radiat Oncol Biol Phys 59:665–673
77. Mueller-Lisse UG, Vigneron DB, Hricak H et al (2001) Localized prostate cancer: effect of hormone deprivation therapy measured by using combined three-dimensional 1H MR spectroscopy and MR imaging: clinicopathologic case-controlled study. Radiology 221:380–390

78. Low RN, Fuller DB, Muradyan N (2011) Dynamic Gadolinium-Enhanced Perfusion MRI of Prostate Cancer: Assessment of Response to Hypofractionated Robotic Stereotactic Body Radiation Therapy. Am J Roentgenol 197:10.2214/AJR 10.6356. In press for October Am J Roentgenology
79. Pound CR, Partin AW, Eisenberger MA et al (1999) Natural history of progression after PSA elevation following radical prostatectomy. JAMA 281:1591–1597
80. Laufer M, Pound CR, Carducci MA, Eisenberger MA (2000) Management of patients with rising prostate-specific antigen after radical prostatectomy. Urology 55:309–315
81. Amling CL, Blute ML, Bergstralh EJ et al (2000) Long-term hazard of progression after radical prostatectomy for clinically localized prostate cancer: continued risk of biochemical failure after 5 years. J Urol 164:101–105
82. Catalona WJ, Smith DS (1994) 5-year tumor recurrence rates after anatomical radical retropubic prostatectomy for prostate cancer. J Urol 152:1837–1842
83. Freedland SJ, Mangold LA, Walsh PC et al (2005) The prostatic specific antigen era is alive and well: prostatic specific antigen and biochemical progression following radical prostatectomy. J Urol 174:1276–1281; discussion 1281; author reply 1281
84. Zincke H, Oesterling JE, Blute ML et al (1994) Long-term (15 years) results after radical prostatectomy for clinically localized (stage T2c or lower) prostate cancer. J Urol 152:1850–1857
85. Trapasso JG, deKernion JB, Smith RB et al (1994) The incidence and significance of detectable levels of serum prostate specific antigen after radical prostatectomy. J Urol 152:1821–1825
86. Kattan MW, Wheeler TM, Scardino PT (1999) Postoperative nomogram for disease recurrence after radical prostatectomy for prostate cancer. J Clin Oncol 17:1499–1507
87. D'Amico AV, Crook J, Beard CJ, DeWeese TL, Hurwitz M, Kaplan I (2002) Campbell's urology, 8th edn. Saunders, Philadelphia
88. Pollack A, Smith LG, von Eschenbach AC (2000) External beam radiotherapy dose response characteristics of 1127 men with prostate cancer treated in the PSA era. Int J Radiat Oncol Biol Phys 48:507–512
89. Kramer S, Gorich J, Gottfried HW et al (1997) Sensitivity of computed tomography in detecting local recurrence of prostatic carcinoma following radical prostatectomy. Br J Radiol 70:995–999
90. Silverman JM, Krebs TL (1997) MR imaging evaluation with a transrectal surface coil of local recurrence of prostatic cancer in men who have undergone radical prostatectomy. AJR Am J Roentgenol 168:379–385
91. Sella T, Schwartz LH, Swindle PW et al (2004) Suspected local recurrence after radical prostatectomy: endorectal coil MR imaging. Radiology 231:379–385
92. Sala E, Eberhardt SC, Akin O et al (2006) Endorectal MR imaging before salvage prostatectomy: tumor localization and staging. Radiology 238:176–183
93. Pucar D, Shukla-Dave A, Hricak H et al (2005) Prostate cancer: correlation of MR imaging and MR spectroscopy with pathologic findings after radiation therapy-initial experience. Radiology 236:545–553
94. Haider MA, Chung P, Sweet J et al (2008) Dynamic contrast-enhanced magnetic resonance imaging for localization of recurrent prostate cancer after external beam radiotherapy. Int J Radiat Oncol Biol Phys 70:425–430
95. Casciani E, Polettini E, Carmenini E et al (2008) Endorectal and dynamic contrast-enhanced MRI for detection of local recurrence after radical prostatectomy. AJR Am J Roentgenol 190:1187–1192
96. Cheikh AB, Girouin N, Colombel M et al (2009) Evaluation of T2-weighted and dynamic contrast-enhanced MRI in localizing prostate cancer before repeat biopsy. Eur Radiol 19:770–778
97. Langer DL, van der Kwast TH, Evans AJ et al (2010) Prostate tissue composition and MR measurements: investigating the relationships between ADC, T2, K(trans), v(e), and corresponding histologic features. Radiology 255:485–494
98. Kurhanewicz J, Vigneron D, Carroll P, Coakley F (2008) Multiparametric magnetic resonance imaging in prostate cancer: present and future. Curr Opin Urol 18:71–77
99. Riches SF, Payne GS, Morgan VA et al (2009) MRI in the detection of prostate cancer: combined apparent diffusion coefficient, metabolite ratio, and vascular parameters. AJR Am J Roentgenol 193:1583–1591
100. Tukbey B, Pinto PA, Mani H et al (2010) Prostate cancer: value of multiparametric MR Imaging at 3T for detection - histopathologic correlation. Radiology 255:89–99

List of Contributors

Shafak Aluwini, M.D.
Departments of Radiation Oncology and Urology
Erasmus Medical Centre
Daniel den Hoed Cancer Center
Rotterdam, The Netherlands

Mohammad Attar, M.D.
Radiotherapy Unit, Radiology Department
King Abdulaziz University Hospital
Jeddah, KSA

William Chen, M.D.
Department of Radiation Oncology
Case Western Reserve University
School of Medicine
Cleveland, OH, USA

Brian T. Collins, M.D.
Department of Radiation Medicine
Georgetown University Hospital
Georgetown University School of Medicine
Washington, DC, USA

Sean P. Collins, M.D., Ph.D.
Department of Radiation Medicine
Georgetown University Hospital
Georgetown University School of Medicine
Washington, DC, USA

Alexandru Daşu, M.Sc., Ph.D.
Department of Radiation Physics
Linköping University Hospital
and Linköping University
Linköping, Sweden

Nancy Dawson, M.D.
Department of Radiation Medicine
Georgetown University Hospital
Georgetown University School of Medicine
Washington, DC, USA

Anatoly Dritschilo, M.D.
Department of Radiation Medicine
Georgetown University Hospital
Georgetown University School of Medicine
Washington, DC, USA

Rodney J. Ellis, M.D.
Department of Radiation Oncology
Case Western Reserve University
School of Medicine
Cleveland, OH, USA

Debra Freeman, M.D.
Clinical Programs, Accuray Incorporated
Naples, FL, USA

Donald B. Fuller, M.D.
Radiosurgery Medical Group, Inc.
San Diego CyberKnife Center
San Diego, CA, USA

Matthew Gettman, M.D.
Department of Urology
Mayo Medical School and Mayo Clinic
Rochester, MN, USA

Mihai Ghilezan, M.D.
Department of Radiation Oncology
William Beaumont Hospital
Royal Oak, MI, USA

L.E. Ponsky et al. (eds.), *Treating Prostate Cancer and Related Genitourinary Applications*, Robotic Radiosurgery,
DOI 10.1007/978-3-642-11495-3,

Heather Hanscom
Department of Radiation Medicine
Georgetown University Hospital
Georgetown University School of Medicine
Washington, DC, USA

Daniel S. Higginson, M.D.
Department of Radiation Oncology
University of North Carolina at Chapel Hill
Chapel Hill, NC, USA

Martin Housset, M.D.
Department of Radiation Oncology
Hôpital euroṕeen Georges-Pompidou
Paris, France

Alan J. Katz, M.D.
Flushing Radiation Oncology
Flushing, NY, USA

Vincent Khoo
Department of Radiotherapy
The Royal Marsden NHS Foundation Trust
London, UK

Joy Kim
Department of Radiation Medicine
Georgetown University Hospital
Georgetown University School of Medicine
Washington, DC, USA

Christopher R. King, Ph.D., M.D.
Department of Radiation Oncology
UCLA School of Medicine
Los Angeles, CA, USA

Eric Lartigau, M.D.
Department of Radiotherapy
Centre Oscar Lambret, Lille Cedex, France

Siyan Lie
Department of Radiation Medicine
Georgetown University Hospital
Georgetown University School of Medicine
Washington, DC, USA

Russell N. Low, M.D.
Sharp and Children's MRI Center
and San Diego Imaging, Inc.
San Diego, CA, USA

John H. Lynch, M.D.
Sharp and Children's MRI Center
and San Diego Imaging, Inc.,
San Diego, CA, USA

Víctor Macias Hernandez, M.D., Ph.D.
Department of Radiation Medicine,
Georgetown University Hospital,
Georgetown University School of Medicine,
Washington, DC, USA

Alvaro Martinez, M.D.
Department of Radiation Oncology
William Beaumont Hospital
Royal Oak, MI, USA

Mary Ellen Masterson-McGary, M.S.
CyberKnife Center of Tampa Bay
Tampa, FL, USA

Kevin McGeagh, M.D.
Department of Radiation Medicine
Georgetown University Hospital
Georgetown University School of Medicine
Washington, DC, USA

Mackenzie McGee, M.D.
Department of Radiation Oncology
William Beaumont Hospital
Royal Oak, MI, USA

David E. Morris, M.D.
Department of Radiation Oncology
University of North Carolina at Chapel Hill
Chapel Hill, NC, USA

Alexander Muacevic, M. D.
European CyberKnife Center Munich
Munich, Germany

Eric Oermann
Department of Radiation Medicine
Georgetown University Hospital
Georgetown University School of Medicine
Washington, DC, USA

Hyeon U. Park, Ph.D.
Department of Radiation Medicine
Georgetown University Hospital
Georgetown University School of Medicine
Washington, DC, USA

Lee E. Ponsky, M.D.
Center for Urologic Oncology
and Minimally Invasive Therapies
Urology Institute
University Hospitals Case Medical Center Case
Western Reserve University School of Medicine
Cleveland, OH, USA

Benjamin Sherer
Department of Radiation Medicine
Georgetown University Hospital
Georgetown University School of Medicine
Washington, DC, USA

Mark Shimko, M.D.
Department of Urology
Mayo Medical School and Mayo Clinic
Rochester, MN, USA

Simeng Suy, Ph.D.
Department of Radiation Medicine
Georgetown University Hospital
Georgetown University School of Medicine
Washington, DC, USA

Juliette Thariat, M.D.
Department of Radiation
Oncology/IBDC CNRS UMR 6543
Cancer Center Antoine-Lacassagne
University Nice Sophia
Nice Cedex, France

Alison Tree
Department of Radiotherapy
The Royal Marsden NHS Foundation Trust
London, UK

Eric Umbreit, M.D.
Department of Urology
Mayo Medical School and Mayo Clinic
Rochester, MN, USA

Nick van As, M.D.
Department of Radiotherapy
The Royal Marsden NHS Foundation Trust
London, UK

Mahesh A. Varia, M.D.
Department of Radiation Oncology
University of North Carolina at Chapel Hill
Chapel Hill, NC, USA

Gino Vricella, M.D.
Division of Oncology
Urology Institute and
Center for Urologic Oncology
and Minimally Invasive Therapies
Urology Institute
University Hospitals Case Medical Center Case
Western Reserve University School of Medicine
Cleveland, OH, USA

Xia Yu, Ph.D.,
Department of Radiation Medicine
Georgetown University Hospital
Georgetown University School of Medicine
Washington, DC, USA

Index

L.E. Ponsky et al. (eds.), *Treating Prostate Cancer and Related Genitourinary Applications*, Robotic Radiosurgery, DOI 10.1007/978-3-642-11495-3, © Springer-Verlag Berlin Heidelberg 2012

MIX
Papier aus verantwortungsvollen Quellen
Paper from responsible sources
FSC® C105338

If you have any concerns about our products,
you can contact us on
ProductSafety@springernature.com

In case Publisher is established outside the EU,
the EU authorized representative is:
Springer Nature Customer Service Center GmbH
Europaplatz 3, 69115 Heidelberg, Germany

Printed by Libri Plureos GmbH
in Hamburg, Germany